The Effects on Human Health of Subtherapeutic Use of Antimicrobials in Animal Feeds

Committee to Study the Human Health Effects
of Subtherapeutic Antibiotic Use in Animal Feeds
Division of Medical Sciences
Assembly of Life Sciences
National Research Council

NATIONAL ACADEMY OF SCIENCES
WASHINGTON, D.C. 1980

NOTICE

The project that is the subject of this report was approved by the Governing Board of the National Research Council, whose members are drawn from the Councils of the National Academy of Sciences, the National Academy of Engineering, and the Institute of Medicine. The members of the committee responsible for the report were chosen for their special competences and with regard for appropriate balance.

This report has been reviewed by a group other than the authors according to procedures approved by a Report Review Committee consisting of members of the National Academy of Sciences, the National Academy of Engineering, and the Institute of Medicine.

The work on which this report is based was performed pursuant to Contract No. 282-78-0163, T. O. 8, with the Food and Drug Administration.

Library of Congress Catalog Card Number 80-81486

International Standard Book Number 0-309-03044-7

Available from

Office of Publications
National Academy of Sciences
2101 Constitution Avenue, N.W.
Washington, D. C. 20418

Printed in the United States of America

COMMITTEE TO STUDY THE HUMAN HEALTH EFFECTS OF SUBTHERAPEUTIC ANTIBIOTIC USE IN ANIMAL FEEDS

Reuel A. Stallones, *Chairman*
University of Texas School of Public Health
Houston, Texas

E. Russell Alexander
University of Arizona Health Sciences Center
Tucson, Arizona

Charles E. Antle
Pennsylvania State University
University Park, Pennsylvania

Pierce Gardner
The Pritzker School of Medicine
Chicago, Illinois

Edward H. Kass
Channing Laboratory
Harvard Medical School and Peter Bent Brigham Hospital
Boston, Massachusetts

Carl A. Keller
National Institute for Child Health and Human Development
National Institutes of Health
Bethesda, Maryland

J. Michael Lane
Center for Disease Control,
Atlanta, Georgia

Frank J. Massey, Jr.
University of California School of Public Health
Los Angeles, California

Robert H. Rownd
University of Wisconsin
Madison, Wisconsin

Paul R. Sheehe
Upstate Medical Center
State University of New York
Syracuse, New York

Vernon L. Tharp
Ohio State University,
Columbis, Ohio

Assembly of Life Sciences Staff:

Enriqueta C. Bond
Alvin G. Lazen
Councilman Morgan
Frances M. Peter
Daniel L. Weiss
Roy Widdus

CONSULTANTS

N. Franklin Adkinson, Jr.
Good Samaritan Hospital
Baltimore, Maryland

Board on Agriculture and
Renewable Resources (BARR/CNR),
National Academy of Sciences
National Research Council
Washington, D.C.
See page v.

Robert N. Goodman
University of Missouri
Columbia, Missouri

George A. Jacoby
Massachusetts General Hospital
Boston, Massachusetts

Stanley E. Katz
Rutgers University
New Brunswick, New Jersey

Jackson S. Kiser
Consultant, Agricultural
Division of American
Cyanamid Co.
Princeton, New Jersey

K. Brooks Low
Yale University Medical School
New Haven, Connecticut

Thomas F. O'Brien
Peter Bent Brigham Hospital
Boston, Massachusetts

William E. Pace
Bolling Air Force Base
Washington, D.C.

Dwayne C. Savage
University of Illinois
Urbana, Illinois

John F. Timoney
Cornell University,
Ithaca, New York

John P. Utz
Georgetown University Hospital
Washington, D.C.

ADVISORY PANEL ON ANTIBIOTICS IN ANIMAL FEEDS
BOARD ON AGRICULTURE AND RENEWABLE RESOURCES
COMMISSION ON NATURAL RESOURCES

Joseph P. Fontenot, *Cochairman*
Virginia Polytechnic Institute
and State University
Blacksburg, Virginia

George C. Poppensiek, *Cochairman*
New York State College of
Veterinary Medicine
Ithaca, New York

David P. Anderson
University of Georgia
Athens, Georgia

Ernest L. Biberstein
University of California
Davis, California

James L. Bittle
Pitman-Moore, Inc.
Washington Crossing, New Jersey

William Hale
University of Arizona
Tucson, Arizona

Leo S. Jensen
University of Georgia
Athens, Georgia

Vaughn C. Speer
Iowa State University
Ames, Iowa

Clarence M. Stowe
University of Minnesota
St. Paul, Minnesota

Howard S. Teague, *Liaison Member*
U.S. Department of Agriculture
Washington, D.C.

BARR/CNR Staff:

Philip Ross
Selma P. Baron

PREFACE

In 1978, the Congress of the United States provided to the Food and Drug Administration (FDA) an appropriation designated for the National Academy of Sciences to evaluate epidemiological approaches to the effects on human health of subtherapeutic[1,2] use of antimicrobials in animal feeds as defined by the FDA.[3]

The task accepted by the committee was:

"1. To study the human health effects of subtherapeutic use of penicillin and tetracycline (chlortetracycline and oxytetracycline) in animal feeds.

"2. To review and analyze published and unpublished epidemiological data and other data as necessary in order to assess the human health consequences of subtherapeutic use of penicillin and tetracycline in animal feeds.

"3. To assess the scientific feasibility of additional epidemiological studies, and, if needed, to make recommendations about what kinds of research should be carried out, the estimated cost and time required to complete such research and the possible mechanism to be used to conduct such studies."

To complete this task, the committee decided that it should:

1. define and evaluate the effects on human health that are associated with bacterial resistance to antimicrobials,
2. measure changes in numbers of pathogens and define changes in their virulence and in the prevalence of antimicrobial resistance resulting from the use of antimicrobials in animals, and

---

[1] 200 g or less/ton for 2 weeks or longer.
[2] Throughout this report, use of the word ton denotes the "short" ton (2,000 lb), which is most commonly used in the United States. Exceptions to this are noted in the text.
[3] Including milk replacers, medicated blocks, and liquid feeds, but not as used in water alone. FDA does not have jurisdiction over drinking water.

3. differentiate the effects attributable to subtherapeutic levels of antimicrobials from those due to other uses in animal husbandry and in medical applications to animals and human beings.

Because of insufficient data in certain areas, the committee was not able to accomplish all of the above.

The significance of possible effects on human health due to the use of antimicrobials in animal feeds has been the subject of exhaustive reviews by several groups of distinguished scientists in the United States and Europe. Controversy surrounding the restriction of subtherapeutic uses of antimicrobials in animals can be expected to continue until more definitive epidemiological evidence confirms or refutes the potential hazards to human health postulated by these review groups.

The formulation of policy concerning such restriction requires that both benefits and adverse effects be weighed. This committee, however, was not asked to determine policy. Rather, it was charged with and undertook a more limited responsibility: evaluation of existing evidence and development of recommendations pertaining to the kinds of research needed to provide a clearer view of the effects on human health.

COMMITTEE PROCEDURE

An extensive bibliography of the research reports relating to the subtherapeutic use of antimicrobials in animal feeds has been prepared. Plans are being made to publish the bibliography in the near future.

Selected consultants and a special advisory panel from the National Academy of Sciences Board on Agriculture and Renewable Resources were asked to write papers on certain aspects of the problem for use by the committee. These papers are attached to this report as appendixes.

1. The Clinical Use of Antimicrobials and the Development of Resistance--John P. Utz (Appendix A)

2. Possible Human Health Effects of Subtherapeutic Antimicrobial Use as Pesticides--Robert N. Goodman (Appendix B)

3. Genetics of Antimicrobial Resistance--George A. Jacoby and K. Brooks Low (Appendix C)

4. Impact of Antimicrobials on the Microbial Ecology of the Gut--Dwayne C. Savage (Appendix D)

5. Antimicrobial Residues and Resistant Organisms: Their Occurrence, Significance, and Stability--Stanley E. Katz (Appendix E)

6. Zoonotic Aspects of Subtherapeutic Antimicrobials in Feed--John F. Timoney (Appendix F)

7. Transmission of Food-Borne Diseases--Implications of the Subtherapeutic Use of Antimicrobials --Jackson S. Kiser (Appendix G)

8. Food Contamination--William E. Pace (Appendix H)

9. Infectious Disease: Effect of Antimicrobials on Bacterial Populations--Thomas F. O'Brien (Appendix I)

10. Immunological Consequences of Antimicrobials in Animal Feeds--N. Franklin Adkinson, Jr. (Appendix J)

11. Antibiotics in Animal Feed. A report prepared by the Committee on Animal Health and the Committee on Animal Nutrition, Board on Agriculture and Renewable Resources, Commission on Natural Resources, National Research Council, National Academy of Sciences (Appendix K).

On August 22, 1979, the committee met in Washington, D.C. to hear presentations by its consultants and to exchange information and opinions. On the following day, August 23, 1979, a public meeting was held to receive information from persons and organizations. The members of the committee reviewed and evaluated pertinent epidemiological research and, during the week of September 16-21, 1979, convened to develop proposals for further epidemiological studies.

ACKNOWLEDGMENTS

It is a pleasure to express, on behalf of the entire committee, a special note of thanks to the staff: Dr. Enriqueta C. Bond, Dr. Roy Widdus, Mrs. Frances Peter, and Mrs. Susan Barron, whose informed and tireless efforts ably supported the committee. We are grateful for the assistance of those consultants who supplied information and critical reviews of a vast literature and for the help of many members of the staff of the Food and Drug Administration, the Department of Agriculture, the Center for Disease Control, and the Office of Technology Assessment, especially Mr. Philip Frappaolo, Dr. Norman Tufts, Dr. Lester Crawford, Dr. Howard Teague, Dr. John Spaulding, Dr. Robert Brown, Dr. John Bennett, and Dr. Roger Feldman. The committee appreciates the cooperation and information provided by American Cyanamid Company, Pfizer Inc., National Pork Producers Council, representatives of the poultry industry, the Animal Health Institute, and other organizations and individuals too numerous to list.

Last, but not least, we thank the members of the public and the international community of scientists who submitted suggestions and information for our consideration.

Reuel A. Stallones
Chairman
Committee to Study the Human
Health Effects of Subtherapeutic Antibiotic Use in
Animal Feeds

TABLE OF CONTENTS

TABLE OF CONTENTS
(Continued)

SUMMARY

Soon after antimicrobials were introduced into medical practice, the selection pressure exerted by their use caused an increase in the prevalence of microorganisms with resistance to antimicrobials, thereby reducing the effectiveness of therapy. The expanding array of antimicrobial drugs has provided alternative agents in most cases, but control of infections is sometimes delayed because resistance may not be recognized initially. Moreover, the alternative drugs may be more toxic, more expensive, or less effective than those that would be used if the infecting organisms were not resistant.

Most clinically significant antimicrobial-resistant bacterial strains are selected during the administration of antimicrobials to humans, but concern has been expressed that the continuous use of antimicrobials in the feed or drinking water of animals is also responsible for the emergence of resistant strains that may endanger human health. Penicillin and the tetracyclines are effective as additives to animal feed, but since they are also particularly effective and widely used in the therapy of human disease, the Food and Drug Administration has proposed to restrict their use in animal feeds at subtherapeutic doses.

Bacterial resistance to antimicrobials is a genetically determined characteristic, and genes for resistance may be carried either on chromosomes or on extrachromosomal elements called resistance (R) plasmids or R factors. Microorganisms possessing plasmid-mediated resistance to antimicrobials are designated R^+. R factors may be transferred from some bacterial species to certain other species, and resistance to several different antimicrobials is often linked on the same plasmid. Consequently, administration of one antimicrobial may result in the appearance of bacteria with resistance not only to the administered drug but also to one or more others.

The use of antimicrobials in animal husbandry for the improvement of growth and efficiency of feed conversion, for prophylaxis, and for the treatment of diseases has steadily increased since 1950, as has animal production. In 1978, approximately 48% of the antibiotics produced were designated for addition to animal feeds or for other (minor) uses. Antimicrobials are perceived as especially beneficial when animals are stressed either by intensive husbandry or shipment (BARR, Appendix K).

Data demonstrate that the use of antimicrobials in animal husbandry increases the prevalence of R^+ enteric organisms in animals. Some of these organisms may be pathogenic for humans. A number of investigators have asserted that the administration of antimicrobials in subtherapeutic doses to animals raised for human consumption increases the total numbers of R^+ bacteria above that resulting from therapeutic uses of antimicrobials in animals and both therapeutic and prophylactic uses in humans. If this is true and if resistant bacteria are carried through the food processing system to the retail store, animal handlers, meat processors, and consumers would be at increased risk of infection by antimicrobial-resistant pathogens or have an increased likelihood of acquiring a nonpathogenic resistant organism capable of transferring such resistance to pathogens. The committee concluded that not enough information is available on these issues to determine the effects on human health.

Several generalizations can be made:

1. Little is known about the composition of the gastrointestinal flora of humans or animals, especially their anaerobic components (Savage, Appendix D). In those studies of R factors that have been conducted on the enteric flora of animals or humans, investigators have observed changes in the populations of *Escherichia coli* or those of its close relative *Salmonella* because these organisms are easy to culture and manipulate and because they are pervasive pathogens of both animals and humans.

2. The subtherapeutic use of antimicrobials does increase the prevalence of resistance among the *E. coli* and *Salmonella* of treated animals.

3. Persons in close contact with animals receiving antimicrobials are more likely to harbor antimicrobial-resistant *E. coli* than are persons not so exposed. However, studies do not usually indicate the type, duration, and dose levels of the antimicrobials received by the animals. Subtherapeutic use is generally not distinguished from therapeutic use.

4. Abattoir workers carry some of the same phage types[1] that occur in the slaughterhouse environment and in slaughtered animals. Because this information was generated by a study of a small number of people, the comparisons are not conclu-

---

[1]Phage typing is a procedure used by diagnostic laboratories to characterize and identify strains of bacteria according to their pattern of lysis by bacterial viruses (phage).

sive. Furthermore, these workers were exposed to animals that had probably received therapeutic as well as subtherapeutic doses of antimicrobials.

5. There are no data from which to assess the relationship between consumption of meat from animals that received subtherapeutic amounts of antimicrobials and the prevalence of antimicrobial-resistant *E. coli* in the general human population. Limited observations suggest that vegetarians do not harbor fewer resistant *E. coli* than do meat eaters.

6. No data exist to establish a relationship between illness caused by antimicrobial-resistant, pathogenic bacteria, and contact with animals or meat from animals given only subtherapeutic amounts of antimicrobials.

7. No data exist to quantitate the frequency of transfer of antimicrobial-resistance factors from the bacterial flora of animals to the flora of humans or of the transfer within the flora of humans.

8. The therapeutic or prophylactic use of antimicrobials in humans results in a greater prevalence of R^+ strains in the bacterial flora of treated people and their immediate contacts.

9. The disadvantages of using an alternative drug where antimicrobial resistance is present depend on the drugs chosen and each clinical situation. Thus, precise quantitation of the threat of potential "compromise of therapy" posed by an increased prevalence of antimicrobial resistance is exceedingly difficult. However, information on nosocomial infections (which are often resistant) does illustrate the magnitude of the problem.

10. Restrictions on the use of antimicrobials in other countries may well have altered the pattern of their use without significant reduction in the total amount used or in the apparent consequences for humans.

After reviewing the evidence, the committee concluded that the postulated hazards to human health from the subtherapeutic use of antimicrobials in animal feeds were neither proven nor disproven. The lack of data linking human illness with this subtherapeutic use must not be equated with proof that the proposed hazards do not exist. The research necessary to establish and measure a definite risk has not been conducted.

The committee also concluded that it is not possible to conduct a feasible, comprehensive epidemiological study of the effects on human health arising from the subtherapeutic use of antimicrobials in animal feeds, partly because it is impossible to determine the antimicrobial history of the animal from which a particular piece of meat came. However, the committee does present several study possibilities to investigate certain aspects of the problem. These include (1) a study to determine the contribution of subtherapeutic and therapeutic antimicrobial dosing regimens to the prevalence of R^+ enteric organisms in meat animals; (2) a study to measure the extent to which carriage of bacteria having R factors is associated with meat consumption by comparing the enteric flora of vegetarians and meat eaters; (3) a study to measure the extent to which occupational exposure of humans to bacteria from animals in abattoirs is associated with carriage of bacteria having R factors and secondarily to gauge the spread of R factors among close contacts of abattoir workers; (4) a comparison of controls with subjects having urinary tract infections to determine if carriage of antimicrobial-resistant fecal flora is associated with increased morbidity or mortality from the infection.

The committee recommends further research on the mechanisms by which subtherapeutic levels of antimicrobials promote growth of animals. Understanding of this mechanism may lead to the development of other substances or procedures (e.g., immunizations) that provide the same effect, thereby rendering moot the question of possible effects on human health. However, the committee also recommends continued monitoring and occasional review of the possible effects on humans resulting from the subtherapeutic use of antimicrobials in animal feeds.

CHAPTER 1

THE USE OF ANTIMICROBIAL AGENTS[1]

The discovery of the first selective antimicrobial agent approximately four decades ago was a major milestone in the history of medicine and human health. The subsequent development of antimicrobial therapy largely centered on the search for drugs with effectiveness against microbial species that were not susceptible to drugs then in use.

These powerful new drugs have been shown to save lives when used to treat some severe infections and to reduce the burden of illness when used prophylactically in certain clinical situations (Utz, Appendix A). Since antibiotics[1] are isolated from microorganisms, strains of some microbial species have predictably evolved the capacity to inactivate them or become impermeable to them, i.e., these strains have developed resistance to these antibiotics. Resistance to synthetic antimicrobial agents arises from the variation normally displayed by individual microorganisms within species. Thus, the consequence of expanded use of antimicrobial drugs has been an increased prevalence of resistant organisms resulting from the selection process. In certain places, such as hospitals, contact between individuals has facilitated the spread of these resistant bacteria.

Consequently, researchers sought agents that were active against strains in which resistance had become prevalent. The expanding array of antimicrobials, particularly antibiotics, provided alternatives in most cases. But control of infections is sometimes delayed if the resistance of the infecting organism is not recognized immediately, and physicians may need to use drugs that are more toxic, more expensive, or less effective than those that would be selected if the infecting organisms were not resistant (Utz, Appendix A).

Trends in the antimicrobial resistance patterns of a number of clinically important pathogens have been reviewed by Finland (1979) and Stollerman (1978). The prevalence of multiply antimicrobial-resistant *Staphylococcus aureus* increased until 1960 but subsequently declined in association with a change in phage types. Recently, strains of *Streptococcus pneumoniae* with multiple resistance have been found in a number of countries. Strains of *Haemophilus*

---

[1]An antibiotic is a chemical substance produced by microorganisms that has the capacity at low concentrations to inhibit the growth of or to destroy bacteria and other microorganisms. An antimicrobial is any agent that destroys microorganisms or suppresses their multiplication or growth.

influenzae producing β-lactamase and occasional strains with resistance to chloramphenicol have also been observed, as have strains of *Neisseria gonorrhoeae* producing plasmid-mediated β-lactamase. Other changes are noted by Finland (1979).

Differences in resistance encountered in certain pathogens of humans are often observed in separated geographical areas (Finland, 1979), in different hospitals (O'Brien, Appendix I), or in local outbreaks, e.g., of chloramphenicol-resistant strains of *Salmonella typhi* in Vietnam and Mexico (Finland, 1979). The committee could find no comparable assessments of the trends in resistance to antimicrobials that might have occurred in the major pathogens of food animals over the last three decades.

The prevalence of clinically significant antimicrobial-resistant bacterial strains correlates with the increasing use of antimicrobial agents in the course of clinical practice (Finland, 1955a,b,c; 1979).

The necessity for therapeutic use of antimicrobial agents in the treatment of overt disease in animals has not been questioned. However, the continuous use of subtherapeutic levels of antimicrobials in animal feeds for growth promotion, improvement of feed efficiency, and disease prophylaxis has been criticized as posing dangers to human health by making an important quantitative contribution to the pool of antimicrobial-resistant bacteria that may be transferred to the human population. Possible "qualitative" effects of the selection pressure imposed by subtherapeutic usage on resistance profiles or transfer mechanisms are discussed below and by O'Brien (Appendix I).

For regulatory purposes, the Food and Drug Administration (FDA) defines subtherapeutic use as the administration of doses less than or equal to 200 g of antimicrobial per ton of feed for 2 weeks or longer. However, the FDA has approved the marketing of some antimicrobial agents for use at levels below 200 g/ton to treat certain diseases (Animal Health Institute, 1979). Therefore, the current definition of subtherapeutic use in animal feeds encompasses certain uses that are therapeutic in intent in addition to those for prophylaxis and the improvement of growth and efficiency of feed conversion.

In the hope of preserving the effectiveness of the antimicrobial agents that are important in the therapy of human diseases, some governments (e.g., the United Kingdom) have regulated the use of these agents as growth promotants in animal feeds (Swann *et al.*, 1969). Antimicrobials used to treat humans are still approved in those countries for use in animals on veterinary prescription.

Similar actions have been under consideration in many other countries, including the United States. Since penicillin and the tetracyclines are effective and widely used in the therapy of human disease, the FDA has proposed restriction of their subtherapeutic use in animal feeds.

This committee has attempted to determine if human health is affected by the subtherapeutic use of antimicrobials in animal feeds and to ascertain what additional information is needed to make a more definitive determination.

NATURE OF THE SELECTION PRESSURE IMPOSED BY ANTIMICROBIALS

It is important to distinguish between the effects of an antimicrobial drug on a single antimicrobial-sensitive microbial strain and the effects on a heterogeneous mixture of species or strains. When antimicrobial drugs are brought into contact with multiplying susceptible microorganisms, the organisms are generally inhibited from multiplying further or are killed. When the susceptible organisms constitute a portion of the total microbial flora that is exposed to the drugs, the elimination of the susceptible organisms is generally followed by some degree of compensatory multiplication of the more resistant or nonsusceptible strains. Such a shift in the composition of the enteric flora may facilitate infection by a pathogen (Seelig, 1966).

Another important consideration in the evaluation of possible effects on human health is the possibility of "qualitative" as well as quantitative changes in resistance brought about by the continuing selection pressure exerted by subtherapeutic levels of antimicrobials in animal feeds. To date, most research has been focused on quantitative changes, i.e., changes in the prevalence of resistance, primarily because techniques to study qualitative changes have only recently been developed. Qualitative changes could include the development of new combinations of resistance genes, combination with genes for other characteristics, e.g., toxins, the spread of such plasmids to new hosts and, possibly most seriously, the evolution of more efficient, wider host-range transfer mechanisms. The evidence for such changes is discussed by Jacoby and Low (Appendix C). The implications of this "molecular epidemiology of plasmids" are considered by O'Brien (Appendix I). Another change that could be regarded as qualitative is the shift in the composition of the gastrointestinal flora under the selection pressure of subtherapeutic dosages of antimicrobials. This shift will produce changes in the interactions of the flora components with each other and with the host. Little is known about the composition of the gastrointestinal flora in either humans or animals, especially the anaerobic components (Savage, Appendix D). Therefore, because of the lack of data and methodology to carry out *in-vivo* experiments, it is not possible to assess the significance for human health of such shifts.

Investigators who have studied resistance in the gastrointestinal flora of humans or animals have generally observed changes in the prevalence of R factors in *E. coli* or its close relative *Salmonella* because these organisms are easy to culture and manipulate and because they can be pervasive pathogens in both humans and animals. The significance of resistance in these two species may not be the same since their "ecology" is different. This is discussed briefly in the next section.

A thorough assessment of the significance for human health of various uses of antimicrobials requires knowledge of the consequences of the selection pressures imposed by intermittent, therapeutic doses versus subtherapeutic continuous feeding and of different routes of administration. Unfortunately, there are insufficient data comparing these regimens. Such data would have been of invaluable assistance to the committee during its deliberations.

MECHANISMS AND TRANSFER OF RESISTANCE

In most instances bacterial resistance to antimicrobial agents is conferred by extrachromosomal genetic elements called plasmids. Those conferring resistance are called R factors or R plasmids (Jacoby and Low, Appendix C). These plasmids are widely distributed among bacterial species, including those that are pathogenic in humans and animals. Some plasmids transfer between species of different genera.

Two general types of R plasmids have been identified on the basis of their transmissibility characteristics:

Large R plasmids harbor approximately 100 genes and are transmissible to other cells by a process called conjugation or bacterial mating. Approximately 25 plasmid genes code for functions that are required for transmissibility, several other genes code for replication functions, and from four to six genes generally code for resistance to antimicrobials. The functions of other genes on the larger R plasmids have not been identified.

Small R plasmids usually harbor approximately 10 genes. These plasmids do not carry the genes for transmissibility and are not transmissible when by themselves. However, a transmissible plasmid may sometimes mediate the transfer of an otherwise untransmissible one when present simultaneously in the same cell.

Some pairs of R plasmids cannot coexist stably in the same host cell, a phenomenon referred to as "incompatibility." This simple criterion has enabled investigators to differentiate R plasmids into more than 40 incompatibility groups. The mechanism of incompatibility is not yet understood. It may be related to the control of plasmid replication.

Different R plasmids may represent a group of genetic elements of diverse origin. However, even if located on plasmids in different incompatibility groups, the genes that confer resistance to specific antimicrobials are very similar. This may be explained by recent observations that certain antimicrobial resistance genes are located on segments of DNA (transposons) that may spontaneously translocate from one plasmid to another, thereby disseminating the resistance gene(s) among various plasmids (Kleckner, 1977). Factors that promote or inhibit the transfer of R factors *in vivo* are not completely understood (Jacoby and Low, Appendix C).

The biochemical mechanisms of resistance are known in most instances. R plasmids confer resistance to antimicrobials either by encoding for enzymes that chemically modify and thus inactivate the agent, by specifying a substitute metabolic enzyme that is insensitive to the agent, or by specifying a decrease in cell permeability to the agent. All three types of resistance mechanisms may be determined by the same plasmid, whether transmissible or nontransmissible. Thus, R plasmids are endowed with genes that increase the probability of survival of host cells in the presence of combinations of antimicrobials. The continued spread among bacteria of resistance to more than one antimicrobial and the further acquisition of additional resistance genes by individual R plasmids results from the selection pressure imposed by the use of antimicrobials.

A number of factors affect the transfer rates of plasmids between species, e.g., the frequency with which R^+ enteric bacteria come into contact with other bacteria and the environment in which they meet. The logistics of transfer of bacteria from animals to humans and of interbacterial transfer of plasmids may be different for different organisms. Salmonellae are generally infrequent, abnormal components of the flora of animals and humans, but when present they occur in enormous numbers that increase the potential for transfer at such times. *E. coli*, compared to the anaerobic flora, usually constitute a numerically small proportion of the gastrointestinal flora of animals and humans, but its continuous presence (Savage, Appendix D) offers a different potential for transfer.

Bacterial genetic aspects of drug resistance have been reviewed by Jacoby and Low (Appendix C). The dissemination of drug-resistance genes among diverse bacterial genera is also discussed by these authors as well as by O'Brien (Appendix I). The epidemiology of plasmid transfer has not been studied in sufficient detail.

Whatever motivation lies behind the use of antimicrobial agents in any specific situation, the consequences will be the same. Administration of an antimicrobial will result in a selection pressure favoring an increase in the prevalence of resistant organisms.

THE USE OF ANTIMICROBIALS IN HUMAN MEDICINE

The use of antimicrobials in both hospitalized and ambulatory patients is extensive. Kunin (1979) reported that between 23% to 37.8% of hospitalized individuals receive them. Finkel (1978) estimated from dispensed prescription data and FDA certification records that approximately 190 million prescriptions for the major antimicrobials were filled for ambulatory patients in the United States in 1977. This is nearly one course of treatment per year for each person in the United States and includes approximately 43 million prescriptions for tetracycline.

The consequences resulting from the administration of antimicrobials to humans have been examined by Finland (1979). Hartley and Richmond (1975) reported that oral intake of tetracycline leads to the emergence of a predominantly tetracycline-resistant coliform gastrointestinal flora within 48 hours in those treated. The excretion of resistant organisms continues at least 10 days after the treatment is terminated (Richmond, 1975).

A complete evaluation of the increased prevalence of resistance to antimicrobials would require consideration of not only the contributions from subtherapeutic and therapeutic use in animals but also the extent to which these agents are administered to humans. Richmond and Linton (1980) studied the use of tetracyclines in the County of Avon in England and its possible relation to the excretion of tetracycline-resistant bacteria. They estimated that one in 130 individuals in the county carried a large proportion of tetracycline-resistant organisms in their alimentary tracts. Examination of swabs from sewers in predominantly residential areas of Bristol (in Avon) (Linton *et al.*, 1974) indicated that approximately 3% of the isolated coliforms were resistant to tetracycline. Richmond and Linton (1980) concluded that, ". . . there hardly seems a need to postulate a veterinary source for the resistant coliforms encountered in the human population. This is not to say that resistant *E. coli* of animal and poultry origin cannot reach the human population: clearly they can and do (Linton *et al.*, 1977). And some resistant salmonellae of animal origin certainly seem to have caused serious human epidemic disease (Anderson, 1968[b]). But whether the use of antibiotics in the animal and poultry rearing industries has a major quantitative impact must be questionable; . . ."

The approach adopted by Linton and Richmond is necessarily indirect and requires a number of approximations and assumptions. Although no similar studies have been conducted in the United States, the data reported by Kunin (1979) and Finkel (1978) on prescriptions in this country indicate that the administration of antimicrobials to humans is widespread.

THE USE OF ANTIMICROBIALS IN AGRICULTURE

The livestock and poultry industry has undergone dramatic changes since 1950. Operations that were extensive became more intensive. There were increases in the size of facilities, the number of animals reared, and a move toward centralization. Socioeconomic changes, as well as advances in biomedical sciences, nutrition, engineering, and management, have all contributed to this evolution.

Shortly after antimicrobials had been discovered and their therapeutic use in humans and animals had begun, investigators learned that the addition of antimicrobials to animal feed was effective in growth promotion, improvement of feed conversion, prophylaxis, and treatment of certain diseases. These effects of antimicrobials are especially useful when animals are stressed either by intensive husbandry practices or shipment.

The use of antibiotics (and most probably sulfonamides) in animal husbandry has steadily increased since 1950 as has animal production (Table 1). In 1978 approximately 48% of the antibiotics produced were designated for addition to animal feeds or for other (minor) uses (U.S. International Trade Commission, 1979). The motivation for such use and the economic consequences of restricting subtherapeutic concentrations of antimicrobials in feed have been dealt with in reports by the National Academy of Sciences Board on Agriculture and Renewable Resources (BARR, Appendix K) and the U.S. Department of Agriculture (1978).

TABLE 1

Antibiotic Production from 1950 to 1978 (millions of kg)[a,b]

Year	Total	Medicinal Use in Humans and Animals	Added to Animal Feed and Other Applications
1978	11.66	6.08	5.58
1977	10.48	6.35	4.58
1976	9.30	4.72	4.54
1975	8.30	4.26	4.04
1974	9.30	5.99	3.36
1973	9.43	5.72	3.72
1972	7.53	4.45	3.08
1971	8.12	4.90	3.22
1970	7.67	4.35	3.31
1969	5.99	3.36	2.63
1968	4.67	2.72	1.95
1967	4.29	2.36	1.91
1966	4.40	2.45	1.91
1965	3.40	2.13	1.27
1964	2.95	1.77	1.18
1963	3.04	1.91	1.13
1962	2.86	1.81	1.04
1961	2.31	1.50	0.82
1960	2.13	1.36	0.77
1959	1.68	1.04	0.64
1958	1.59	1.18	0.41
1957	1.47	1.08	0.39
1956	1.24	0.89	0.35
1955	0.95	0.71	0.24
1954	1.05	0.83	0.22
1953	0.94	0.74	0.20
1952	0.79	0.67	0.12
1951	0.69	0.58	0.11
1950	0.39	0.39	Mentioned, but no figure

[a]Data extracted from reports of the U.S. International Trade Commission (1951-1979).

[b]Values exclude production of sulfonamides.

The mechanisms by which antimicrobials improve growth and the efficiency of feed conversion are not fully understood. Some suggested effects include modification of host metabolism, nutrient sparing or alteration of nutrient absorption, and selective activity against microorganisms (BARR, Appendix K).

Total amounts used and patterns of usage, which vary with species and geographic location, are described in reports by BARR (Appendix K) and the Animal Health Institute (1979). Information on the total amount of specific antimicrobials administered for each application listed above does not appear to be available.

Certain antimicrobials (streptomycin, tetracyclines, penicillin) are also used to control plant pathogens. Although this application might also have consequences for human health, the amounts used are much smaller (Goodman, Appendix B).

The addition of subtherapeutic amounts of antimicrobials to animal feeds continues to be of concern because of its implications for human health and because some believe that this use is unessential. In the United States therapeutic concentrations of drugs are given to livestock extensively, with or without veterinary prescription. Treated animals are not always isolated from untreated ones, and animal-to-animal transfer of R^+ organisms is known to occur (Levy, 1978). Since most herds and flocks receive antimicrobials somewhere in the production chain either for growth promotion, prophylaxis, or therapy, it is difficult to identify slaughtered livestock that have not been given antimicrobials or have not been exposed to animals that had.

DEFINITION OF HUMAN HEALTH HAZARD

The difficulty of determining whether human health is affected by the subtherapeutic use of antimicrobials in feeds is compounded by the diversity of opinions concerning the definition of a hazard to human health. Some view an increase in the pool of antimicrobial-resistant bacteria or an increase in *Salmonella* shedding by food animals as a source of danger. Others maintain that a significant hazard to health exists only if antimicrobial-resistant organisms can be shown to be transmitted to animal handlers or to meat processors. Others attach importance only to the passage of resistant microorganisms to meat consumers. Still others view these circumstances as unrealized, potential hazards. These scientists insist that incremental morbidity and, perhaps, excess mortality that can reasonably be attributed to resistant organisms resulting from subtherapeutic use of antimicrobials must be documented before risk to human health from this cause can be substantiated. This divergence of opinion was reflected in the committee itself.

There are no data from which to predict quantitatively the change in the morbidity and mortality of humans that might result from an increased prevalence of resistant bacteria in animals or from the transfer of these organisms to humans. Although a measurable risk to human health cannot be ascribed to these phenonema, they remain plausible potential hazards since some of the individual steps in the transmission chain to humans have been independently demonstrated but not quantified (see Chapter 3).

An increased prevalence of resistant bacteria may result from the administration of both therapeutic and subtherapeutic levels of antimicrobials to animals and human beings. Thus, the question is raised whether antimicrobials used subtherapeutically in the meat industry add measurably to the carriage of resistant organisms, the incidence of clinical illness, or the number of complications resulting from antimicrobial resistance in the treatment of diseases. The committee could find little relevant information on the relative selection pressures for antimicrobial resistance exerted by continuous low-dose feeding versus intermittent higher, therapeutic doses. This subject is examined later in this report.

Other possible hazards to health (also discussed below) received committee attention but were eliminated from further deliberations because they were not central to the major issue or because there was insufficient information.

Katz (Appendix E) prepared for committee consideration an assessment of the potential hazards to humans presented by residues of antimicrobials in livestock and poultry meat products. Surveys have shown that slaughtered animals may contain residues of penicillin or tetracycline that probably resulted from inadequate withdrawal times or large dosages (Huber, 1971). More recent surveys (Katz, Appendix E; Mussman, 1975; USDA, 1979) indicate that the residues resulting from penicillin or tetracycline used as feed additives were generally below the limits currently permitted by the FDA. Residues of tetracyclines were undetectable in animals slaughtered 1 to 5 days after withdrawal of antimicrobial-containing feed. The small amounts of these residues in the muscle tissues of animals do not survive normal food preparation because of heat inactivation during cooking (Katz, Appendix E).

Katz (Appendix E) reported that there has been concern that the therapeutic use of penicillin has resulted in significant residues. However, he noted that current regulations governing the subtherapeutic use of penicillin as a feed additive appear to result in very low or infrequent residues in meat.

Katz concluded, "It is doubtful that antibiotic residues or their degradation products will provide any selective pressure on enteric bacteria contaminating the carcasses of animals." The committee concurs with this assessment. It believes that further studies of the effect on human health resulting from penicillin and tetracycline residues in meat would not elucidate the hazard from subtherapeutic levels of antimicrobials in animal feeds.

The committee also viewed an assessment of the immunological consequences to humans resulting from penicillin and tetracycline residues in livestock and poultry meat products (Adkinson, Appendix J). Although pertinent information is limited, the committee concurs with Adkinson's conclusion that "there is little reason to believe that foodstuffs obtained from animals fattened with antibiotic-supplemented feed impose a significant risk to human health by contributing to antibiotic-induced allergic reactions."

Adkinson indicated that further investigations in several areas could provide information that would be useful in clinical situations. However, the committee believes that immunological problems arising from the use of antimicrobials in animal feeds are not a serious health risk for the general population.

In attempting to define the possible hazards to human health, the committee wished to know how the acquisition of antimicrobial resistance affected the virulence of pathogens infecting humans and animals. Since limited conclusive information appeared to be available (Jacoby and Low, Appendix C), the committee decided not to review this topic in depth.

CHAPTER 2

MEASURING EFFECTS ON HUMAN HEALTH FROM THE SUBTHERAPEUTIC USE OF ANTIMICROBIALS IN ANIMAL FEEDS

A complex chain of events begins with the addition of subtherapeutic levels of antimicrobials to animal feed, proceeds to the selection of bacteria bearing R plasmids in the animal gut and the transfer of these bacteria to humans (or their plasmids into the flora of humans), and ends with possibly adverse effects on human health.

The entire chain can be thought of as a stochastic process. All steps of the chain are apparently possible, but have not been quantified. For example, the extent of the normal transfer of R^+ organisms between animals or between animals and humans has not been adequately measured.

The entire length of this chain is germane to this study, i.e., how does a change in the addition of antimicrobials to animal feed at the beginning of the chain alter the probability or severity of diseases or the ability to treat them at the end of the chain?

A number of complications can arise when attempting to resolve this question. This is illustrated by the following series of questions that should be addressed when treating a hospitalized patient suffering from septicemia due to *Salmonella*.

1. Is the *Salmonella* strain resistant to antimicrobials?

2. Is the resistance plasmid mediated?

3. Was the *Salmonella* resistant to drugs when the infection occurred or did it acquire resistance through transfer of an R factor from the patient's resident microbial flora?

4. Did the patient acquire the *Salmonella* infection from contaminated meat or from another person?

5. If the infection was acquired from meat, had the animal received an antimicrobial?

6. Was the antimicrobial given to the animal for growth promotion, for prophylaxis, or for treatment of an illness?

7. If the *Salmonella* acquired resistance by R-factor transfer from *E. coli*, was the resistant *E. coli* selected by an antimicrobial used in previous treatment or did the patient acquire a resistant *E. coli* strain from another person or from ingestion of contaminated meat? If the resistant strain was acquired from another person, was that person infected via the food chain and did the food chain begin with an animal that had received subtherapeutic doses of antimicrobials?

Determination of the answers to all of these questions for an individual patient is obviously very difficult and may well be impossible.

Antimicrobial use varies greatly among producers of cattle, swine, and poultry, within each of these subsets of the industry, and among different parts of the country. Moreover, the distribution channels are long and complex. Consequently, a consumer may purchase meat that was processed in a distant plant from animals raised in a still more distant place.

The beef consumed by a household may have come from a feedlot in which antimicrobials were used only to treat sick animals, but its pork may have come from pigs fed tetracycline for growth promotion. Even if *Salmonella* may be judged more likely to have come from one source than from another, it may have acquired resistance by plasmid transfer from *E. coli* derived from either source.

EPIDEMIOLOGICAL STUDIES

The definitive epidemiological study of effects related to the subtherapeutic use of antimicrobials in animal feeds should encompass all aspects of meat production from animal breeding to consumption.

Methods

The committee examined the approaches that could be taken to relate the subtherapeutic use of antimicrobials in animal feed to the risk of increased morbidity and mortality in humans. It then grouped these approaches into six categories.

Cross-Sectional Studies (Population or Prevalence Surveys). Total communities, random samples of a total community, or selected subsets of a population may be identified and asked to provide answers to questions, undergo laboratory or clinical procedures, or both. Such surveys are conducted once, and the findings are customarily presented as prevalence ratios of a disease or condition between populations. Differences in the prevalence of the disease or condition in demographic subgroups may be interpreted as reflecting differences in risk caused by the exposure under study. Specifically, populations that have had considerable exposure and others with minimal exposure to animals receiving antimicrobials via their feed could be surveyed to determine the prevalence of some specific conditions, e.g., urinary tract infection caused by R^+ organisms. The results of such surveys may be confounded by differences in prevalence of some associated causal or risk factors, such as socioeconomic status. For instance, elevated rates of diarrheal disease in farm workers handling feed containing antimicrobials, when compared to rates in nonfarm groups, may be due as much to differences in sanitation in the work and home environments as to the acquisition of resistant pathogens from animals.

Surveys are conducted frequently because they are relatively inexpensive and generally quite rapid. Survey data are generally unreliable in identifying the differences between statistical association and cause and effect, partly because the effects of time are difficult to incorporate into a cross-sectional survey. This weakness presents a particular disadvantage in any situation that changes over time.

Case-Comparison Studies. The characteristics of patients with a disease or other condition may be compared with those of a group of people who are free of the disease or condition, but whose other characteristics, such as age, sex, race, and history of exposure to therapeutic levels of antimicrobials, are similar. The comparison subjects are often selected from the same clinical setting in which the cases were discovered, but may be selected from groups living in the same neighborhood or perhaps by a random sampling of the general community. The characteristics of both groups and the exposure to which they have been subjected are surveyed retrospectively. For instance, patients with a disease believed to be attributable to resistant microorganisms can be matched with comparison subjects. Exposure to animals, to animal products, or to feed containing antimicrobial agents is the determined retrospectively. The efficiency of such a study may be improved by careful selection of comparison subjects to match the characteristics of the cases. The relative risk associated with certain characteristics, such as degrees of exposure to antimicrobials in animal feed, may be estimated by calculating odds ratios. Such studies may be relatively inexpensive and can be conducted rapidly, but they require careful predetermination of the characteristics to be matched and investigated retrospectively. If important variables are missed or mismatching occurs, results may be interpreted incorrectly.

Cohort Studies. Variables related to risk of a population or a selected subset of a population may be identified and characterized, and the study group followed over time to observe new cases of illness. For instance, generally healthy individuals with high exposure to animal feeds containing antimicrobials, or to meat from animals that consumed such feed, and other members of the same community without such exposure may be followed for a year or longer. Populations with different exposures can be examined for differences in incidence or severity of diseases or for difficulties encountered during their treatment. The differences in these measurements will reflect the risk associated with the different exposures.

Cohort studies are generally considered to be the most effective approach to establishing differences in risk associated with various conditions, but they are expensive and time-consuming. Moreover, they require careful recordkeeping, meticulous followup of the cohort, and attentiveness to ensure that differences in medical care or inaccurate definitions of morbid events do not confound the study.

Experimental Studies. After a defined study population is identified and characterized, an appropriate subgroup is subjected to an experimental procedure. The test group is then followed to observe the effects of the procedure. The remainder of the initial group serves as a control. Experimental studies, particularly when the exposed group is randomly selected, are very effective in establishing the cause-and-effect relationship between the experimental variable and the observed outcome. Thus, if it were possible to select a large number of subjects and randomly assign them to groups that are or are not exposed to animals fed antimicrobials or to the products of those animals, useful information would undoubtedly accrue.

The performance of experimental studies with humans may be questioned on ethical grounds if there is any known or theorized hazard of the exposure being investigated. Moreover, such controlled trials are frequently very difficult to conduct because the subjects may not adhere to the regimen to which they have been randomly assigned. Experimental studies cannot yield definitive information on the likelihood that similar effects would result at similar frequencies under natural conditions.

Investigation of Epidemics. Outbreaks of a disease may be investigated retrospectively with epidemiological methods. Such investigations cannot quantitate the prevalence of diseases since only reported cases can be investigated. Nevertheless, they can be useful in establishing a probable chain of transmission.

Case Reports/Case Series. Although not an epidemiological method, reports of individual cases or series of cases may also establish that a particular sequence or chain of events is possible. They cannot be used to predict the prevalence of a disease or condition or the risk of any practice.

WHAT IS THE IDEAL STUDY?

The ideal study would start with the selection of animal-rearing facilities marked by sharply different practices in antimicrobial use--i.e., no use; subtherapeutic use in feeds for improving growth and feed conversion and for prophylaxis; intermittent therapeutic use; and both subtherapeutic and therapeutic use. A substantial number of facilities in each selected category should be studied to ensure that any observed differences in flora are more likely to be related to differences in antimicrobial use rather than to other confounding variables.

Fecal specimens should be examined from a large enough sample of animals in each flock or herd to monitor changes in the proportion of animals carrying *Salmonella* spp. and *E. coli* with resistance and the percentage of these resistant organisms in each animal's flora. Ideally, full microbiological characterization of the flora, both aerobic and anaerobic, should be performed for both animals and humans. Special attention should be given to changes in those indices associated with intermittent therapeutic applications of antimicrobials.

Similar studies should be conducted of employees, their families, and a comparison group of neighbors employed in other occupations to determine whether their microflora follow patterns like those observed in animals.

At the next several steps in the production chain--the slaughterhouses and wholesale and retail butcher shops--bacteriological studies of carcasses, the work environments, employees, their families, and their neighbors should be pursued over time to determine whether changes in the indices of drug resistance occurring in the production facilities can be traced through the processing plants. The processing plants should, of course, receive meats from only one of the specified categories of animal producers.

Finally, these same investigative techniques should be used in comparable communities where the meats and meat products are sold, prepared, and consumed, still separated by the type of antimicrobial use in animal feeds at their sources. Selecting comparable communities may be difficult since many factors need to be matched, e.g., the degree of hygiene in butcher shops. Samples of households should be selected, and the enteric bacteria of the family members should be characterized. The sampling would permit community-wide estimates of the prevalence of both resistant and susceptible Salmonella infection, as well as the prevalence of colonization with resistant E. coli. A system of defining, identifying, and recording illnesses should be established in order to compute the rates of disease caused by Salmonella and to determine the special problems that result from illnesses attributable to resistant strains.

Attempts should be made to trace the spread of Salmonella infection in these communities, identifying wherever possible cases attributable to contact with or consumption of contaminated meat and those due to secondary spread from person to person.

The nature of antimicrobial resistance in other pathogens causing illness in these communities should also be investigated to ascertain the extent to which R factors arising from therapeutic and subtherapeutic antimicrobial use in animals are transferred between microbial species and constitute a health problem.

A characterization of the R plasmids, which can be achieved by physical, genetic, or enzyme techniques (Jacoby and Low, Appendix C; O'Brien, Appendix I), could provide corroborative evidence of the direction of transmission and information on qualitative changes in resistance.

If the inquiries conducted on the breeding farms and the feedlots reveal no differences in the prevalence of resistant organisms in animals related to the differing use of antimicrobials, the study could be terminated. If such differences are apparent, further work would be needed. The second phase of the study would determine the occupationally associated risk of acquisition of resistant organisms and provide some information on the likelihood of spread from these foci. The carrier rates in samples from the neighborhoods of the abattoir workers should provide data on the prevalence of resistant enteric bacteria in general communities, as would the information derived from the household samples in the third phase. The community-based studies would relate the carrier rates in a community to the use of antimicrobials in animals and measure the associated burden of disease (see Table 2-1).

TABLE 2-1

The Ideal Comprehensive Study Design

PHASE 1: BREEDING FARMS AND FEEDLOTS

Study Groups	Study Procedures
Herds and flocks in four categories of antimicrobial use:	Bacteriological indices:
no antimicrobial use subtherapeutic use only therapeutic use only both subtherapeutic and therapeutic use	Prevalence of carriage of antimicrobial-resistant *Salmonella* spp./relative frequency of resistant organisms in each specimen
Animal handlers Family members	Prevalence of carriage of antimicrobial-resistant *E. coli*/relative frequency of resistant organisms in each specimen
Neighbors	Characterization of fecal flora and plasmids

PHASE 2: SLAUGHTERHOUSES, PROCESSING PLANTS, AND RETAIL BUTCHER SHOPS

Study Groups	Study Procedures
Carcasses	Bacteriological indices (as above)
Meat handlers	Human illness caused by bacteria
Family members	
Neighbors	

PHASE 3: COMMUNITIES

Study Groups	Study Procedures
Households selected on the basis of probability sample	Bacteriological indices (as above)
Cases of salmonellosis	Tracing of source of infection
Other cases of infectious diseases caused by bacteria	

FEASIBILITY OF A COMPREHENSIVE STUDY

The committee reviewed methods for gathering information on the effects of various exposures on subsequent morbidity and mortality and for determining the specific needs for information on the subtherapeutic use of antimicrobials in animal feeds. It concluded that the comprehensive study described above could not be realized or even approximated. This decision reflects a number of facts, which are discussed below:

The use of antimicrobials differs markedly for the three major meat animals--cattle, swine, and poultry. Moreover, for each type of animal the use of antimicrobials varies in various parts of the country and at different times, e.g., with seasons or weather conditions. Moreover, it is often not possible to differentiate whether the antimicrobials had been given for growth promotion, prophylaxis, or treatment of manifest illness. In much of the industry, only insignificant numbers of animals have never received any antimicrobials, and in normal rearing and processing operations, it is not practical to identify these animals. During shipment from breeding farms to feedlots, groups of animals with different exposures to antimicrobials are often combined. The likely exchange of bacteria between animals under these circumstances further hinders the identification of the origin of any observed R^+ organisms.

The processing of meats and meat products also contributes to the mixing of meats from animals with different antimicrobial histories. Cross-contamination can also occur in these processes, e.g., via cutting boards and instruments. Currently, there is no hope of identifying communities in which residents can purchase only the meat of animals that had been exposed to only one regimen of antimicrobial usage.

The diseases and conditions likely to result from resistant microorganisms in the general population exposed to meat are relatively rare. Overt diarrhea caused by *Salmonella*, acute urinary tract infections in young women, and other illnesses related to infections with enteric pathogens all have extremely low incidence rates. Thus, any study attempting to relate an increase (possibly a small increase) in morbidity or mortality to exposure to R^+ organisms on meat (whether selected by subtherapeutic or therapeutic antimicrobial use) would be so massive that it would probably be unmanageable. Additionally, the chain of events linking antimicrobial-resistant bacteria in the animal gut to overt human infections is extraordinarily difficult to trace in any given case. This difficulty would increase the uncertainty in the study and jeopardize the validity of any risk estimates that might be developed.

ALTERNATIVES TO A COMPREHENSIVE STUDY AND THEIR DEFICIENCIES

Less comprehensive approaches, although more realistic, cannot provide direct evidence of a consistent chain of causation from subtherapeutic antimicrobial use in animal feeds to human illness. Moreover, the fragmentary data that are available (discussed below) not only suffer from deficiencies of method and design but also leave gaps that can be bridged only by conjecture or speculation. Better research may repair the former, but little can be done about the latter. Some deficiencies of the narrower studies are listed below:

- Studies of the prevalence of antimicrobial-resistant bacteria in animals cannot be used to determine the extent of the transmission of R^+ enteric organisms from animals to human populations.

- In studies of the prevalence of R^+ organisms in farm workers, the R^+ bacteria acquired directly from animals cannot easily be distinguished from those R^+ organisms resulting from the selection pressure exerted by ingested or inhaled antimicrobials from the feeds.

- Studies of the prevalence of resistant organisms on carcasses or in abattoir workers do not provide direct measurements of the extent to which these organisms are transmitted to the general population, nor can they distinguish the effects of subtherapeutic use from the therapeutic use of antimicrobials.

- Studies comparing the prevalence of R^+ organisms in meat-eaters and vegetarians cannot differentiate whether observed differences in the meat-eaters can be attributed to the selective pressure for resistance exerted by the subtherapeutic use or by the therapeutic use of antimicrobials in the animals consumed. Such studies would also need to take into account the use of antimicrobials in the subjects themselves or in persons in their immediate environment.

- Studies on the prevalence rates of R^+ organisms in different populations can only imply the causes for differences in rates. They do not relate R^+ prevalence rates to increases in morbidity, mortality, or complications in therapy caused by resistance in the pathogen.

The foregoing discussion makes it clear that isolated studies on parts of the transmission chain cannot be used to quantitate the overall effects on human health resulting from the subtherapeutic use of antimicrobials in animal feeds.

This committee therefore concludes that it is not possible to conduct a feasible, comprehensive direct study of the effects on human health arising from the subtherapeutic use of antimicrobials in animal feeds. However, after examining some of the issues and the research conducted to date, the committee outlined several studies that might quantitate some of the stages in the chain of causation on which speculation of hazard is based.

The studies are presented as an indication of what the committee believes to be the most fruitful approaches. They will not provide a direct assessment of the effects on human health resulting from subtherapeutic levels of antimicrobials. Chapter 4 contains descriptions of these studies and some caveats on the interpretation of their results.

CHAPTER 3

CRITICAL REVIEW OF THE EPIDEMIOLOGICAL LITERATURE

Effects on human health resulting from the use of antimicrobials in animal feeds have been reviewed by distinguished scientists in the United States and Europe. Reports prepared by the Swann Committee (Swann *et al.*, 1969), the Food and Drug Administration (FDA) Task Force (FDA, 1972), the FDA Environmental Impact Statement staff (FDA, 1978), the Office of Technology Assessment (1979), and the World Health Organization (1974, 1976, 1978) provide extensive coverage of the issues and background information. The majority opinion expressed in each report was that an increased prevalence of antimicrobial-resistant organisms presents a threat to human health and that the subtherapeutic use of antimicrobials increases the prevalence of R^+ organisms in animals. In all of the reports authors were not able or did not attempt to quantitate or estimate the relative contribution of the subtherapeutic use of antimicrobials in animals to health problems in humans caused by R^+ organisms--one of the objectives of this study. Majorities of the individuals involved in these various studies recommended policies aimed at restricting the subtherapeutic use of antimicrobials in animal feeds, particularly for those agents used in the therapy of diseases in humans.

The therapeutic use of antimicrobials in both animals and humans has been shown to result in an increased prevalence of resistant bacteria (Anderson, 1968a; Finland, 1979; Mercer *et al.*, 1971). Similar results have been demonstrated for subtherapeutic use in both animals and humans (Goldberg *et al.*, 1961; Savage, Appendix D; Siegel, 1976; Sprunt, 1977).

There is little evidence to indicate the quantitative contributions of these usages to effects on human health attributable to antimicrobial-resistant bacteria. The epidemiological literature on this topic is reviewed below.

INVESTIGATIONS OF EPIDEMICS

A number of investigations of epidemics have indicated that antimicrobial-resistant bacteria from animals can cause infections in humans (Anderson, 1968a; Anderson and Datta, 1965; Center for Disease Control, 1977; Fish *et al.*, 1967; Lyons *et al.*, 1980; Rowe *et al.*, 1979; Threlfall *et al.*, 1978a, b). Some of these epidemics, involving *Salmonella typhimurium* phage type 1 (Anderson and Datta, 1965), phage type 29 (Anderson, 1968a), and phage types 204 and 193

(Rowe *et al.*, 1979; Threlfall, 1978a,b), took place in the United Kingdom. One case in Canada was also caused by *S. typhimurium* (Fish *et al.*, 1967). Another outbreak, which took place in Connecticut, involved *S. heidelberg* (Center for Disease Control, 1977; Lyons *et al.*, 1980).

In the earlier outbreaks in the United Kingdom, there was substantial evidence indicating that the resistant bacteria were selected by indiscriminate therapeutic use of antimicrobials in animals (Anderson, 1968a; Anderson and Datta, 1965). The value of phage typing, as it is used in the United Kingdom, is its clear demonstration that the entire sequence of events involved in transmission of R^+ organisms to humans via food is possible. In the Connecticut outbreak, the investigators demonstrated that the reservoir of the multiply resistant *Salmonella* infection was likely to have been harbored by a group of 1-week-old calves owned by one of the ill persons. Lyons *et al.* (1980) indicate that these calves had been treated by their owner for the diarrhea that they had when brought to the owner's farm. In the Canadian case, the patient became ill approximately 1 week after illness was observed in a cow with which he had had direct physical contact. The cow had been treated therapeutically with antimicrobials by the owner at the onset of the illness. Organisms identified as *S. typhimurium* phage type 10 with identical antimicrobial-resistance profiles were isolated initially from the cow and later from the patient. Although reports of these epidemics document the transfer of resistant bacteria from animals to humans, there are no studies to quantitate the frequency of that occurrence.

Furthermore, not all observations have reinforced the suggestion that a reservoir of resistant bacteria in animals provides the major source of resistant bacteria in humans. In a study conducted in Omaha, Nebraska between 1968 and 1978, Meyer and Lerman (1980) documented the rise and fall in prevalence of resistant strains of *Shigella sonnei*, which was a predominant pathogen in humans during that period. In 1973, they observed a peak in the prevalence of resistance to ampicillin and a similar pattern of resistance to five other antimicrobials. There was no evidence that the use of ampicillin in humans had changed during the course of the study.

Cherubin *et al.* (1980) reported a very similar pattern of rise and fall of resistance to ampicillin for *Salmonella typhimurium* isolated in New York City from 1965 to 1968. He attributed this pattern in humans to an epidemic of a resistant strain but pointed out that isolates from calves and other animals in New York State did not exhibit a similar change. Calves continued to harbor ampicillin-resistant strains at a prevalence that increased annually from 1972 to 1978. Thus, there is evidence for waves of resistant enteric flora in humans and in animals that do not correlate with each other or with patterns of antimicrobial usage in humans. This suggests a substantial degree of separation of reservoirs in humans and animals.

POPULATION SURVEYS

By conducting retrospective health surveys of farm families, rural families with no animals, and urban families, all having had a recent hospital admission, Smith _et al._ (1974) attempted to determine whether association with farm animals was connected with greater risk of disease. Comparing admission diagnoses, they found no significant differences and no preponderance of antimicrobial-resistant bacterial disease. However, since there were insufficient numbers of subjects in the survey and the study design was not satisfactory, no general conclusion can be drawn.

In other attempts to determine the possible consequences to human health from the subtherapeutic use of antimicrobials in animal feeds, investigators have studied the relative prevalence of antimicrobial-resistant bacteria among various groups or have attempted to demonstrate the possibility of particular steps in the chain connecting the antimicrobials in animal feeds to increased carriage of R^+ bacteria in humans. Discussions of many of these studies are contained in the consultant reports to the committee (Appendixes A-J). Those that deal with the epidemiological aspects of the question are reviewed briefly below. Limitations on the inferences that can be drawn from these narrow studies are detailed in Chapter 2.

As far as the committee could determine, there have been no adequate attempts to relate an increased carriage of R^+ organisms to putative increased morbidity and mortality or dilemmas caused by resistance in the treatment of infection. Thus, predictions of the magnitude of any possible risk cannot be made from results of studies on particular stages or steps in the transmission chain.

The prevalence of resistant enterobacteria in groups with varying exposure to domestic livestock has been investigated by Betinovå (1972), Dorn _et al._ (1975), Fein _et al._ (1974), Linton _et al._ (1972), Siegel (1976), Siegel _et al._ (1975), Smith and Crabb (1961), Smith _et al._ (1974), Wells and James (1973), Wiedemann and Knothe (1971), and Woods _et al._ (1972).

Smith *et al.* (1974) compared the proportion of *E. coli* with resistance to antimicrobials among several groups of Iowa families and their livestock. They compared rural families with and without livestock, urban families, and both urban and rural families in which one member had recently been discharged from hospital inpatient status. Results generally indicated that the proportion of *E. coli* with resistance to four or more antimicrobials was greatest among families with livestock, regardless of their recent association with hospitals, and lowest among both urban and rural groups without a recent hospital association or proximity to livestock. These results include neither quantification of the transfer of resistance between animals and humans nor specification of resistance patterns. Since all livestock raised by these families had received some antimicrobials, some members of these families had been exposed to both the livestock fed antimicrobials and the feed containing the antimicrobials. However, the study does suggest that persons working with livestock that are receiving antimicrobials do harbor more resistant *E. coli* than do families not exposed to livestock, independent of recent hospital exposures. Unfortunately, the history of antimicrobial use by these humans was not documented.

Comparing rural and urban dwellers in England, Linton *et al.* (1972) found a much higher proportion of drug-resistant coliform bacilli in the feces of rural adults working with livestock than in rural adults not so employed. Urban adults harbored an intermediate proportion of resistant organisms. Both urban and rural children less than 5 years old harbored the highest proportion of all groups tested. Although this finding suggests an association between working with livestock and increased levels of resistant organisms, the authors supplied no information on antimicrobial usage in either animals or humans nor was there a comparison of specific resistance patterns between the flora of the animals and that of the humans exposed to them.

Dorn *et al.* (1975) conducted a small study comparing the specific resistance patterns between Missouri farm families raising beef and hogs and their animals and between families both raising and consuming home-raised meat and their animals. They found a significant association between resistance patterns in animals and families who consumed home-raised meat but not between patterns in animals and families who did not consume meat they raised. They concluded that the exposure of humans to *E. coli* from animals through consumption of meat was more plausible than mere contact with animals as an explanation for interspecific crossover of transferable drug resistance.

Siegel et al. (1975) compared the proportion of antimicrobial-resistant coliforms in five groups of Illinois persons with varying exposure to antimicrobials and animals fed antimicrobials. They found that the proportion of the enteric flora with resistance to antimicrobials in these groups ranked in the following decreasing order: (1) people working on farms in contact with farm animals receiving antimicrobials in feed, (2) people residing on the same farms but not in contact with the animals, (3) people treated with antimicrobial drugs, (4) untreated people residing with treated individuals, and (5) untreated people not residing on livestock farms. In general, groups 1, 2, and 3 had similarly high proportions of coliforms with resistance to oxytetracyclines, dihydrostreptomycin, and ampicillin, group 5 had the lowest proportion, and group 4 was usually intermediate. These results indicate that living on farms, raising livestock fed antimicrobials, or being treated with antimicrobials resulted in approximately equivalent proportions of organisms with resistance to these three antimicrobials and that persons without direct exposure to antimicrobials or animals fed antimicrobials have fewer resistant organisms. Since Siegel and his colleagues presented few data concerning specific antimicrobials used in humans or animals or specific matching resistance patterns, it is not possible to evaluate the role of feed containing subtherapeutic levels of antimicrobials in increasing the prevalence of resistant bacteria in either animals or people.

From studies conducted in the Federal Republic of Germany, Wiedemann and Knothe (1971) indicated that both farm workers and city dwellers carried enterobacteria with resistance to antimicrobials (in some cases plasmid-mediated), but that the proportion of the total enterobacterial flora with resistance was higher in farm workers. The significance of the results they obtained by comparing the percentages of farm workers, their relatives, feed handlers, city dwellers, slaughterhouse workers, chickens, calves, and pigs carrying resistant Enterobacteriaceae cannot be evaluated since the number of subjects in each category was not reported.

Each of the studies noted above suffers from various methodologic deficiencies that should be avoided in future efforts. None adequately quantitates the nature and extent of exposure to antimicrobials. Particularly lacking are data pertaining to those drugs given therapeutically to the study subjects. Moreover, the studies do not specify the type of antimicrobial given to the animals. Most of the investigators do not adequately describe the contact between the animals and the subjects. Since these studies are cross-sectional, they can indicate whether an association exists between an increased prevalence of resistant bacteria in humans and contact with animals, or direct contact with feeds containing antimicrobials, but cannot establish that such contacts cause the increase. In only one study was there an attempt to match the specific resistance patterns of *E. coli* from animals to those from exposed humans. None of the studies adequately documents the health status of the study subjects.

Despite their limitations, these studies lead to certain conclusions. Animals fed antimicrobial agents for extended periods or treated with antimicrobials develop resistant enterobacteria. People in close contact with those animals and their antimicrobial-containing feed are more likely to harbor resistant organisms in their gut flora than those without contact with animals. Patients who have received therapeutic drugs have a similar or even greater likelihood of carrying resistant organisms. Children who have not personally received antimicrobials also seem to have a high prevalence of R^+ organisms in their flora for reasons that are currently not clear. Future studies can be based on the assumption that these conclusions have been reasonably well established.

Two more surveys that deserve attention compared the prevalence of resistant *E. coli* in meat-eaters and in those who did not eat meat. Such a comparison would indicate if eating meat from animals that were presumed to have received antimicrobials was associated with an increased carriage of R^+ organisms. In a study by Guinée *et al.* (1970) the groups selected as meat-eaters were military kitchen personnel and office workers; those who did not eat meat were vegetarians and infants less than 6 months of age. Because the groups were relatively small and not strictly comparable, the conclusions drawn from these studies are questionable. But the percentages of the 77 vegetarians and 87 infants yielding resistant *E. coli* were not significantly lower than those in the meat-eating groups. This study does not provide evidence that eating meat is associated with an increased intestinal carriage of resistant coliforms.

Lebek (1972) reported the distribution of R factors among *E. coli* isolated from feces of healthy and ill human subjects. The percentages of various groups studied having R^+ organisms in their fecal flora were: hospital patients, 84% (74 of 88); healthy nurses, 82% (82 of 100); healthy soldiers, 51% (26 of 51); healthy 6-9 year olds, 65% (66 of 101); and healthy vegetarians, 57% (16 of 28). The vegetarians were described as "belonging to a religious community" that "takes no drugs and lives on a vegetarian diet," and the children, according to their parents, had not received antimicrobial drugs during the 2 years preceding the investigation. Although it is difficult to determine if the groups were strictly comparable, the results again do not support the concept that eating meat is associated with an increased intestinal carriage of resistant coliforms.

EXPERIMENTAL STUDIES

In the experimental studies described below, investigators have examined aspects of the transfer of resistant bacterial strains from animals to humans. By themselves these studies do not allow quantitative prediction of risk for the general population.

Hirsh and coworkers (Burton *et al.*, 1974; Hirsh *et al.*, 1974) examined the effects of varying doses of oxytetracycline (OTC) on colonization of the gut in humans following ingestion of resistant *E. coli* of bovine origin. No differences were found in length of time the organisms were excreted by those fed either 0 or 50 mg OTC/day, but 1,000 mg/day did potentiate the establishment of tetracycline-resistant *E. coli*.

In more direct experiments, Smith (1969) fed to a human various doses of resistant *E. coli* of animal origin containing unique resistance markers. The resident strains occasionally acquired resistance from the animal donor strains but the resistance was not maintained.

In an experiment that simulated the most likely exposure to be encountered by the general public, Linton (1977) studied five humans who, over a period of 3 months, handled, cooked, and ingested 15 chickens that had been sampled for *E. coli*. One of the five subjects was clearly colonized after handling but before eating. The colonization was transient. As in the experiment by Smith, plasmid-mediated resistance from *E. coli* in chickens was transferred to a strain of *E. coli* in the original resident flora of the human host.

In "feeding" studies, highly artificial conditions are sometimes created, e.g., huge doses are sometimes fed to a subject in a medium such as bicarbonate. Hence, results must be extrapolated with caution.

In two more experiments, investigators attempted to determine whether the administration of low doses of tetracycline to animals resulted in the transfer of resistant bacteria to humans. Hirsh and Wiger (1977) studied the fecal flora from 30 calves, 16 of which were fed 350 mg/day of tetracycline, and from their 20 handlers. A low level of transfer was found irrespective of whether the calves were receiving tetracycline.

Levy and coworkers (Levy, 1978; Levy *et al.*, 1976a,b) observed an increased prevalence of antimicrobial-resistant intestinal bacteria in a farm family in contact with chickens fed tetracycline and the tetracycline-containing feed. Later, they detected resistance in organisms isolated from chickens not fed antimicrobials and from farm personnel other than the family. Of particular interest was the reversibility of the apparent selection for resistant organisms after 9 months of usage. This was indicated by the finding that resistant organisms were not observed 6 months after discontinuance of the supplement. Furthermore, the use of only one antimicrobial (tetracycline) did lead to selection of strains with multiple resistance. There were some problems with the design of this study. More appropriate controls could have been used, and the sampling frequencies could have been more nearly equal. Resistance patterns reported in the earlier paper by Levy et al. (1976a) did not always include resistance to tetracycline, the agent in the chicken feed exerting the selection pressure.

When the results of these studies are examined together, they suggest that supplementation of animal feeds with antimicrobials can select for resistance in the enteric organisms of animals. This resistance can be transferred to humans who are in contact with these animals and their feeds or to those who handle the carcasses, e.g., those who prepare food for cooking. The resistance profiles selected may include resistance to agents in addition to those added to the feed since resistance genes are often linked. In some studies the prevalence of resistance has been shown to decline when supplementation is discontinued. In other instances herds receiving feed believed to be free of antimicrobials and with no recent history of antimicrobial therapy have a high prevalence of R^+ organisms (Smith et al., 1974). This may be attributable to contamination of the feed (Siegel, 1976). In January 1980, this topic was discussed at a conference sponsored by the U.S. Department of Agriculture on the contamination of feed by the sulfonamides. However, it cannot be predicted with certainty that the overall prevalence of antimicrobial-resistant organisms in animals will decrease to low levels if the subtherapeutic use of antimicrobials in feed is ended.

A large and complicated study was designed and conducted by Siegel (1976). He attempted to use bacteriophage typing to identify E. coli strains so that he could follow their transfer from various animal sources to humans--on the farm, in the slaughterhouse, or in the surrounding community. Despite some methodological problems, the study indicates that swine were the probable source of bacterial phage types that were found in poultry and beef cattle. These phage types were the same as those found most often in humans on farms. Presumably, they also originated from the pigs. Some of the farm strains that were prevalent on the carcasses were also found in slaughterhouse workers and in the slaughterhouse. There was evidence that other strains--some of which were carried by the workers or were present in the slaughterhouse--were transferred onto the carcasses at this point. Analysis of the flora of the consumers of the pork products was more difficult. Although pork consumers shared some common phage types with the workers in the slaughterhouse and on the farm, the route and extent of transfer was impossible to measure. This type of observational study is limited in what it can demonstrate, since it cannot indicate the direction in which organisms transfer. Genetically marked organisms, such as those used by Smith (1969) and Hirsh *et al.* (1974), might provide a better technique for following transmission.

CASE REPORTS

Some case reports provide evidence for the transfer of plasmid-mediated resistance under normal conditions. Petrocheilou and coworkers (1977, 1979) described tetracycline-resistant plasmids found in a number of *E. coli* strains from a woman who had received prolonged tetracycline treatment for acne vulgaris. Her husband, who had received no antimicrobial therapy, also harbored such strains. The two *E. coli* strains were indistinguishable as were the plasmids they carried. This observation suggests that *E. coli* carrying R plasmids may spread from individuals under treatment to untreated close contacts.

The study by Neu *et al.* (1973) suggested that specific resistance patterns could be transferred (in the intestines of one patient and in the urinary tract of another) from one organism to another. The transfer was suggested by the similar spectra of antimicrobial resistance. Corroboration of the transfer by plasmid DNA homology studies, such as those reported by Petrocheilou and coworkers (1977, 1979), was not attempted in the study of Neu *et al.* (1973).

Brumfitt and coworkers (1971) studied urinary tract infections caused by *E. coli* in patients living at home. Seven (19%) of 37 female patients had infections characterized by resistant *E. coli* and 23 (62%) carried some resistant *E. coli* in their fecal flora. In eight patients who had predominantly resistant (> 60%) *E. coli* fecal flora, five had urinary tract infections characterized by resistant *E. coli*. In 15 patients whose fecal flora contained a lower proportion of resistant *E. coli* (0-50%), only one patient had a urinary tract infection characterized by a resistant strain. From these findings, the investigators concluded that resistant strains of *E. coli*, when carried in the intestine, were neither more nor less likely to infect the urinary tract than were nonresistant strains.

SUBTHERAPEUTIC USE IN HUMANS

The committee also examined reports pertaining to the consequences of long-term administration of subtherapeutic levels of antimicrobials to humans to learn if there were adequate data which, upon extrapolation, might allow conclusions to be drawn about the effects on human health that could result from subtherapeutic levels of antimicrobials in animal feeds.

Goldberg et al. (1961) demonstrated that low dosages (10 mg per day) of OTC increased the prevalence of resistant bacteria in prison volunteers. Some subjects who did not receive OTC shed resistant coliforms. In those individuals whose resistant bacterial flora was increased by OTC, the prevalence of resistant coliforms returned to normal within 2 months after the OTC treatment was stopped.

Haight and Pierce (1954) reported a study in which naval recruits were given 250 mg of chlortetracycline or 100,000 units of procaine penicillin per day orally for 7 weeks. Those receiving antimicrobials gained more weight than did the controls.

There are a number of categories of infections for which antimicrobials have been used prophylactically in humans (Utz, Appendix A). A major use is the administration of tetracyclines to control acne in adolescents (Schmidt et al., 1973). Antimicrobials are also used in the prevention of endocarditis subsequent to rheumatic fever (McVay and Sprunt, 1953). Valtonen et al. (1977) have described the effects on enteric bacterial flora that result from neomycin prophylaxis in patients with hypercholesterolemia.

The committee examined many original research reports and a number of review articles on the subtherapeutic use of antimicrobials in humans including the following. Many papers on the use of tetracyclines to control acne have been reviewed by the American Academy of Dermatology (1975). Jukes (1973) described a variety of reports on the long-term administration of antimicrobials to infant and children or to patients with tropical sprue. Reports on the subtherapeutic and prophylactic use of antimicrobials in humans have been reviewed extensively by the Council for Agricultural Science and Technology (in press) and Pfizer, Inc. (1978).

The subtherapeutic or prophylactic administration of antimicrobials to humans generally results in an increased prevalence of resistant organisms in the recipient. Sprunt (1977) demonstrated that this increase is lower when intermittent doses are injected intramuscularly than when prophylaxis is administered orally. Moreover, she reported that lower doses eliminate only a small portion of the resident flora, thereby permitting fewer resistant organisms to survive and multiply.

In most of these studies no added health risk attributable to resistant organisms was recorded. However, the number of individuals involved in any one study of prophylaxis was small, and the study designs did not have as their primary objective the detection of adverse health effects of antimicrobial use. Thus, it is not possible to quantify the risk of infection from resistant bacteria resulting from such antimicrobial usage. Risks from prophylactic use are indicated in a recent report of two patients who developed endocarditis due to resistant viridans streptococci after undergoing oral penicillin prophylaxis subsequent to rheumatic fever (Parrillo *et al.*, 1979). How commonly this happens is not known. Since reports of such occurrences are rare, the committee believes that they probably occur infrequently.

EXPERIENCE WITH REGULATIONS IN OTHER COUNTRIES

Surveys of resistance in isolates from animals and humans have been conducted in several countries following the institution of various regulations governing the addition of antimicrobials to animal feeds. The reports of these surveys should be reviewed although they contain information that is far from conclusive. Moreover, surveys of the prevalence of resistance do not necessarily indicate "qualitative" changes in resistance, e.g., new combinations of resistance, more efficient transfer mechanisms, or a wider potential host range for a new plasmid.

In the United Kingdom the regulations recommended by the Swann committee (Swann *et al.*, 1969) were implemented in 1971 although no baseline data on antimicrobial use or resistance patterns had been collected. The development of the regulations and their effects have been reviewed by Braude (1978), Linton *et al.* (1977), and Smith (1977). The "Swann regulations" restricted primarily feed supplementation with antimicrobials that have value in the therapy of infections in humans. However, the restricted antimicrobials have remained available through veterinary prescription for use in animals. Smith (1977) reported that "in the four years since [the 'Swann'] prohibition, the *amount* of tetracycline-resistant *E. coli* in the pig population might have decreased slightly but the incidence of pigs excreting these organisms (100% in 1975) had not." In the United Kingdom, Sojka *et al.* (1977) reported that from 1971 to 1974 there was no evidence of a consistent decline in total resistance; however, they reported a small increase in resistance to tetracycline in salmonellae isolated from animals.

Since 1974, 30%-35% of the *Salmonella* isolates from humans in the United Kingdom have been resistant to antimicrobials. Recently, there has been a rise in multiple resistance due to a particular prevalent phage type. In 1965, also in the United Kingdom, approximately 40% of the *Salmonella* isolates from bovines were resistant. By 1978 this had risen considerably: approximately 70% of the *Salmonella* isolates from bovines were resistant (L. Ward, Central Public Health Laboratory, United Kingdom, personal communication). Linton *et al*. (1977) and Braude (1978) point out that there is little indication that the overall sales of antimicrobials for veterinary use have declined as a consequence of the Swann regulations. Farm animals may well be receiving the same amounts of antimicrobials as in the past, ostensibly for different purposes, i.e., prophylaxis or treatment of disease rather than for growth promotion, and possibly by alternative routes of administration (Braude, 1978).

Regulations developed by the European Economic Community to control the use of antimicrobials in animal feeds came into force in 1974. They proscribed the addition of tetracyclines to feed, a practice that had been increasing in the Netherlands since the 1960's. Subsequent to this prohibition, a decrease in the prevalence of tetracycline-resistant strains of *Salmonella* in pigs and humans was reported by van Leeuwen *et al*. (1979). It is difficult to attribute this decrease unequivocally to the ban on tetracyclines as feed additives since an epidemic of one antimicrobial-resistant phage type (505) of *Salmonella typhimurium* contributed greatly to the prevalence of resistant strains in the early 1970's. It is questionable whether the decrease in resistance to tetracycline after 1974 was due to the change in regulations or to the cessation of the epidemic of this particular resistant strain in both humans and pigs. The prevalence of resistant strains before that epidemic was similar to the levels after regulations came into force. A similar decrease in resistance was not observed in isolates from calves for which tetracycline is still used therapeutically. Phage type 505 of *S. typhimurium* was not prevalent in this species. There are no data to show if the use of tetracycline has in fact decreased during the period studied by van Leeuwen and colleagues (1974-1978).

In the Federal Republic of Germany, Bulling and coworkers (1973) and Stephan *et al*. (1976a,b, 1977a,b) reported a decline in tetracycline-resistant *S. typhimurium* and *S. panama* in calves and pigs since the 1974 ban. There are no comparable data on isolates from humans in Germany nor on antimicrobial use in that country.

A specific strain of *S. typhimurium* (phage type 505) was a major contributor to the resistance pattern in the Netherlands and the Federal Republic of Germany. Since the epidemic caused by that strain has now dissipated, it remains to be seen whether the trend of reduced prevalence of resistance will continue.

Data from Europe do not indicate whether restrictive regulations have actually reduced or averted hazards to human health.

CONCLUSIONS DRAWN FROM THE LITERATURE

Relatively little research on the subtherapeutic use of antimicrobials in animal feeds and the use of antimicrobials in animals generally is truly epidemiological. Reports are often based on regrettably few subjects observed for brief periods. The findings of such research are fragmented bits of information concerning isolated sections of the meat production system. Therefore, they do little to resolve the question: does the subtherapeutic use of antimicrobials in animal feeds relate to excessive morbidity and mortality of humans? However, the data indicate that antimicrobial-resistant organisms transfer from animals to humans who have been in contact with them on farms. Moreover, abattoir workers have been shown to harbor the same phage types as found in farm animals. The extent of subsequent person-to-person exchange has not been adequately determined. Furthermore, there is no evidence to prove that resistant bacteria are more prevalent among people consuming meat and meat products than among other groups.

There are no data linking human illness with the subtherapeutic use of antimicrobials in any aspect of animal husbandry, but the absence of information is certainly not to be equated with proof that the proposed hazards do not exist. For many questions pertaining to the subtherapeutic use of antimicrobials, the research is inadequate or nonexistent. The committee discussed in detail how this situation might be remedied. Its suggestions are contained in Chapter 4.

CHAPTER 4

STUDY POSSIBILITIES

The committee considered ways to remedy deficiencies in the information that has been used to support claims that the subtherapeutic use of antimicrobials in animal feeds creates a hazard to the health of humans. The studies suggested in this chapter are not to be interpreted as proposals of work that would provide a sufficient basis for an acceptable quantitative assessment of any risk to human health since the remaining gaps in knowledge would still have to be bridged by conjecture or speculation. Rather, the committee believes these studies to be the most fruitful approaches to quantifying some of the stages in the chain of events from which health hazards might result (see Chapter 2) so that speculations concerning such hazards may be more firmly based.

Study 1 should identify relative contributions of subtherapeutic and therapeutic antimicrobial regimens to the emergence of resistant enteric flora in animals. Studies 2 and 3 are designed to assess the extent to which carriage by humans of bacteria having R factors is associated with meat consumption or occupational exposure to bacteria from animals in abattoirs. Study 4 addresses the relationships between carriage of or occupational exposure to R^+ organisms and increased morbidity from urinary tract infections. Each proposal points out the limitations of the study and indicates what conclusions can be drawn from the data to be collected. Before these studies commence more detailed protocols should be evaluated by groups of individuals with expertise in the disciplines that are relevant to each study.

STUDY 1--THE EFFECTS OF SUBTHERAPEUTIC AND THERAPEUTIC DOSES OF ANTIMICROBIALS ON THE PREVALENCE OF R^+ ENTERIC ORGANISMS IN ANIMALS

In this study, the relationship between the appearance of resistant Enterobacteriaceae and the pattern and dose of antimicrobials used in the feed of food animals or otherwise administered to them could be examined. The proportion of *E. coli*, salmonellae, and other Enterobacteriaceae carrying R plasmids should be measured in beef cattle, hogs, and chickens before, during, and after they are fed and/or treated with various doses of tetracycline at growth promotional, prophylactic, and/or therapeutic levels. This study will clarify the contribution of subtherapeutic and therapeutic dosing regimens to the emergence of resistant enteric flora in animals.

Experimental Study Design

The committee regards the ability to obtain animals with a very low, preferably zero, incidence and proportion of R^+ enteric bacteria in their gut flora as central to the usefulness of this study. Alternative strategies, which could be adopted if it proves impossible to meet this criterion, are discussed under "Interpretation of Results."

Within each animal species, individual animals not previously exposed to antimicrobials should be allocated randomly to pens, and the pens should be assigned randomly to treatment groups, each of which contains more than one pen of animals. The number of animals in each pen and the number of pens may differ among the three animal species and should be specified so that the samples are of sufficient size for investigators to detect meaningful differences in the proportions of animals carrying tetracycline-resistant organisms among the various treatment groups.

Prior to random allocation, several fecal samples should be collected from each animal to establish the baseline for total flora, for the prevalence of R^+ organisms, and for the rate at which such pathogens as Salmonella are shed. Fecal specimens should be examined for a short period after penning in order to monitor exchange of bacteria among animals in each pen. Specimens should be examined at regular intervals thereafter to monitor the changes occurring during the feeding period. Bacteriological procedures should be determined on the advice of persons with expertise in the field of veterinary microbiology.

Animals should be divided into treatment groups as follows:

1. No antimicrobials. These animals should be given no antimicrobials of any sort during the feeding period.

2. Subtherapeutic levels of tetracyclines. These animals should receive tetracyclines for a period similar to that during which the antimicrobials are administered during typical rearing conditions for that species. Three dose levels should be given to different groups:

    a. A level no greater than the minimum regarded as necessary to elicit growth promotion or more efficient feed conversion.

    b. The usual level of antimicrobials fed to the particular animal species for growth promotion, improvement of feed conversion, and disease prophylaxis.

c. A level substantially above the usual feeding level but not above regulatory definition of a maximum subtherapeutic dose.

3. Therapeutic doses of tetracycline. These animals should not receive subtherapeutic antimicrobials. A simulated typical course of tetracycline therapy should be administered to the group at a specified time during the feeding period in accordance with accepted veterinary practices for the test species. If it is decided that tetracycline should be given to only some animals in the group, this must be recorded.

4. Subtherapeutic plus therapeutic doses of tetracyclines. These animals should be fed the usual subtherapeutic levels (2b) of tetracycline during the entire feeding period and should be treated with a simulated therapeutic course of tetracycline, thus combining 2b and 3 above.

In the event of sickness requiring the use of therapeutic doses of antimicrobials in any treatment group, all animals judged (on predetermined criteria) to be sick should be permanently removed from the experiment and from contact with the remaining test animals and should be treated as indicated by prudent veterinary practice.

Antimicrobials should be discontinued in all animals prior to slaughter at the time designated by current regulations to ensure that residual levels do not exceed those permitted in carcasses. Monitoring of R^+ bacteria should be continued in some animals for a period after the animals normally would have been slaughtered to observe all changes in R^+ prevalence after antimicrobials are withdrawn.

Design of data acquisition. The design of the quantitative culture techniques should enable investigators to detect a biologically important difference in the number of tetracycline-resistant organisms in fecal specimens from the various treatment groups. These techniques should be designed by persons with expertise in microbiology and in biostatistics as it relates to the analysis of microbiological data. The protocols and analytical methods should be specified in advance.

Data to be collected:

1. The number of animals in each group carrying Enterobacteriaceae with R factors mediating tetracycline resistance should

be recorded. For each stool specimen, the Enterobacteriaceae should be enumerated and serotyped, and the percentage carrying R factors mediating resistance to tetracycline should be ascertained by quantitative culture techniques.

2. Salmonellae shed by each animal should be enumerated and serotyped.

3. The weight of each animal should be recorded at the beginning, at the end, and at regular intervals during the experiment.

4. Feed should be analyzed chemically for a range of antimicrobials prior to use to avoid contamination and to ensure that the desired levels of tetracycline are achieved when supplementation is intended. Contaminated feed should be discarded to avoid the selection (by antimicrobial agents other than tetracycline) of organisms carrying plasmids on which resistance to tetracycline is linked to other resistances. The feed consumed in each pen should be recorded, and the consumption of antimicrobials by individual animals should be calculated.

Site conditions: One or more sites, such as an agriculture experiment station or veterinary college, should be selected. They should enable investigators to meet the following criteria:

1. Test animals should be maintained in a controlled experimental environment, but they should be handled in a manner that simulates current growing and finishing practices before marketing.

2. The sites should contain isolation facilities to prevent transfer of bacteria among pens. Different personnel will be needed for each pen to prevent cross-infection between pens.

3. Direct veterinary supervision during the course of the experiment should be available.

4. There should be local slaughtering facilities in which the bacteriological characteristics of carcasses produced during this experiment can be monitored.

Observational Studies

These studies require the cooperation of commercial operations that use antimicrobials in a pattern similar to some or all of those used in the experimental study design described above. Fecal samples and feed samples should be collected, and the feeding history and weight gains of the animals throughout the feeding period should be recorded. Fecal samples should be analyzed microbiologically with the same methods that were proposed in the experimental study design. The data obtained from these groups should be analyzed in a manner that will enable investigators to compare the appearance of R^+ organisms in these groups to that of the groups in the experimental study design.

Costs

The numbers of animals used in the following calculations are for illustrative purposes only. They should not be interpreted as the committee's recommendation for quantities needed to obtain statistically meaningful results. Investigators should determine the number to be used in accordance with the principles indicated in the study design outlined above. Animals should be observed past the usual marketing time in order to assess the full consequences of antimicrobial withdrawal on the microbial flora. The costs of acquiring specimens are included under Veterinary Supervision estimates. Partial costs may be recovered by sale of the animals.

EXPERIMENTAL STUDY: BOVINES

Costs are based on six groups of 20 animals.

Purchase of Animals:

In order to acquire animals with known antimicrobial exposure histories, it may be necessary to pay more than the going market rate, which varies with time.

Acquisition of 120 400-lb calves at approximately $1.25/lb will cost:

120 x 400 lb x $1.25/lb	=	$ 60,000	
Feed and Care Costs:			
120 x 240 days x $5.00/day	=	144,000	
Veterinary Supervision (2 h/day):			
2 h x 240 days x $30/h	=	14,400	
Animal Husbandry: Total Direct Cost	=		$218,400
Laboratory Services (based on one specimen/animal every 3 days):			
80 specimens/animal x 120 animals x $25/specimen	=		240,000
Total Direct Costs	=		458,400
Overhead (estimated 50%)	=		229,200
BOVINES, TOTAL COST			$687,600

EXPERIMENTAL STUDY: SWINE

Costs are based on six groups of 20 animals.

Purchase of Animals:

Acquisition of 120 specific pathogen-free animals, approximately 4 weeks old, will cost:

120 x $180/animal	= $ 21,600	
Feed and Care Costs:		
120 x 180 days x $2.00/day	= 43,200	
Veterinary Supervision (2 h/day):		
180 days x 2 h x $30/h	= 10,800	
Animal Husbandry: Total Direct Cost =		$75,600
Laboratory Services (based on one specimen/animal every 3 days):		
60 specimens/animal x 120 animals x $25/specimen	=	180,000
Total Direct Costs	=	$255,600
Overhead (estimated 50%)	=	127,800
SWINE, TOTAL COST		$383,400

EXPERIMENTAL STUDY: CHICKENS

Costs are based on six groups of 50 chickens.

Purchase of Animals:

Acquisition of 300 specific pathogen-free chicks will cost:

300 x $15	=	$ 4,500	

Purchase cost may be lower if chicks are reared from eggs rather than obtained already hatched.

Feed and Care Costs:

300 chickens x $0.50/day x 100 days	=	15,000	

Veterinary Supervision (2 h/day):

100 days x 2 h/day x $30/h	=	6,000	
Animal Husbandry: Total Direct Cost	=		$ 25,500

Laboratory Services (based on one specimen/animal every 3 days):

34 specimens/animal x 300 animals x $25/specimen	=		255,000
Total Direct Costs	=		280,500
Overhead (estimated 50%)	=		140,250
CHICKENS, TOTAL COST			$420,750

TOTAL COSTS - STUDY PROPOSAL 1: EXPERIMENTAL STUDY

Bovines	=	$687,600
Swine	=	383,400
Chickens	=	420,750
		$1,491,750

Any costs recovered from the sale of the animals could be returned to the contractor.

OBSERVATIONAL STUDY

Cost for the observational study will be dependent upon the arrangements that can be made with those commercial concerns willing to cooperate in the study and the sizes of the groups to be observed.

Interpretation of Results

There are a number of possible results from this study:

Animals receiving antimicrobials may have no greater prevalence of R^+ organisms and no more Salmonella with pathogenicity for humans than animals not receiving antimicrobials. This is an unlikely result, given data to the contrary. However, if such a result did occur, there would be no evidence to indicate that the subtherapeutic use of antimicrobials might affect human health.

The prevalence of R^+ organisms or Salmonella with pathogenicity for humans may be similar in animals on subtherapeutic regimens of antimicrobials and those on therapeutic regimens, and these prevalences might be greater than that in the untreated animals. In this instance there would be no evidence to indicate that subtherapeutic use of antimicrobials increases the possible hazard to humans over that from the therapeutic use of antimicrobials.

If the prevalence of either R^+ organisms or of pathogenic Salmonella resulting from the subtherapeutic use of antimicrobials significantly exceeds that from therapeutic use, then one still cannot infer that the subtherapeutic use of antimicrobials represents a definite risk of human disease. Further studies would be required to measure the effects on human health resulting from increased prevalence in animals of R^+ organisms or of Salmonella with pathogenicity for humans.

If animals with a low initial prevalence of R^+ enteric organisms cannot be obtained, the study should be modified to determine if the feeding of strictly monitored antimicrobial-free feed results in a decline in R^+ prevalence.

The validity of such conclusions depends upon the degree to which the experimental conditions, antimicrobial regimens, etc., actually parallel production practices. This can be ascertained by including the observational study in the overall design.

STUDY 2--STUDIES OF VEGETARIANS AND NONVEGETARIANS

This study would measure the extent to which carriage of bacteria with R factors is associated with meat consumption. It begins with the hypothesis that consumption of meat contaminated with antimicrobial-resistant bacteria from animals would result in meat-eaters having a higher prevalence of antimicrobial-resistant enteric bacteria than do vegetarians. Two related studies are described in Chapter 3.

Study Design

Groups of vegetarians and nonvegetarians should be compared for prevalence of resistant Enterobacteriaceae in their fecal flora. The groups must be carefully controlled for factors such as antimicrobial usage, age, socioeconomic status, family size, age of children, and pets. Seventh Day Adventists and Mormons would provide two convenient study groups. In this study the prevalence of R^+ factors is monitored by the use of resistance to tetracycline because of its likely frequency in the population and its therapeutic significance. Moreover, it is the subject of the proposed restrictions by the Food and Drug Administration (FDA).

Data to be Collected

The number of persons in each group carrying Enterobacteriaceae with R factors mediating resistance to tetracycline should be determined. The sample size should be sufficiently large for investigators to identify a meaningful difference, if it exists, in the rate of colonization by organisms with resistance to tetracycline.

The percentage of Enterobacteriaceae that carry R factors mediating resistance to tetracycline in each fecal specimen should be ascertained by quantitative culture techniques. These techniques should be designed to detect a biologically important difference in the prevalence of tetracycline resistance factors in stool specimens obtained from the groups being compared.

Costs

A preliminary survey should be conducted to ascertain approximate prevalence rates of R^+ carriage. A pilot study of 100 vegetarians and 100 nonvegetarians would cost approximately $100,000 for epidemiological and laboratory services. The size and desirability of the full survey should be decided on the basis of the results of the preliminary survey.

Interpretation of Results

If the prevalence of organisms with R factors is the same in vegetarians as in meat-eaters, there would be no support from this study for the belief that either the therapeutic or subtherapeutic use of antimicrobials in animals affects human health via R^+ organisms on or in meat.

If meat-eaters have a greater prevalence of R^+ bacteria than do vegetarians, it is possible to infer that the excess of antimicrobial-resistant bacteria is associated with the ingestion of meat, but it is not possible to differentiate between the effects of subtherapeutic and therapeutic uses of antimicrobials in meat sources. Other confounding variables would include the handling of meat products and contamination of cooking utensils or work surfaces. If meat-eating is associated with a greater R^+ prevalence, then further studies would be needed to determine if the excess of R^+ organisms results in excess morbidity or mortality or complicates the treatment of diseases and to determine the influence on R^+ prevalence of other aspects of diet.

STUDY 3--STUDIES OF ABATTOIR WORKERS, THEIR FAMILIES, AND NEIGHBORHOOD CONTROLS

This study would measure the extent to which occupational exposure of humans to bacteria from animals is associated with carriage by humans of bacteria with R factors. Secondarily, it would gauge the spread of these bacteria or R factors among humans who are in close contact with one another.

Abattoir workers are exposed to large numbers of bacteria from animals but are not exposed to antimicrobial-containing feeds. Consequently, they are exposed to the organisms (which are likely to be resistant in animals fed antimicrobials), but unlike farm workers they are not exposed to dusts containing antimicrobials that might be ingested or inhaled, thereby exerting a selective pressure favoring resistant enteric or respiratory tract bacteria. Thus, abattoir workers can be used productively to evaluate the propensity of bacteria from animals to colonize humans and to study the secondary spread of such bacteria and/or R factors via contact spread to family members. If secondary spread occurs, family members would be expected to have an intermediate but increased R factor carriage rate compared to controls.

Study Design

Groups of abattoir workers involved in the processing of poultry, pork, and cattle, their household contacts, and neighborhood controls should be compared for the prevalence of R^+ Enterobacteriaceae in their stool flora. The groups must be carefully controlled for factors such as antimicrobial usage, age, socioeconomic status, family size, age of children, and household pets. In this study the prevalence of R factors is monitored by the use of resistance to tetracycline as a marker for the same reasons given under Study 2.

Data to be Collected

The number of persons in each group carrying Enterobacteriaceae with R factors mediating resistance to tetracycline should be determined. The population groups studied should be large enough to provide a high probability for identifying a meaningful difference, if one exists, in the carriage rate for the tetracycline resistance factor. Information on the task performed by the abattoir workers should be collected in order to determine their potential for exposure to enteric organisms.

For each stool specimen, quantitative culture techniques should be used to determine the percentage of Enterobacteriaceae that carry R factors mediating resistance to tetracycline. These techniques should be designed to detect a biologically important difference in prevalence.

Costs

A preliminary survey should be conducted to ascertain approximate prevalence rates of R^+ carriage. The rates found in such a survey would determine the size and desirability of a full survey. A pilot study of 100 abattoir workers and 100 controls would cost approximately $100,000 for epidemiological and laboratory services. The size and desirability of the full survey should be decided on the basis of the results of the preliminary survey.

Interpretation of Results

By comparing rates at which R^+ bacteria are carried by abattoir workers with those of their families and neighborhood controls, one can determine if any association exists between occupational exposure to bacteria from animals and an increased prevalence of R factors in the human enteric flora. Such comparisons would also allow one to evaluate spread of R factors among humans in close contact with one another.

If the prevalence of organisms with R factors is the same in abattoir workers and controls, this study would provide no support for the belief that resistant bacteria, resulting from either the therapeutic or subtherapeutic use of antimicrobials in animals, significantly affects the flora or health of humans.

It would not be possible to attribute a greater prevalence in the abattoir workers solely or in part to the subtherapeutic use of antimicrobials in feeds. Further studies would be needed to determine if any observed excess of R^+ organisms in abattoir workers resulted in excess morbidity or mortality or in complications in the treatment of diseases.

RATIONALE FOR CONDUCTING STUDIES OF MORBIDITY AND MORTALITY IN HUMANS

The three studies described above are intended to serve as indicators of the development and transfer of resistant enteric organisms. If there is no indication of an important association between the exposure of animals to either subtherapeutic or therapeutic levels of antimicrobials and the development of resistant enteric organisms, or if exposure to bacteria from animals fails to influence the flora of humans, the possibility of detrimental effects on human health would not be sufficiently well established to justify widespread changes in the current use of antimicrobials throughout the meat industry. If either the vegetarian study or the abattoir study indicates that the carriage of resistant organisms by humans is associated with meat consumption or occupational exposure to bacteria from animals, more extensive evaluations of morbidity and mortality would be justified. One possible study is detailed below.

STUDY 4--COMPARISON OF CONTROLS WITH SUBJECTS WITH URINARY TRACT INFECTION

Laboratory screening services frequently discover urinary tract infections (UTI) by culturing urine samples obtained from women during routine medical examinations. These screenings can be linked with other microbiological tests to determine the existence of an association between R^+ Enterobacteriaceae in stool flora and the occurrence of primary UTI and to ascertain the proportion of primary UTI infection that is caused by antimicrobial-resistant Enterobacteriaceae. Brumfitt *et al.* (1971) have conducted a small study of these topics.

Study Design

If the results of Studies 1, 2, and 3 indicate that more extensive evaluations of morbidity and mortality are necessary, the committee recommends that a screening for primary UTI be conducted on 5,000 females who work in the meat processing industry (e.g., in poultry dressing plants) and who thus are exposed to high levels of antimicrobial-resistant bacteria. If the screening can be conducted in a processing plant that can provide reliable data concerning the antimicrobials received by the birds that are processed, the antimicrobial-resistant profiles of the flora of the poultry carcasses should be compared with those of the isolates from humans. Such additional sampling would add to the costs of the study but would provide exceedingly useful corroborative information. In conjunction with the screening of meat processors, an equally large group of controls should be studied, e.g., the 9,000 women in East Boston, Massachusetts first studied by Kass (1978) could be resurveyed. These surveys would enable investigators to compare female meat processors who have bacteriuria with similarly infected women in an urban setting far removed from contact with livestock and to match cases and controls for age, race, parity, and antimicrobial history.

Participating screening services should use uniform procedures and criteria to detect UTI's. New cases should be asked to return for a confirmatory urinary culture, at which time a rectal swab should be obtained to determine the carriage of R^+ Enterobacteriaceae.

Women who have not received antimicrobials during the preceding calendar year should then be matched with control (non-UTI) women of comparable age, race, parity, and negative antimicrobial history as determined by the screening service. For each stool specimen from a case or control, all Enterobacteriaceae should be serotyped and the percentage with R factors should be ascertained by quantitative culture techniques. The number of cases and controls required to discriminate between no association and a meaningful difference at acceptably low probabilities for error must be specified in a detailed protocol. The control population of 9,000 should yield approximately 150 cases of bacteriuria, approximately 100-120 of which will be infected with *E. coli* (Kass, 1978).

The role of resistance selected by the therapeutic use of antimicrobials in humans should be rigorously investigated and controlled in this study. Even a negative result with a large group would enable investigators to estimate the upper bound of the risk to human health.

All confirmed cases of UTI should be studied in the following manner.

1. Each isolated infecting strain should be tested for antimicrobial susceptibility patterns, type distribution, and plasmid DNA sequence homology.

2. Each patient should be sent a questionnaire to determine:

Basic demographic data

Basic household composition

Identification of infection as a sporadic case or part of an outbreak

Occupation of patient, spouse, and household contacts

Outcome of illness--expense in terms of workdays lost, medical expenses, etc.

Present health status of subject

Antimicrobial history of subject and household members and pets during past 2 years

Hospitalization history of subject during past 2 years

Major illness of subject and household members during past 2 years

Patients with UTI characterized by bacteria with resistance to antimicrobials should be compared with patients with UTI characterized only by antimicrobial-sensitive bacteria to determine whether there are differences in antimicrobial history, in exposure to animals or carcasses that had been in contact with antimicrobials, or in exposure to feeds containing antimicrobials.

Interpretation of Results

If women with resistant enteric flora have a relatively high risk of a UTI compared to those without resistant fecal flora, the prevalence of R^+ fecal flora among new cases should be greater than that among comparable controls. The observation of such an association would favor the interpretation that the carriage of R^+ organisms, from whatever source, is indicative of an elevated risk of UTI. An insignificant association would indicate that the presence of R^+ enteric flora does not make an important contribution to this form of morbidity. This study would be sensitive to a differential virulence between resistant and susceptible enteric flora causing UTI's, but it would not elucidate the contribution of the subtherapeutic use of antimicrobials in animal feeds to this cause of illness. Whatever the results of this study, they would not provide justification for drawing general conclusions about the likely changes in the virulence of other pathogens gaining resistance to antimicrobials.

The comparison of UTI prevalence between groups with high and low exposure to R^+ enteric organisms would provide some indication of the amount of primary UTI that is attributable to an occupational exposure. With a sufficiently large control group and high risk groups in proximity to animals or carcasses with high levels of R^+ organisms, a positive result would enable some conclusions to be drawn about total antimicrobial use in animals and UTI in humans caused by antimicrobial-resistant bacteria. No conclusion could be drawn about the relative contribution of subtherapeutic use to the increased morbidity.

Costs

If such a study were conducted over 2 years, which would allow time for training of personnel and analyzing results, an estimated $150,000 per year would be required. If the study were spread over 3 years, the total annual cost would be reduced by approximately 15%. If the information concerning the antimicrobials received by poultry passing through the processing plant can be obtained and the flora of the carcass is subsequently sampled, then additional costs will be incurred.

CHAPTER 5

CONCLUSIONS AND RECOMMENDATIONS

CONCLUSIONS

A relatively small proportion of the research that has been conducted on the subtherapeutic or therapeutic use of antimicrobials in animal feeds is truly epidemiological. Much of the information on this subject has been generated by poorly controlled studies of small numbers of subjects observed for brief periods.

An ideal study of the effects on human health resulting from the subtherapeutic use of antimicrobials in animal feeds would be able to relate, without conjecture or speculation, antimicrobials in feed to changes in morbidity or mortality or to treatment complications caused by resistance to antimicrobials in humans who had been exposed to animals or meat products during processing, handling, or, especially, consumption. Changes in morbidity and mortality could be used to quantitate the risk of the potential hazards posed by increased prevalence of resistant bacteria, by the development of plasmids conferring multiple resistance, or by the evolution of especially efficient transfer mechanisms within the reservoir of bacteria in animals.

Because the literature provides only isolated fragments of information relating to various components of the meat production system, it is insufficient for assessing the direct relationship between the use of subtherapeutic levels of antimicrobials in animal feeds and the health of humans. A major deficiency in much of the literature is the lack of a clear differentiation between the consequences of subtherapeutic and therapeutic uses of antimicrobials in animals. Moreover, data gathered in the United Kingdom, the Federal Republic of Germany, and the Netherlands do not indicate clearly whether restrictive regulations have actually reduced or averted the postulated hazards to human health. Restrictions on the use of antimicrobials in the United Kingdom may well have altered the patterns of their use without significant alteration in the total amounts used or their consequences. Therefore, it is not possible to conclude from the literature that restricting only the subtherapeutic use of antimicrobials will cause a decrease in the overall prevalence of R^+ organisms in humans or animals. Furthermore, there is little information on qualitative changes in resistance in the enteric bacteria of animals or humans. For example, no data exist to indicate the extent to which new resistance combinations or more efficient transfer mechanisms have been brought about by the subtherapeutic use of antimicrobials in feeds.

After reviewing the evidence, the committee concluded that the postulations concerning the hazards to human health that might result from the addition of subtherapeutic antimicrobials to feeds have been neither proven nor disproven. The lack of data linking human illness with subtherapeutic levels of antimicrobials must not be equated with proof that the proposed hazards do not exist. The research necessary to establish and measure a definite risk has not been conducted and, indeed, may not be possible.

The committee gave considerable thought to the necessary elements of the ideal study to measure accurately the effects on human health resulting from the subtherapeutic use of antimicrobials in animal feeds and how such a study should be designed.

It concluded that a comprehensive, all-encompassing study could not be realized or even approximated because of insurmountable technical difficulties. This decision reflected a number of facts:

- There are marked differences in both the therapeutic and subtherapeutic use of antimicrobials in the various major species of animals raised for their meat and in the different regions of the country.

- It is not clear how much the subtherapeutic use of antimicrobials, as compared to the therapeutic use, contributes to the prevalence of resistant bacteria in animals.

- Animals with different histories of exposure to antimicrobials are known to exchange bacteria during normal rearing and shipping prior to slaughter. Consequently, the types and amounts of antimicrobials received by a particular slaughterbound animal or its companions cannot be determined.

- Household members consume meats from animals that have been exposed to different antimicrobial agents during the course of different regimens, both subtherapeutic and therapeutic. Thus, it is not practical to determine the original selective pressure for resistant bacteria that may occur on a particular piece of meat.

- It is difficult to determine the relative contributions made by subtherapeutic and therapeutic levels of antimicrobials in animals or in humans to the pool of resistant bacteria that may affect human health.

The committee concluded that less comprehensive approaches, although more feasible, could not provide direct evidence of a consistent chain of events from animal production to meat consumption. However, it did outline a sequence of four possible studies on individual aspects of the transmission chain. The results of these studies, if interpreted with the recommended precautions, would provide a useful scientific background for policymakers. At best, however, the remaining gaps in our knowledge will still have to be bridged by conjecture or speculation.

The committee also discussed some nonepidemiological aspects of the subtherapeutic use of antimicrobials. A better understanding of the mechanisms through which subtherapeutic levels of antimicrobials produce beneficial effects may lead to development of other substances or other treatments of equal or greater effectiveness, thereby rendering this entire issue moot. For example, if the beneficial effect is caused primarily by controlling infections, then other preventive techniques such as new vaccines may yield equal benefit. If the mechanism is nutritional, i.e., nutrient sparing or an alteration of nutrient absorption, then new nutritional supplements may yield the desired result.

Plasmids in isolates from animals and humans must be characterized to assess the possibility that subtherapeutic levels of antimicrobials in animals produce qualitative changes in resistance to antimicrobials in the enteric flora of animals, changes that might subsequently affect human health.

RECOMMENDATIONS

The committee RECOMMENDS that future epidemiological studies, whether the ones suggested here or others, be carefully planned to fill gaps in our present knowledge and, especially, to avoid the errors of ambiguous design and small sample size that have caused such difficulties in interpretating the data. The proportionate contributions to resistance made by subtherapeutic and therapeutic uses of antimicrobials in animals and in humans urgently need resolution.

The committee RECOMMENDS increased and continued monitoring and surveillance of the occurrence of antimicrobial resistance in bacteria in animals, in meat and meat products, and in humans, especially in cases of human illness due to *Salmonella* and pathogenic *E. coli*. If restrictions on antimicrobial use are adopted, the committee RECOMMENDS that monitoring be continued in order to determine the effect of such restrictions.

The committee RECOMMENDS further research on:

- the mechanism of action of subtherapeutic levels of antimicrobials in feed (BARR, Appendix K) including characterization of the composition and interactions of the gastrointestinal flora (Savage, Appendix D),

- factors that inhibit the development and transfer of resistance *in vivo* (Jacoby and Low, Appendix C), and

- studies on the epidemiology of plasmid-mediated resistance to antimicrobials in both animals and humans (O'Brien, Appendix I).

REFERENCES

American Academy of Dermatology. 1975. Systemic antibiotics for treatment of acne vulgaris. Efficacy and safety. Compiled by the Ad Hoc Committee on the Use of Antibiotics in Dermatology, Division of Research, National Program for Dermatology. Arch. Dermatol. 111:1630-1636.

Anderson, E. S. 1968a. Drug resistance in Salmonella typhimurium and its implications. Br. Med. J. 3:333-339.

Anderson, E. S. 1968b. The ecology of transferable drug resistance in the enterobacteria. Annu. Rev. Microbiol. 22:131-180.

Anderson, E. S., and N. Datta. 1965. Resistance to penicillins and its transfer in Enterobacteriaceae. Lancet 1:407-409.

Animal Health Institute. 1979. 1979 Feed Additive Compendium. The Miller Publishing Company, Minneapolis, Mn. 366 pp.

Betinová, M. 1972. Incidence of antibiotic resistant staphylococci in humans from different environments in Slovakia. Pp. 385-390 in V. Krčméry, L. Rosival, and T. Watanabe, eds. Bacterial Plasmids and Antibiotic Resistance. First International Symposium. Infectious Antibiotic Resistance. Castle of Smolenice, Czechoslovakia, 1971. Springer-Verlag, Berlin, Heidelberg, and New York.

Braude, R. 1978. Antibiotics in animal feeds in Great Britain. J. Anim. Sci. 46:1425-1436.

Brumfitt, W., D. S. Reeves, M. C. Faiers, and N. Datta. 1971. Antibiotic-resistant Escherichia coli causing urinary-tract infection in general practice: Relation to faecal flora. Lancet 1:315-317.

Bulling, E., R. Stephan, and V. Sebek. 1973. [In German; English abstract.] Die Entwicklung der Antibiotika-resistenz von Salmonellabakterien tierischer Herkunft in der Bundesrepublik Deutschland einschl. Berlin (West). 1. Mitteiling: Ein Vergleich Zwischen 1961 und 1970-71. Zentralbl. Bakteriol. Parasitenkd. Infektionskr. Hyg., I. Abt. Orig Reihe A 225:245-256.

Burton, G. C., D. C. Hirsh, D. C. Blenden, and J. L. Zeigler. 1974. The effects of tetracycline on the establishment of Escherichia coli of animal origin, and in vivo transfer of antibiotic resistance, in the intestinal tract of man. Pp. 241-253 in F. A. Skinner and J. G. Carr, eds. The Society for Applied Bacteriology Symposium Series No. 3. The Normal Microbial Flora of Man. Academic Press, London and New York.

Center for Disease Control. 1977. An Outbreak of Multiple Drug-Resistant Salmonella heidelberg, Connecticut. Reported by M. L. Cohen, J. G. Wells, C. L. Samples, P. A. Blake, J. L. Conrad, and E. J. Gangarosa. Report Number EPI-77-13-2. Center for Disease Control, Atlanta, Ga. 8 pp.

Cherubin, C.E., J. F. Timoney, M. F. Sierra, P. Ma, J. Marr, and S. Shin. 1980. A sudden decline in ampicillin resistance in Salmonella typhimurium. J. Am. Med. Assoc. 243:439-442.

Council for Agricultural Science and Technology. In press. Antibiotics in Animal Feeds. Council for Agricultural Science and Technology, Ames, Ia.

Dorn, C. R., R. K. Tsutakawa, D. Fein, G. C. Burton, and D. C. Blenden. 1975. Antibiotic resistance patterns of Escherichia coli isolated from farm families consuming home-raised meat. Am. J. Epidemiol. 102:319-326.

Fein, D., G. Burton, R. Tsutakawa, and D. Blenden. 1974. Matching of antibiotic resistance patterns of Escherichia coli of farm families and their animals. J. Infect. Dis. 130:274-279.

Finkel, M. J. 1978. Magnitude of antibiotic use. Ann. Intern. Med. 89:791-792.

Finland, M. 1955a. Emergence of antibiotic-resistant bacteria. N. Engl. J. Med. 253:909-922.

Finland, M. 1955b. Emergence of antibiotic-resistant bacteria (continued). N. Engl. J. Med. 253:969-979.

Finland, M. 1955c. Emergence of antibiotic-resistant bacteria (concluded). N. Engl. J. Med. 253:1019-1028.

Finland, M. 1979. Emergence of antibiotic resistance in hospitals, 1935-1975. Rev. Infect. Dis. 1:4-21.

Fish, N. A., M. C. Finlayson, and R. P. Carere. 1967. Salmonellosis: Report of a human case following direct contact with infected cattle. Can. Med. Assoc. J. 96:1163-1165.

Food and Drug Administration. 1972. Report to the Commissioner of the Food and Drug Administration by the FDA Task Force on the Use of Antibiotics in Animal Feeds. Bureau of Veterinary Medicine, Food and Drug Administration, Department of Health, Education, and Welfare, Rockville, Md. 21 pp.

Food and Drug Administration. 1978. Draft Environmental Impact Statement--Subtherapeutic Antibacterial Agents in Animal Feeds. Bureau of Veterinary Medicine, Food and Drug Administration, Department of Health, Education, and Welfare, Rockville, Md. [371 + xviii] pp.

Goldberg, H. S., R. N. Goodman, J. T. Logue, and F. P. Handler. 1961. Long-term, low-level antibiotics and the emergence of antibiotic-resistant bacteria in human volunteers. Antimicrob. Agents Chemother. 80-88.

Guinée, P., N. Ugueto, and N. van Leeuwen. 1970. Escherichia coli with resistance factors in vegetarians, babies, and nonvegetarians. Appl. Microbiol. 20:531-535.

Haight, T. H., and W. E. Pierce. 1954. Influence of small doses of antibiotics on the weight behavior of young males. J. Lab. Clin. Med. 44:807-808.

Hartley, C. L., and M. H. Richmond. 1975. Antibiotic resistance and survival of E. coli in the alimentary tract. Br. J. Med. 4:71-74.

Hirsh, D. C., and N. Wiger. 1977. Effect of tetracycline upon transfer of an R plasmid from calves to human beings. Am. J. Vet. Res. 38:1137-1139.

Hirsh, D. C., G. C. Burton, and D. C. Blenden. 1974. The effect of tetracycline upon establishment of Escherichia coli of bovine origin in the enteric tract of man. J. Appl. Bacteriol. 37:327-333.

Huber, W. G. 1971. The impact of antibiotic drugs and their residues. Adv. Vet. Sci. Comp. Med. 15:101-132.

Jukes, T. H. 1973. Public health significance of feeding low levels of antibiotics to animals. Adv. Appl. Microbiol. 16:1-30.

Kass, E. H. 1978. Horatio at the orifice: The significance of bacteriuria. J. Infect. Dis. 138:546-557.

Kleckner, N. 1977. Translocatable elements in procaryotes. Cell 11:11-23.

Kunin, C. M. 1979. Problems in antibiotic usage. Pp. 383-395 in J. L. Mandell, R. G. Douglas, Jr., and J. E. Bennett, eds. Principles and Practice of Infectious Diseases. John Wiley & Sons, New York, N.Y.

Lebek, G. 1972. Epidemiological investigations of R-factors in man and animals in Switzerland. Pp. 47-54 in V. Krčméry, L. Rosival, and T. Watanabe, eds. Bacterial Plasmids and Antibiotic Resistance. First International Symposium. Infectious Antibiotic Resistance. Castle of Smolenice, Czechoslovakia, 1971. Avicenum, Czechoslovak Medical Press, Prague and Springer-Verlag, Berlin, Heidelberg, and New York.

Levy, S. B. 1978. Emergence of antibiotic-resistant bacteria in the intestinal flora of farm inhabitants. J. Infect. Dis. 137: 688-690.

Levy, S. B., G. B. FitzGerald, and A. B. Macone. 1976a. Changes in intestinal flora of farm personnel after introduction of a tetracycline-supplemented feed on a farm. N. Engl. J. Med. 295:583-588.

Levy, S. B., G. B. FitzGerald, and A. B. Macone. 1976b. Spread of antibiotic-resistant plasmids from chicken to chicken and from chicken to man. Nature 260:40-42.

Linton, A. H., K. Howe, P. M. Bennett, M. H. Richmond, and E. J. Whiteside. 1977. The colonization of the human gut by antibiotic resistant Escherichia coli from chickens. J. Appl. Bacteriol. 43:465-469.

Linton, K. B., P. A. Lee, M. H. Richmond, W. A. Gillespie, A. J. Rowland, and V. N. Baker. 1972. Antibiotic resistance and transmissible R-factors in the intestinal coliform flora of healthy adults and children in an urban and a rural community. J. Hyg., Camb. 70:99-104.

Linton, K. B., M. H. Richmond, R. Bevan, and W. A. Gillespie. 1974. Antibiotic resistance and R factors in coliform bacilli isolated from hospital and domestic sewage. J. Med. Microbiol. 7:91-103.

Lyons, R. W., C. L. Samples, H. N. DeSilva, K. A. Ross, E. M. Julian, and P. J. Checko. 1980. An epidemic of resistant Salmonella in a nursery. J. Am. Med. Assoc. 243:546-547.

McVay, L. V., Jr., and D. H. Sprunt. 1953. Aureomycin in the prophylaxis of rheumatic fever. N. Engl. J. Med. 249:387-393.

Mercer, H. D., D. Pocurull, S. Gaines, S. Wilson, and J. V. Bennett. 1971. Characteristics of antimicrobial resistance of Escherichia coli from animals: Relationship to veterinary and management uses of antimicrobial agents. Appl. Microbiol. 22:700-705.

Meyer, P. W., and S. J. Lerman. 1980. Rise and fall of Shigella antibiotic resistance. Antimicrob. Agents Chemother. 17:101-102.

Mussman, H. C. 1975. Drug and chemical residues in domestic animals. Fed. Proc. 34:197-201.

Neu, H. C., P. J. Huber, and E. B. Winshell. 1973. Interbacterial transfer of R factor in humans. Antimicrob. Agents Chemother. 3:542-544.

Office of Technology Assessment. 1979. Drugs in Livestock Feed. Volume I: Technical Report. Office of Technology Assessment, Congress of the United States, Washington, D.C. 67 pp.

Parrillo, J. E., G. C. Borst, M. H. Mazur, P. Iannini, M. S. Klempner, R. C. Moellering, Jr., and S. E. Anderson. 1979. Endocarditis due to resistant viridans streptococci during oral penicillin chemoprophylaxis. N. Engl. J. Med. 30:296-300.

Petrocheilou, V., M. H. Richmond, and P. M. Bennett. 1977. Spread of a single plasmid clone to an untreated individual from a person receiving prolonged tetracycline therapy. Antimicrob. Agents Chemother. 12:219-225.

Petrocheilou, V., M. H. Richmond, and P. M. Bennett. 1979. The persistence of plasmid-carrying tetracycline-resistant Escherichia coli in a married couple, one of whom was receiving antibiotics. Antimicrob. Agents Chemother. 16:225-230.

Pfizer, Inc. 1978. Material submitted to the Food and Drug Administration Hearing Clerk under Docket Numbers 77N-0230 (penicillin) and 77N-0316 (tetracyclines). Food and Drug Administration, Department of Health, Education, and Welfare, Rockville, Md.

Richmond, M. H. 1975. R factors in man and his environment. Pp. 27-35 in D. Schlessinger, ed. Microbiology--1974. American Society for Microbiology, Washington, D.C.

Richmond, M. H., and K. B. Linton. 1980. The use of tetracycline in the community and its possible relation to the excretion of tetracycline-resistant bacteria. J. Antimicrob. Chemother. 6:33-41.

Rowe, B., E. J. Threlfall, L. R. Ward, and A. S. Ashley. 1979. International spread of multiresistent strains of Salmonella typhimurium phage types 204 and 193 from Britain to Europe. Vet. Rec. 105:468-469.

Schmidt, H., E. From, and G. Heydenreich. 1973. Bacteriological examination of rectal specimens during long-term oxytetracycline treatment for acne vulgaris. Acta Dermatol. Venereol. 53:153-156.

Seelig, M. S. 1966. Mechanisms by which antibiotics increase the incidence and severity of candidiasis and alter the immunological defenses. Bacteriol. Revs. 30:442-459.

Siegel, D. 1976. The Ecological Effects of Antimicrobial Agents on Enteric Florae of Animals and Man. Final Technical Report, FDA Contract Number 71-269. Food and Drug Administration, Department of Health, Education, and Welfare, Rockville, Md. 404 pp.

Siegel, D., W. G. Huber, and S. Drysdale. 1975. Human therapeutic and agricultural uses of antibacterial drugs and resistance of the enteric flora of humans. Antimicrob. Agents Chemother. 8:538-543.

Smith, H. W. 1969. Transfer of antibiotic resistance from animal and human strains of Escherichia coli to resident E. coli in the alimentary tract of man. Lancet 1:1174-1176.

Smith, H. W. 1977. Antibiotic resistance in bacteria and associated problems in farm animals before and after the 1969 Swann report. Pp. 344-357 in M. Woodbine, ed. Antibiotics and Antibiosis in Agriculture with Special Reference to Synergism. Butterworth, Boston, Mass. 386 pp.

Smith, H. W., and W. E. Crabb. 1961. The faecal bacterial flora of animals and man: Its development in the young. J. Pathol. Bacteriol. 82:53-66.

Smith, I. M., E. Habte-Gabr, F. W. Gutzman, D. W. Pearson, and L. F. Burmeister. 1974. Antibiotic Resistance of Animal and Human Bacteria and Human Disease in Relation to the Use of Animal Antibiotic Feed Supplements. Paper presented at the 14th Interscience Conference on Antimicrobial Agents and Chemotherapy, September 11-13. 30 pp.

Sojka, W. J., C. Wray, and E. B. Hudson. 1977. A survey of drug resistance in salmonellae isolated from animals in England and Wales during 1973 and 1974. Br. Vet. J. 133:292-311.

Sprunt, K. 1977. Role of antibiotic resistance in bacterial endocarditis. Pp. 17-19 in E. L. Kaplan and A. V. Taranta, eds. Infective Endocarditis. American Heart Association Symposium. Proceedings of a Seminar, Dallas, Texas, May 14-15, 1976. The American Heart Association, Inc., Dallas, Tx.

Stephan, R., E. Bulling, and A. Steinbeck. 1976a. [In German; English summary.] Die Entwicklung der Antibiotikaresistenz von Salmonellabakterien tierischer Herkunft in der Bundesrepublik Deutschland einschliesslich Berlin (West). 3. Mitteilung: Jahresbericht 1972. Zentralbl. Bakteriol. Parasitenkd. Infektionskr. Hyg., I. Abt. Orig. Reihe A 234:29-36.

Stephan, R., E. Bulling, and A. Steinbeck. 1976b. [In German; English summary.] Die Entwicklung der Antibiotikaresistenz von Salmonellabakterien tierischer Herkunft in der Bundesrepublik Deutschland einschliesslich Berlin (West). 4. Mitteilung: Jahresbericht 1973. Zentralbl. Bakteriol. Parasitenkd. Infektionskr. Hyg., I. Abt. Orig. Reihe A 234:37-45.

Stephan, R., E. Bulling, and A. Steinbeck. 1977a. [In German; English summary.] Die Entwicklung der Antibiotikaresistenz von Salmonellabakterien tierischer Herkunft in der Bundesrepublik Deutschland einschleisslich Berlin (West). 5. Mitteilung: Jahresbericht 1974. Zentralbl. Bakteriol. Parasitenkd. Infektionskr. Hyg., I. Abt. Orig. Reihe A 237:254-263.

Stephan, R., E. Bulling, and A. Steinbeck. 1977b. [In German; English summary.] Die Entwicklung der Antibiotikaresistenz von Salmonellabakterien tierischer Herkunft in der Bundesrepublik Deutschland einschliesslich Berlin (West). 6. Mitteilung: Jahresbericht 1975. Zentralbl. Bakteriol. Parasitenkd. Infektionskr. Hyg., I Abt. Orig. Reihe A 237:264-273.

Stollerman, G. H. 1978. Trends in bacterial virulence and antibiotic susceptibility: Streptococci, pneumococci, and gonococci. Ann. Intern. Med. 89:746-748.

Swann, M. M., K. L. Blaxter, H. I. Field, J. W. Howie, I. A. M. Lucas, E. L. M. Millar, J. C. Murdoch, J. H. Parsons, and E. G. White. 1969. Report of the Joint Committee on the Use of Antibiotics in Animal Husbandry and Veterinary Medicine. Cmnd. 4190. Her Majesty's Stationery Office, London. 83 pp.

Threlfall, E. J., L. R. Ward, and B. Rowe. 1978a. Epidemic spread of a chloramphenicol-resistant strain of Salmonella typhimurium phage type 204 in bovine animals in Britain. Vet. Rec. 103: 438-440.

Threlfall, E. J., L. R. Ward, and B. Rowe. 1978b. Spread of multiresistant strains of Salmonella typhimurium phage types 204 and 193 in Britain. Br. Med. J. 2:997.

U. S. Department of Agriculture. 1978. Economic Effects of a Prohibition on the Use of Selected Animal Drugs. Agricultural Economic Report No. 414, Econonic, Statistics, and Cooperatives Service, U.S. Department of Agriculture, Washington, D.C. 68 pp.

U. S. Department of Agriculture. 1979. Monitoring Phase Biological Residue Report, January 1978 through December 1978. Data from Residue Monitoring Program, Food Safety and Quality Service, U. S. Department of Agriculture, Washington, D.C.

U. S. International Trade Commission. 1951-1979. Synthetic Organic Chemicals. United States Production and Sales, 1950-1978. U.S. Government Printing Office, Washington, D.C.

U. S. International Trade Commission. 1979. Section VI. Medicinal chemicals. Pp. 150-176 in Synthetic Organic Chemicals, 1978. United States Production and Sales, 1978. USITC Publication 1001. U.S. Government Printing Office, Washington, D.C.

Valtonen, M. V., R. H. Ylikahri, R. J. Suomalainen, and V. V. Valtonen. 1977. Selection of multiresistant coliforms by long-term treatment of hypercholesterolaemia with neomycin. Br. Med. J. 1:683-684.

Van Leeuwen, W. J., J. Van Embden, P. Guinee, E. H. Kampelmacher, A. Manten, M. Van Schothorst, and C. E. Voogd. 1979. Decrease of drug resistance in Salmonella in the Netherlands. Antimicrob. Agents Chemother. 16:237-239.

Wells, D. M., and O. B. James. 1973. Transmission of infectious drug resistance from animals to man. J. Hyg., Camb. 71:209-215.

Wiedemann, B., and H. Knothe. 1971. Epidemiological investigations of R factor bearing enterobacteria in man and animal in Germany. Ann. N.Y. Acad. Sci. 182:380-382.

Woods, D. R., D. Marcos, and D. A. Hendry. 1972. The incidence of R factors among coliform bacteria. S. Afr. Med. J. 46:189-191.

World Health Organization. 1974. Long-Term Programme in Environmental Pollution Control in Europe. Control of Harmful Residues in Food for Human and Animal Consumption. The Public Health Aspects of Antibiotics in Feedstuffs. Report of a Working Group convened by the Regional Office for Europe of the World Health Organization, Bremen, 1-5 October 1973. EURO 3604(2). Regional Office for Europe, World Health Organization, Copenhagen. 35 pp.

World Health Organization. 1976. Public Health Aspects of Antibiotic-Resistant Bacteria in the Environment. Report on a consultation meeting, Brussels, 9-12 December 1975. ICP/FSP 002. Regional Office for Europe, World Health Organization, Copenhagen. 13 pp.

World Health Organization. 1978. Surveillance for the Prevention and Control of Health Hazards Due to Antibiotic-Resistant Enterobacteria. Report of a WHO Meeting. Tech. Rep. Series 624. World Health Organization, Geneva. 57 pp.

CONSULTANTS' PAPERS

THE APPENDIXES

The following papers, Appendixes A through K, were commissioned by the Committee to Study the Human Health Effects of Subtherapeutic Antibiotic Use in Animal Feeds. They were used by the committee as working papers and are attached to the committee's report for information only. They do not constitute part of the foregoing report prepared by the committee. All references to these papers should be attributed to the authors, not to the committee.

A transcription of the public meeting held August 23, 1979 also formed part of the working papers used by the committee. These records may be obtained on loan from Dr. Enriqueta C. Bond, National Academy of Sciences, 2101 Constitution Ave., N.W., Room 347, Washington, D.C. 20418.

APPENDIX A
THE CLINICAL USE OF ANTIMICROBIALS AND THE DEVELOPMENT OF RESISTANCE

John P. Utz[1]

Infectious diseases are the most common cause of absence from school or work, are the most frequent of the known causes of birth defects, and, as pneumonia and influenza, are the fourth most common cause of death in the United States.

CONTROL OF DISEASE

Immunization with vaccines is the major technique used in the United States to prevent infectious diseases. The oral polio vaccine, as the ultimate example, is clearly responsible for the world-wide control of poliomyelitis, despite an outbreak of the disease, which spread from the Netherlands to Canada and the United States in 1979 (Center for Disease Control, 1979a). Similarly, the tetanus vaccine is solely responsible for the elimination of tetanus, as observed in the Armed Forces during World War II and the conflicts in Korea and Vietnam. Other live virus vaccines are used primarily in children to prevent rubella, rubeola, and mumps. Vaccination with killed bacteria (pertussis) or their toxic products (diphtheria toxoid) is also an effective preventive measure.

Antimicrobials are used to prevent approximately a dozen categories of infection. Some of these uses are described below.

Between 1960 and 1976 there were 131 published studies of the prophylactic use of antimicrobials to reduce the possibility of infection after surgical procedures. Although only 24 of these studies describe controlled, prospective, double-blind studies, they report striking statistically significant reductions in various types of wound infections when antimicrobials were administered in conjunction with repair after hip fracture, hip prosthesis, vaginal hysterectomy, and colon, biliary, and gastrointestinal surgery (Chodak and Plaut, 1977). These procedures are regarded as clean in contrast to compound fractures and gunshot or stab wounds of the abdomen, which are considered already infected. Thus, antimicrobial use in these instances is therapeutic, rather than prophylactic.

---

[1]School of Medicine, Georgetown University, Washington, D.C.

A second category of antimicrobial prophylaxis was first demonstrated in San Francisco where isoniazid was used to prevent overt tuberculosis in populations with delayed cutaneous hypersensitivity to tuberculin (American Thoracic Society, 1974; Ferebee, 1970). The continuing protection demonstrated in the treated group led to the wide use of this drug in patients with a known positive test. The enthusiasm engendered by these successes continued until the recognition in the Washington, D.C. area of the hepatotoxicity of isoniazid (Garibaldi *et al.*, 1972).

Antimicrobials administered prophylactically to immunodeficient patients lacking the benefit of a protected environment have produced variable results. Immunodeficiency may result from a disease state or from the use of drugs. Immunosuppression may be desired, e.g., when drugs are administered to transplant recipients to prevent host-versus graft rejection, or may be an undesired consequence of cancer chemotherapy. Protection afforded by antimicrobial prophylaxis is enhanced by a protected environment.

Studies conducted over many years, beginning early in the antimicrobial era, have shown that oral sulfonamides and penicillin G or intramuscular benzathine penicillin G protect against recurrence of rheumatic fever by preventing infection by Group A *Streptococcus pyogenes*. Failure of such prophylaxis is not usually related to the development of resistance, but instead to a lack of compliance on the part of patient or parents. Hence, benzathine penicillin G injected by a medical professional is the most successful drug and route, since patient cooperation--except for travel to a doctor's office or clinic--is not required.

An even earlier practice was the prevention of ophthalmia neonatorum by the routine use of silver nitrate and, later, penicillin G, in all newborn infants.

Scrub typhus (tsutsugamushi disease) occurs rarely in this country, and then only in people who have once spent time near or in northern Australia, Pakistan, or Japan. This disease can be prevented by 1 g of chloramphenicol every other day for a month after exposure, but because the disease is infrequent, this prophylactic application of chloramphenicol is little known.

At various times and during different epidemics, sulfonamides, rifampin, or minocycline given to family members or other groups have prevented the spread of meningococcal infections from patients or carriers of Neisseria meningitidis. Since this species is frequently a commensal of humans, it has virtually always resulted in later recolonization and the carrier state following prophylaxis.

Chemoprophylaxis is probably effective in the prevention of syphilis and shigellosis, but is rarely used for this purpose. More commonly it is practiced in the hope of preventing bacterial endocarditis, but there are no data demonstrating the efficacy of this use.

Controlled trials indicate that either a tetracycline or ampicillin is effective in preventing febrile disease and loss of time from work for patients with chronic obstructive pulmonary disease (Batten, 1976). However, the magnitude of that population and the cost-benefit ratio are so great that this method of preventing recurrent infection has not been widespread.

The elimination of smallpox (variola) by the use of vaccination (cowpox or vaccinia) has overshadowed the demonstration of methisazone as a chemoprophylactic agent. Field trials in Madras, India showed that the use of methisazone in 1,101 exposed persons resulted in only three cases of mild smallpox, in contrast to 78 cases (with 12 deaths) among 1,126 controls who did not receive the drug (Bauer *et al.*, 1963).

Enthusiasm for amantadine in the prevention of influenzas has been tempered by the limited spectrum of its antiviral activity--type A_2 (Asian) influenza only--and by the limited period of effectiveness (immediately before or after the exposure, the time of which is always uncertain).

Since World War II chemoprophylaxis has been an accepted practice in malarial areas. The development of chloroquine-resistant strains in Southeast Asia and Africa has lessened the effectiveness of that antimalarial drug and has led to the requirement for other drugs (Anonymous, 1978a).

Specific Agents

With the exception of the arsenicals and bismuth, the antimicrobial era began in the mid-1930's with the use of the sulfonamides. Even today members of this family are the first choice in the treatment of uncomplicated urinary tract infections, nocardiosis, some Chlamydia trachomatis infections, and chancroid. Resistance of N. meningitidis to the sulfonamides has been encountered principally in prophylaxis of family members or in active treatment of meningitis. The more recent combination of a sulfonamide, sulfamethoxazole, with trimethoprim has resulted in an oral preparation that is useful in the treatment of an even wider range of infections, e.g., pneumonia caused by Pneumocystis carinii.

The antibiotic era began in the mid-1940's with the rediscovery of the activity of penicillin G and its use in severe human disease. This drug remains the first choice in the treatment of infection by Group A S. pyogenes (e.g., rheumatic fever), S. pneumoniae (pneumonia), N. meningitidis (meningococcal diseases), Pasteurella multocida (e.g., skin ulcer, osteomyelitis, pleuritis, sinusitis, leptomeningitis), Treponema pallidum (syphilis), Actinomyces israelii (actinomycosis), Leptospira spp. (leptospirosis), Bacillus anthracis (anthrax), and Streptobacillus moniliformis (streptobacillary rat-bite fever).

However, by 1947 Weinstein had reported superinfection by Haemophilus influenzae, which produced septicemia in a patient treated with penicillin G for pneumonia. This first report is the prototype of the truism that the use of any antimicrobial agent ultimately results in the appearance of, or colonization by, microorganisms that are resistant to or not susceptible to that agent. However, this is not always detrimental if the pathogenicity of the new microorganism is less or nonexistent. Indeed, were this not usually the case, antimicrobial therapy could rarely, if ever, be justified.

Streptomycin, first used in 1945, remains as a single drug treatment for one infection by Francisella tularensis (tularemia). In combination with penicillin G it is optimal therapy for Enterococcus (Group D streptococcal infections), with a tetracycline for Malleomyces mallei (glanders) and Yersinia pestis (plague), with ampicillin for more resistant Listeria monocytogenes (listeriosis), and with other antituberculous drugs for tuberculosis.

The tetracyclines and chloramphenicol became available almost simultaneously in 1948. The former are active against many of the Gram-negative Enterobacteriaceae that are resistant to streptomycin and are optimal therapy for Calymmatobacterium granulomatis (granuloma inguinale), Brucella spp. (brucellosis), Vibrio cholerae (cholera), and Borrelia recurrentis (relapsing fever). Tetracyclines are also the first choice in the treatment of another group of infections caused by Rickettsia. Infections caused by Chlamydia, both C. psittaci and C. trachomatis, are similarly treated.

Despite the rare, but commonly fatal, idiosyncratic pancytopenic reactions, chloramphenicol is indicated for H. influenzae (meningitis) and Salmonella typhi (typhoid). Decisions on whether to use antimicrobials for salmonellosis, often acquired from meats and eggs, should be based upon the studies of Woodward and Smadel (1964). These authors defined the precise benefits of such therapy as well as the unaffected factors, e.g., metastases, carrier state, and bowel perforations, and its ill effects, e.g., enhanced relapse rate.

Tricarcillin, usually in combination with an aminoglycoside, is used to treat Pseudomonas aeruginosa infections. Among the aminoglycoside antibiotics, tobramycin appears to have both greater efficacy and less toxicity than gentamicin, kanamycin, or amikacin.

The development of the penicillinase-resistant penicillins methicillin, oxacillin, cloxacillin, dicloxacillin, and nafcillin has resulted in the preferential use of the last two for any Staphyloccus aureus infection when the sensitivity to penicillin G is unknown.

In addition to streptomycin, the most active and best tolerated among the antituberculous drugs are rifampin, ethambutol, and isoniazid. The latter three drugs are generally preferred because they can be administered orally, which is more convenient than the intramuscular route for both long-term use and therapy administered in the home or to ambulatory patients. A study by Phillipon et al. (1977) indicates that rifampin may be preferable to tetracycline in the treatment of brucellosis, especially in its ability to reduce residual infections. But further confirmatory studies are needed before its widespread use can be recommended.

Erythromycin is indicated for the Corynebacterium diphtheriae carrier state (but is not adequate for active diphtheria, which requires antitoxin) and for Mycoplasma spp. and Legionella pneumophila infections because the drug lacks serious side-effects.

For the anaerobic infections, which commonly cause intracerebral, pulmonary, peritoneal, or pelvic infections (usually with abscesses), one has a choice of four drugs: chloramphenicol, clindamycin, metronidazole, or cefoxitin, depending upon which side-effect is less disturbing to the physician, e.g., enterocolitis from clindamycin or the idiosyncratic pancytopenic reactions from chloramphenicol.

Although the activity of amoxicillin or ampicillin is similar to that of penicillin G, the drugs are especially effective in the treatment of infection from *Proteus mirabilis*, *Salmonella* (except *typhi*), *Shigella* spp., and *Listeria monocytogenes*.

When none of the preceding microorganisms is the pathogen, or occasionally, when one after another has been progressively selected, fungal infection or superinfection may occur. Agents for these are amphotericin B, flucytosine, or miconazole, depending on the species or occasionally on the sensitivity of the isolated strain.

Other useful agents include vancomycin, which is enjoying a resurgence of interest because it is so helpful in patients on dialysis, with *Clostridium difficile* in necrotizing, pseudomembranous enterocolitis and in Gram-positive coccal infections that are resistant to penicillin. A special mention must be made of the cephalosporins because there are so many of them, because they are remarkably active against many Gram-negative and Gram-positive bacteria, and because minute chemical changes have resulted in such great activity against previously unsusceptible organisms, e.g., *Enterococcus* and *Pseudomonas aeruginosa*.

BACTERIAL RESISTANCE TO ANTIMICROBIALS

Failure of antimicrobial therapy can be attributed to a number of causes: untreatable infections (e.g., pneumonia due to measles virus), improper dosage (e.g., overdosage increasing risk of superinfection or too low a dose resulting in failure to achieve bactericidal concentrations, as might occur in bacterial meningitis where the level in cerebrospinal fluid may be much lower than that in the blood), improper duration (e.g., failure to treat a Group A streptococcal infection for 10 days), omission of surgical drainage of an intraabdominal or pelvic abscess, or the emergence of microorganisms that are resistant to the antimicrobial.

The development of *S. aureus* that is resistant to penicillin G by means of a penicillinase is of historical importance. From 1955 to 1960 severe disease was caused by such bacteria. These outbreaks were ended by the development of penicillinase-resistant penicillins.

The second instance of resistance to antimicrobial agents that was of major importance was the development of *Streptococcus pneumoniae*, which became resistant to tetracyclines, drugs that were useful at that time for treating pneumonias of uncertain origin, i.e., those now known to to be caused by *Mycoplasma pneumoniae*, *Coxiella burnetii*, and *Legionella pneumophila*. In their studies of Australian aborigines and New Guineans, Hansman *et al*. (1971) found the first isolates of *Streptococcus pneumoniae* with resistance to penicillin. Although strains with intermediate resistance were first reported in New Guinea and Australia and highly resistant ones first in South Africa, resistant organisms were soon thereafter identified in Europe and the United States. Curiously, the highly resistant strains have not been further reported in states other than Minnesota (Center for Disease Control, 1979b).

Fortunately, alternative chemotherapy exists for those bacteria with resistance to both tetracyclines and penicillin. Examples of alternatives to the first-choice drugs usually used for various diseases will be found in the literature (Anonymous, 1978b). The disadvantages in having to use alternatives vary from case to case and are related to the organisms to be combatted, the alternative drug(s), and the patient to be treated. An additional aspect of importance is the 10% to 15% frequency of patients with alleged sensitivity to penicillin and to whom the drug cannot be given. An examination of alternative drugs to combat penicillin- and tetracycline-resistant pneumococci reveals problems in therapy caused by antibiotic resistance quite well. In order of decreasing desirability, alternatives include the cephalosporins, which can be administered orally or parenterally, but are less active; chloramphenicol, which has the danger of fatal aplastic anemia in approximately 1 in 30,000 individuals; vancomycin, which is the most active but can only be administered intravenously and is ototoxic; and erythromycin, which, while being the least toxic, is also the least active.

Resistance to the tetracyclines and penicillins has not been a recognized problem in those patients more prone to infection or more severe disease, e.g., those who have congenital or acquired impairment of antibody- (hypogammaglobulinemia) or cellular- (Hodgkin's disease, sarcoidosis) mediated immunity, or both (chronic lymphatic leukemia). Other patients are susceptible because their defenses are deliberately compromised by azathioprine or prednisone to prevent host-versus-graft reaction, as in kidney or heart transplant patients. Lastly, there are other patients, e.g., those with malignancy, whose antineoplastic therapy, e.g., chemotherapy or radiologic therapy, has the undesired and unpreventable side-effect of such compromise.

Although infants and the elderly are considered fragile and susceptible, one can contend that either group has an advantage over populations of less extreme ages: the infants because they handle stressful procedures well and possess transplacental material antibody, and the elderly because of their past exposure over many years to infectious agents and their development of an imposing immune globulin or other nonantibody defenses. However, one would not question the assertion that there is a distinctive pattern of susceptibility to infections in each group: the infant to the Gram-negative Enterobacteriaceae, *Haemophilus influenzae*, and the Group B *S. pyogenes*, and the elderly, notably those hospitalized, to *S. pneumoniae* and the Gram-negative Enterobacteriaceae.

Increased frequency of infection, especially in those colonized with resistant bacteria, had been anticipated. There have been many studies of two groups of patients that have received antimicrobials daily for many years in doses considered suboptimal for treatment of active disease. One group consists of cystic fibrotic patients in whom duration and quality of life have been improved with such drugs as a tetracycline or chloramphenicol (Batten, 1976). Recurrent infection with *P. aeruginosa*, especially the highly mucous variant, is an acknowledged problem, but it is difficult to attribute this directly to chemotherapy (Mearns *et al.*, 1972). The second group is composed of patients taking tetracycline for either acne vulgaris (adolescents) or acne rosacea (middle-aged and elderly patients). Although tetracycline-resistant organisms can be isolated readily from these patients, more frequent or more resistant disease has not been documented (Schmidt *et al.*, 1973).

Resistance in microorganisms occurs in four patterns, which may overlap:

- Bacteria are unaltered in their pathogenicity or other characteristics (e.g., resistance to streptomycin or sulfonamide).

- Some bacteria lose special enzymes (e.g., catalase and peroxidase) and pathogenicity (e.g., resistance to isoniazid).

- Plasmid-mediated (nonchromosomal) antibiotic resistance may be acquired by and transferred among many Enterobacteriaceae. This is the most recently observed pattern and the most alarming one.

- Development of a specific enzyme (beta-lactamase) by Enterobacteriaceae and *S. aureus* that inactivates penicillin.

Resistant strains become more prevalent when antibiotics are used frequently and/or in high doses (Finland, 1979). Often a resistant strain may develop during the course of antibiotic treatment given to a patient originally infected with a sensitive strain. It is well known that a patient entering a hospital with a urinary tract infection usually has sensitive *E. coli*, whereas the patient hospitalized for only 3 or 4 days who develops such an infection has a much more resistant isolate, presumably acquired from the hospital flora which has been subjected to selection pressure by the use of antimicrobials. To a considerable degree this is a reflection of in-hospital therapy. Surprising, however, is the fact that extensive out-of-hospital use of a drug, e.g., for acne, has not resulted in noticeable increases in diseases from the emergence of resistant organisms. Primary or emergent resistance has not been attributable to antibiotic use in animal feeds. Nor does it seem possible to attribute a hospital outbreak to therapeutic or subtherapeutic use in those feeds.

Lack of response to an antimicrobial may be the result of an inappropriate choice of agent. This is most likely when the causative organism for a disease has not been fully characterized. A number of examples of such diseases whose cause has only recently or has not been recognized come to mind. They include Legionnaires disease (*Legionella pneumophila*), nongonococcal urethritis (*Chlamydia* spp.), infantile pneumonia (*Chlamydia trachomatis*), Lassa fever (Lassa virus), Marburg disease (Marburg virus), infantile botulism (*Clostridium botulinum*), hepatitis (non-A/non-B hepatitis viruses), Norwalk gastroenteritis (Norwalk virus), and enterocolitis caused by *Yersinia enterocolitica*, *Clostridium difficile*, or *Campylobacter fetus*. To choose the optimal therapeutic agent, one must know the cause of a disease or infection and its antibiotic susceptibility.

For these new diseases as well as the older diseases, the selection of antimicrobial agents must be continually reviewed; the pattern of sensitivities of isolates in the hospital or community microbiological laboratory must be evaluated at least yearly, laboratory by laboratory; and the practice of chemotherapy must be monitored, adjusted, and changed continuously. Since the discovery of antimicrobials approximately 40 years ago, the changes in antimicrobial use have been far too numerous to list, but some examples can be cited: the drift toward tetracycline from penicillin to treat *N. gonhorrheae*; the increased use of chloramphenicol and the decreased use of penicillin for acute otitis media owing to the frequency of resistant *H. influenza*; the resurgence of vancomycin after a hiatus of almost 20 years because of newer uses and more resistant microorganisms; and the changing pattern in the immediate treatment of meningitis (i.e., treatment before the causative species are identified). Sulfonamide was the first agent of choice, but it was replaced by penicillin G which was itself replaced by a combination of penicillin, sulfonamide, and chloramphenicol. This combination gave way to ampicillin, then to a combination of ampicillin and chloramphenicol, which is commonly used today.

In many instances the reason for change has been development of a more efficacious and/or less toxic drug by industry. Two examples of such improved drugs are the aminoglycosides and the cephalosporins. The development of the former spans almost 35 years, beginning with streptomycin, neomycin, and dihydrostreptomycin, progressing to kanamycin, then to amikacin, gentamicin, tobramycin, and sisomicin. The history of the cephalosporins covers about half as many years, but the number of new agents is far greater. The two earliest agents, e.g., streptomycin and cephalothin, retain some usefulness. But other drugs, e.g., novobiocin, paromomycin, paraminosalicylic acid, colistimethate, bacitracin, and ristocetin, have disappeared from systemic formularies. But who could predict that they will never reemerge?

There is no reason to anticipate a radical departure from the past in the development of emergent and primary resistant organisms, of new and challenging diseases, of better and better drugs, and of ebbs and flows in drug selection and usage. Thus, we can expect a continuing production of newer vaccines, most imminently for hepatitis B antigen. Most likely vaccines will not replace the need for antimicrobial therapy of overt disease. Rather, both the prophylaxis against and treatment of infectious diseases will continue to be employed, neither replacing the other.

REFERENCES

American Thoracic Society. 1974. Preventive treatment of tuberculosis. A general review. Pp. 29-106 in G. Canetti, ed., H. Birkhäuser and H. Block, co-eds. Advances in Tuberculosis Research. Volume 17. S. Karger, N.Y.

Anonymous. 1978a. Malaria (plasmodia). The Medical Letter 20(1) (Issue 496):20-21.

Anonymous. 1978b. The choice of antimicrobial drugs. The Medical Letter 20(1) (Issue 496):1-8.

Batten, J. 1976. Chemoprophylaxis of respiratory infections. Postgrad. Med. J. 52:571-575.

Bauer, D. J., L. St. Vincent, C. H. Kempe, and A. W. Downie. 1963. Prophylactic treatment of smallpox contacts with N-methylisatin β-thiosemicarbazone. Lancet 2:494-496.

Center for Disease Control. 1979a. Follow-up on poliomyelitis--United States, Canada, Netherlands. Reported by A. van Wezel; [no first initial] van Zermarel; S. Acres; State epidemiologists from Iowa, Missouri, Pennsylvania, and Wisconsin; and the Center for Disease Control. Morbid. Mortal. Weekly Rep. 28:345-346.

Center for Disease Control. 1979b. Isolation of drug-resistant pneumococci--New York. Reported by S. Landesman, V. Ahonkahai, M. Sierra, H. Bernheimer, R. Goetz, A. Josephson, G. Pringle, G. Schiffman, P. Steiner, J. S. Marr, and the Center for Disease Control. Morbid. Mortal. Weekly Rep. 28:225-226.

Chodak, G. W., and M. E. Plaut. 1977. Use of systemic antibiotics for prophylaxis in surgery: A critical review. Arch. Surg. 112:326-334.

Ferebee, S. H. 1970. Controlled chemoprophylaxis trials in tuberculosis. A general review. Pp. 29-106 in G. Canetti, ed., H. Birkhäuser and H. Bloch, co-eds. Advances in Tuberculosis Research. Volume 17. S. Karger, N.Y.

Finland, M. 1979. Emergence of antibiotic resistance in hospitals, 1935-1975. Rev. Infect. Dis. 1:4-21.

Garibaldi, R. A., R. E. Drusin, S. H. Ferebee, and M. B. Gregg. 1972. Isoniazid-associated hepatitis. Report of an outbreak. Am. Rev. Resp. Dis. 106:357-365.

Hansman, D., H. Glasgow, J. Sturt, L. Devitt, and R. Douglas. 1971. Increased resistance to penicillin of pneumococci isolated from man. N. Engl. J. Med. 284:175-177.

Mearns, M. B., G. H. Hunt, and R. Rushworth. 1972. Bacterial flora of respiratory tract in patients with cystic fibrosis, 1950-1971. Arch. Dis. Childhood 47:902-907.

Philippon, A. M., M. G. Plommet, A. Kazmierczak, J. L. Marly, and P. A. Nevot. 1977. Rifampin in the treatment of experimental brucellosis in mice and guinea pigs. J. Infect. Dis. 136:482-488.

Schmidt, H., E. From, and G. Heydenreich. 1973. Bacteriological examination of rectal specimens during long-term oxytetracycline treatment for acne vulgaris. Acta Dermatol. Venerol. 53:153-156.

Weinstein, L. 1947. The spontaneous occurrence of new bacterial infections during the course of treatment with streptomycin or penicillin. Am. J. Med. Sci. 214:56-63.

Woodward, T. E., and J. E. Smadel. 1964. Management of typhoid fever and its complications. Ann. Intern. Med. 60:144-157.

APPENDIX B
POSSIBLE HUMAN HEALTH EFFECTS
OF SUBTHERAPEUTIC ANTIMICROBIAL USE AS PESTICIDES

Robert N. Goodman[1]

The need for antibiotics to control bacterial diseases is greater for perennials than it is for annuals because annual plants (e.g., wheat, soybeans, tomatoes, etc.) can be bred for resistance to diseases more quickly. Consider how few new varieties of apples have appeared on the market during the past 25 years. However, if antibiotics are used to control a disease, the emergence of resistance to that antibiotic is greater when a species remains in place for decades and is treated annually for the same bacterial disease. Therefore, the problem of resistance to antibiotics must be evaluated in these circumstances.

As early as the 1950's, investigators were aware that treatment of plants with antibiotics could result in the emergence of antibiotic-resistant organisms and allergenic effects in people who applied the pesticides as well as in the consumers of the treated plants (Logue _et al._, 1958). Among the earliest studies on the mode of uptake of antibiotics by plants and their mode of action against the organisms causing plant disease were those of Goodman and Dowler (1958) and Goodman and Goldberg (1960). Subsequently, the ease with which resistance to streptomycin might be developed _in vitro_ by the target organism _Erwinia amylovora_ was studied and the resulting antibiotic-resistant organisms were used as markers to study pathogenesis of plant disease (Ayers _et al._, 1979; Goodman, 1963). In further studies, antibiotics were used to develop selective media to isolate specific bacterial species (Crosse and Goodman, 1973).

ANTIBIOTICS AS PESTICIDES

It is difficult to determine the types and quantities of antibiotics used as pesticides since exact production figures are regarded as confidential information by industry. Nonetheless, some estimates can be provided.

The primary antibiotic used to control plant disease is streptomycin. Throughout the United States, approximately 10,000 kg of streptomycin is used in a typical year for various diseases,

[1]Department of Plant Pathology, University of Missouri, Columbia.

predominantly fire blight in apples and pears. The use of streptomycin against bacterial spot of tomatoes and peppers, soft rot of potatoes, bacterial blight of celery, and tobacco pathogens seems to be increasing as does its application to beans to control halo blight.

Approximately 1,000 kg of tetracycline is used annually to control fire blight of apples and pears (when resistance to streptomycin is a problem) nationwide and bacterial spot of peaches in the Eastern United States. This amount also includes administration of tetracycline by infusion to control the infection of palm and other ornamental species by mycoplasmas. These amounts are approximate and vary, often substantially, from year to year with disease prevalence (Pfizer, Inc., personal communication, 1979).

THE USE OF PENICILLIN TO CONTROL PLANT PATHOGENS

There is no evidence to indicate that penicillin is used to any extent to control plant disease.

Most plant pathogens are Gram negative, and only members of the genus *Corynebacterium*, which comprise comparatively few plant pathogenic species, are Gram-variable and sensitive to penicillin. Hence, the value of the penicillins as therapeutic agents for plant diseases is extremely low. This antibiotic might have limited future application since some pathological disorders in plants that were previously believed to be of viral origin have recently been shown to be caused by rickettsia-like organisms (RLO) and to be unexpectedly sensitive to penicillin (Markham *et al.*, 1975; Ulrychová *et al.*, 1975). Where penicillin therapy is being tested experimentally, the most common route of administration is infusion.

THE DISPOSITION OF ANTIBIOTICS USED AS PESTICIDES

Antibiotics applied to plants have a relatively short half-life and undergo a tremendous dilution factor when applied either as a foliar spray or through infusion (Ulrychová *et al.*, 1975). Streptomycin may persist in plant tissues for more than a year (Goodman, 1962, 1963); however, once these tissues are exposed to natural decay processes, antibiotics are quickly degraded.

INGESTION OF ANTIBIOTIC RESIDUES BY ANIMALS AND HUMANS

Both humans and animals could be exposed to antibiotics used as pesticides as a result of ingesting apples, pears, and peaches; however, the levels in pears at harvest are below those detectable by sensitive bioassay (Goodman, 1962).

Antibiotic bioassay procedures were developed for assaying antibiotic residues in fruit and vegetable tissue (Goodman *et al.*, 1958; Morgan *et al.*, 1955). The residual levels determined by these procedures were subsequently used as the basis for feeding trials with volunteers (Goldberg *et al.*, 1961). Ingestion by animals is not a real concern at present since plants used as animal feeds are not being treated with antibiotics for disease control.

There has been a great deal of experimentation to disinfest and disinfect seeds assumed to be contaminated or infected by bacterial pathogens (Lockhart *et al.*, 1976; Sutton and Bell, 1954). Although this type of antibiotic therapy has not been used widely in general practice, this technique is fairly promising and should not contribute a significant hazard to the health of animals or humans. It appears to be the ideal process for controlling plant diseases, particularly when resultant antibiotic residues would be at low levels. The dilution of antibiotic concentrations in the germinating seedlings would continue through growth and maturity of the plant. At harvest, concentrations of the antibiotic in tissue would be beyond detection (Goodman, 1962).

BACTERIAL RESISTANCE

The emergence of resistance in target organisms resulting from prolonged use of antibiotics under field conditions has concerned plant pathologists for some time. In the spring of 1953 streptomycin was first used in Missouri to control *Erwinia amylovora*, a Gram-negative member of Enterobacteriaceae that causes blight in apples and pears (Murneek, 1952). Since that time, streptomycin has been used regularly in the fruit-growing regions of Missouri and other states. There has been no evidence of the emergence of resistant strains of *E. amylovora* in Missouri, although there have been frequent efforts to detect resistance in that state and in New York where streptomycin has been used for almost three decades (Beer and Norelli, 1976). However, in 1971 California investigators found considerable evidence that resistance to streptomycin has emerged in *E. amylovora* (Moller *et al.*,

1972), possibly because there have been significantly more applications of streptomycin per growing season in orchards in the West than in the East.

In apple orchards in Missouri and in the Eastern States streptomycin is used to control fire blight an average of 3 to 4 times (a maximum of 6 times) during the growing season. However, the antibiotic has been applied as many as 13 to 15 times in pear orchards in the Far West where the disease develops continuously over the longer growing season. The selective pressure of 15 applications of streptomycin clearly uncovered those members of the *E. amylovora* population that were resistant to streptomycin, in some cases in concentrations as high as 500 μg/ml (Moller *et al.*, 1972). This has never occurred in orchards in the East. Furthermore, laboratory attempts to develop streptomycin-resistant mutants of *E. amylovora* are successful only with the greatest difficulty (Shaffer and Goodman, 1962).

Using the gradient plate technique, restreaking an inoculum on plates containing streptomycin in increasing concentrations from 0 to 10 μg/l, from 0 to 100 μg/l, and, finally, from 0 to 1,000 μg/ml eventually produces mutants with resistance to 1,000 μg/ml after 35 to 40 days. Apparently, the frequency of mutations with significant resistance to streptomycin in this organism is extremely low.

By far the largest number of species of bacterial plant pathogens with resistance to antibiotics are in the genus *Pseudomonas*, and the second largest number reside in the genus *Xanthomonas* (yellow Pseudomonadaceae). Antibiotics have been used for many years in attempts to control diseases caused by these bacterial species. However, after only two or three applications it became apparent that large proportions of resident populations were not susceptible to concentrations of antibiotics well over 500 μg/ml (Cox and Hayslip, 1957; Crossan and Krupka, 1955). Hence, the efficacy of antibiotics for the control of bacterial diseases has been narrowed to precious few species.

HISTORY OF ANTIBIOTIC USE AS PESTICIDES

The first report of an antibiotic used to control a plant bacterial pathogen appeared as a note in *Phytopathology* in 1952. The antibiotic was thiolutin, and the researcher was Murneek (1952). Since that time, almost all antibiotics with either antibacterial or antifungal activity have been screened at one time or another against a wide spectrum of pathogens affecting plants (Goodman, 1959). Antifungal antibiotics have been successful only upon rare occasions, the most effective being cycloheximide (Whiffin, 1950). However, with the advent of systemic as well as prophylactic organic fungicides, interest in antifungal antibiotics to control fungal plant diseases waned precipitiously. The use of streptomycin has persisted for approximately 26 years and is now an accepted practice in the production of apples and pears and in many parts of this country. Recently, there has been renewed interest in the use of the tetracyclines to control infections of a number of ornamental plants, especially southern palms, by mycoplasma-like organisms (MLO). Experiments have shown that infusion of 1 to 1.5 g of oxytetracycline in 10 to 20 ml of water into a single palm tree causes remission of the disease for more than a year (Arai *et al.*, 1967; Bowyer and Calavan, 1974; McCoy and Gwin, 1977; Rosenberger and Jones, 1977). As mentioned previously, MLO disorders of plants, formerly thought to be viral in origin, seem to be adequately controlled by penicillin (Markham *et al.*, 1975; Ulrychová *et al.*, 1975).

EPIDEMIOLOGICAL STUDIES

Perhaps the single most important question that should be asked in epidemiological studies is whether the transfer of antibiotic resistance genes from the ubiquitous coliforms to plant bacterial pathogens, or vice versa, has resulted from the use of antibiotics to control plant diseases. Experiments that have been conducted *in vitro* clearly show that resistance genes can be transferred from *Escherichia coli* and *Shigella flexneri* to *Erwinia amylovora* under laboratory conditions (Chatterjee and Starr, 1973a) and that reciprocal transfer of resistant genes from *E. amylovora* to *E. coli* and other human and plant pathogens also occur (Chatterjee and Starr, 1973b). One must ask whether the levels of antibiotic titer achieved in the control of plant diseases, either by infusion or spray application, are sufficiently high to support the emergence of the resistant forms of pathogens or epiphytic saprophytic species (U.S. Environmental Protection Agency, 1978).

Rollins *et al.* (1975) reported that in a 44-day feeding experiment more than 2 but less than 10 μg of oxytetracycline per gram of diet is required to increase significantly the proportion of resistant coliform bacteria in the intestine of a dog. The infusion of pear trees with oxytetracycline results in residues of approximately 0.0043 μg/ml oxytetracycline in plant tissue, less than 1/500 of the amount known to select for resistant microflora when administered daily. However, higher levels of streptomycin have been observed (Goodman, 1959). Hence, it is reasonably clear that the treatment of plant tissue with antibiotics to control plant disease can and does result in comprehensive residual levels of these substances.

Concentrations likely to be found in plant tissue can, after prolonged feeding periods, give rise to the development of resistant coliforms in the gut flora of laboratory animals (Goldberg et al., 1958, 1959) and humans (Goldberg et al., 1961). This was observed with both streptomycin and oxytetracycline. The investigators also noted that the resistant organisms were transient in the gut flora of the test subjects. Unfortunately, comprehension of R plasmids at that time was nil, and further study of specific antibiotic-resistant isolates was not attempted.

Recent studies have addressed the emergence of tetracycline resistance in humans exposed to subtherapeutic levels of this antibiotic (Graber et al., 1979). The resulting data are not particularly conclusive (Goldberg et al., 1959) because the study was not as comprehensive as it might have been. Future studies should use larger populations. Perhaps then more meaningful comparisons could be made.

The experiences with oxytetracycline or tetracyclines as pesticides have not been sufficiently long nor have they been sufficiently widespread to provide enough test subjects for comprehensive epidemiological studies among agriculturalists. This is not the case, however, for streptomycin. As indicated earlier in this report, streptomycin has been used in apple orchards for the control of *E. amylovora* on a regular and routine basis since 1953 (Goodman, 1953). The applicators of the antibiotic, at least in Missouri, represent a stable population that can be tested for both the presence of resistant coliforms in their gut flora and inordinate allergenic responses to this antibiotic. The studies of Chatterjee and Starr (1973a, b) clearly show that R factors from coliforms can be transferred to *E. amylovora* and other enterobacteria and that the reverse is also possible. The extent to which resistant coliforms occur in the applicators of streptomycin in Missouri might be reinvestigated (Goldberg et al., 1958, 1960). Research should be conducted to determine categorically that streptomycin does not have some adverse physiological affects on agricultural workers exposed to this drug. The applicator population in Missouri could be examined for an inordinate number demonstrating the clinical symptoms involved. There is little doubt that the examinations could be conducted on between 20 and 25 adult males who have applied streptomycin in apple orchards annually for at least 10 years. The concentrations of the antibiotic sprays (at 150 µg/ml) applied by these men are extremely high. The applicators could be examined in winter prior to the short spraying season, which begins in mid-April and ends in June, and at the termination of the spraying season. Residual levels of streptomycin could be sought in both blood and stool samples, and the latter could also be examined for the presence of resistant coliforms. Patch tests or other procedures for allergenic responses could be performed (Goldberg *et al.*, 1960).

RESISTANT MYCOPLASMAS

There is no evidence to suggest that administration of tetracyclines to plants has resulted in the emergence of antibiotic-resistant mycoplasmas. Failure to detect resistance, however, may be the result of technical problems related to the culturing of mycoplasmas or MLO's found in plants *in vitro*. Consequently, whether resistance, if it occurs, is due to plasmids cannot be determined. The manner in which oxytetracycline is used to control MLO disorders, mainly by infusion or injection procedures (Rosenberger and Jones, 1977), appears to present little risk of hazardous exposure either to the general population or to the applicators. Simple procedures such as the use of rubber gloves and masks should protect the applicator from contamination. The low volatility and small concentrations of these antibiotics in plant tissue suggest that secondary contamination of humans would also be rather rare. Under unusual circumstances, however, such as when animals ingest treated plant tissue in large quantities, resistant microorganisms might be found in their gut flora.

POSSIBLE HEALTH HAZARDS TO HUMANS FROM R-FACTOR TRANSFER

Another point that might be discussed more fully concerns the development of resistance to streptomycin in *Erwinia amylovora*, a species that is currently combatted routinely with this antibiotic. Brief mention was made earlier in this report that the emergence of resistance to streptomycin by this species is rare in nature but when it has occurred it has been widespread. Laboratory studies have shown that streptomycin-resistant mutants of *Erwinia amylovora* are extremely rare (Shaffer and Goodman, 1962). Following are some features of the streptomycin-resistant mutants that have been recovered. First, many are not as well adapted to the natural environment as the wild type virulent forms. They are often completely avirulent, lacking extracellular polysaccharide (EPS) (Ayers et al., 1979), which some investigators believe to be necessary, a priori, for pathogenicity. It also appears that the production of EPS is not controlled by plasmids.

Antibiotic usage to suppress or eradicate bacterial infection in plant cuttings, which are used in vegetative propagation, will probably be expanded. This type of chemotherapy can offer minimal opportunity for the emergence of significant levels of antibiotic resistance in the gut flora of the applicator or of the eventual consumer of the plant. However, plant pathogens carrying the R factor may emerge.

The possible increase in the environment of plant pathogens carrying R factors and their transfer to a ubiquitous plant saprophyte such as *Erwinia herbicola* and vice versa may be possible. Furthermore, human clinical strains of *E. herbicola* appear to possess similar plasmid transfer capabilities (Chatterjee et al., 1978). However, the amount of antibiotics contributed to the environment via plant pesticides must be comparatively small. Unfortunately, R-factor transfer in the field from plant pathogens to saprophytes on human or animal pathogens has not been adequately assessed (Cho et al., 1975). A few well conceived field experiments conducted regionally could provide the necessary answers and the likely assurances that antibiotics as plant pesticides do not constitute a significant hazard to human health.

CONCLUSIONS

Although exceptional progress has been made in the control of fungal diseases of plants, the control of bacterial disorders in plants has been only minimally successful. In general, the use of antibiotics as pesticides represents an extremely small fraction of the total use of antibiotics in therapy of humans and animals and in the production of animal tissues as food. In the few instances when antibiotics have been successful there appear to have been no obvious deleterious effects to either the applicator or the consumer. Experimentation exploring new and improved antibiotics to control bacterial diseases of plants should be synchronized with efforts in laboratories that can adequately test the safety of the new procedures.

REFERENCES

Arai, S., K. Y. Yuri, A. Kudo, M. Kikuchi, K. Kumagai, and N. Ishida. 1967. Effect of antibiotics on the growth of *Mycoplasma*. J. Antibiot. (Tokyo) Series A 20:246-253.

Ayers, A. R., S. B. Ayers, and R. N. Goodman. 1979. Extracellular polysaccharide of *Erwinia amylovora*: A correlation with virulence. Appl. Environ. Microbiol. 38:659-666.

Beer, S. V. 1976. Fire blight control with streptomycin sprays and adjuvants at different application volumes. Plant Dis. Rep. 60:541-544.

Beer, S. V., and J. L. Norelli. 1976. Streptomycin-resistant *Erwinia amylovora* not found in western New York pear and apple orchards. Plant Dis. Rep. 60:624-626.

Bennett, R. A., and E. Billing. 1975. Development and properties of streptomycin resistant cultures of *Erwinia amylovora* derived from English isolates. J. Appl. Bacteriol. 39:307-315.

Bowyer, J. W., and E. C. Calavan. 1974. Antibiotic sensitivity *in vitro* of the mycoplasmalike organism associated with citrus stubborn disease. Phytopathology 64:346-349.

Chatterjee, A. K., and M. P. Starr. 1973a. Gene transmission among strains of *Erwinia amylovora*. J. Bacteriol. 116:1100-1106.

Chatterjee, A. K., and M. P. Starr. 1973b. Transmission of *lac* by the sex factor E in *Erwinia* strains from human clinical sources. Infect. Immun. 8:563-572.

Chatterjee, A. K., M. K. Behrens, and M. P. Starr. 1978. Genetic and molecular properties of E-*lac*$^+$, a transmissible plasmid of *Erwinia herbicola*. Pp. 75-79 in Proceedings of the 4th International Conference on Plant Pathogenic Bacteriology held August 27-September 2, 1978, Angers, France. Phytobacteriology Section, Institut National de la Recherche Agronomique, Angers, France.

Cho, J. J., M. N. Schroth, S. D. Kominos, and S. K. Green. 1975. Ornamental plants as carriers of *Pseudomonas aeruginosa*. Phytopathology 65:425-431.

Cox, R. S., and N. C. Hayslip. 1957. Recent developments on the control of foliar diseases of tomato in south Florida. Plant Dis. Rep. 41:878-883.

Crossan, D. F., and L. R. Krupka. 1955. The use of streptomycin on pepper plants for the control of *Xanthomonas vesicatoria*. Plant Dis. Rep. 39:480-483.

Crosse, J. E., and R. N. Goodman. 1973. A selective medium for, and a definitive colony characteristic of, *Erwinia amylovora*. Phytopathology 63:1425-1426.

Goldberg, H. S., B. E. Read, and R. N. Goodman. 1958. Studies on the emergence of streptomycin-resistant bacteria as a result of low-level, long-term feeding of streptomycin. Pp. 144-148 in H. Welch and F. Marti-Ibañez, eds. Antibiotics Annual, 1957-1958. Medical Encyclopedia, Inc., N.Y.

Goldberg, H. S., R. N. Goodman, and B. Lanning. 1959. Low-level, long-term feeding of chlortetracycline and the emergence of antibiotic-resistant enteric bacteria. Pp. 930-934 in H. Welch and F. Marti-Ibañez, eds. Antibiotics Annual, 1958-1959. Medical Encyclopedia, Inc., N.Y.

Goldberg, H. S., J. T. Logue, and R. N. Goodman. 1960. Untoward reactions in human beings from application of antibiotics in plant disease control. Pp. 531-535 in H. Welch, Chairman of the Symposium, and F. Marti-Ibañez, ed. Antibiotics Annual, 1959-1960. Antibiotica, Inc., N.Y.

Goldberg, H. S., R. N. Goodman, J. T. Logue, and F. P. Handler. 1961. Long-term, low-level antibiotics and the emergence of antibiotic-resistant bacteria in human volunteers. Antimicrob. Agents Chemother. 80-88.

Goodman, R. N. 1953. Antibiotics. A new weapon for fire blight control. Am. Fruit Grower 73(11):7, 16, 17.

Goodman, R. N. 1959. Chapter IV. The influence of antibiotics on plants and plant disease control. Pp. 322-447 in H. S. Goldberg, ed. Antibiotics. Their Chemistry and Non-Medical Uses. D. Van Nostrand Company, Inc., Princeton, N.J.

Goodman, R. N. 1962. The impact of antibiotics upon plant disease control. Pp. 1-46 in R. L. Metcalf, ed. Advances in Pest Control Research, Volume 5. Interscience Publishers, A Division of John Wiley & Sons, New York and London.

Goodman, R. N. 1963. Systemic effects of antibiotics. Pp. 165-184 in M. Woodbine, ed. Antibiotics in Agriculture. Butterworths, London.

Goodman, R. N., and W. M. Dowler. 1958. The absorption of streptomycin by bean plants as influenced by growth regulators and humectants. Plant Dis. Rep. 42:122-126.

Goodman, R. N., and H. S. Goldberg. 1960. The influence of cation competition, time, and temperature on the uptake of streptomycin by foliage. Phytopathology 50:851-854.

Goodman, R. N., M. R. Johnston, and H. S. Goldberg. 1958. Residual quantities of antibiotics detected in treated plant tissue. Pp. 236-240 in H. Welch and F. Marti-Ibañez, eds. Antibiotics Annual, 1957-1958. Medical Encyclopedia, Inc., N.Y.

Graber, C. D., S. H. Sandifer, W. H. Whitlock, C. B. Loadholt, and B. J. Poore. 1979. Acquired resistance of autochthonous *E. coli* in controls and orchardists engaged in the spraying of oxytetracycline. Bull. Environ. Contam. Toxicol. 22:202-207.

Lockhart, C. L., C. O. Gourley, and E. W. Chipman. 1976. Control of *Xanthomonas compestris* in brussels sprouts with hot water and aureomycin seed treatment. Can. Plant Dis. Surv. 56:63-66.

Logue, J. T., H. S. Goldberg, and R. N. Goodman. 1958. The public health significance of antibiotic residues in foods. Pp. 333-335 in H. Welch, ed. Antibiotics Annual, 1957-1958. Medical Encyclopedia, Inc., N.Y.

Markham, P. G., R. Townsend, and K. A. Plaskitt. 1975. A rickettsia-like organism associated with diseased white clover. Ann. Appl. Biol. 81:91-93.

McCoy, R. E., and G. H. Gwin. 1977. Response of mycoplasmalike organism-infected Pritchardia, Trachycarpus and Veitchia palms to oxytetracycline. Plant Dis. Rep. 61:154-158.

Moller, W. J., J. A. Beutel, W. O. Reil, and B. G. Zoller. 1972. Fireblight resistance to streptomycin in California. Phytopathology 62:779.

Morgan, B. S., H. S. Goldberg, and R. N. Goodman. 1955. Residual quantities of a streptomycin-oxytetracycline combination, as determined by a simple microbiologic assay. Pp. 536-539 in H. Welch, ed. Antibiotics Annual, 1954-1955. Medical Encyclopedia, Inc., N.Y.

Murneek, A. E. 1952. Thiolutin as a possible inhibitor of fire blight. Phytopathology 42:57.

Rollins, L. D., S. A. Gaines, D. W. Pocurull, and H. D. Mercer. 1975. Animal model for determining the no-effect level of an antimicrobial drug on drug resistance in the lactose-fermenting enteric flora. Antimicrob. Agents Chemother. 7:661-665.

Rosenberger, D. A., and A. L. Jones. 1977. Symptom remission in x-diseased peach trees as affected by date, method, and rate of application of oxytetracycline-HCl. Plant Dis. Rep. 67: 277-282.

Shaffer, W. H., and R. N. Goodman. 1962. Progression _in vivo_, rate of growth _in vitro_, and resistance to streptomycin, as indices of virulence of _Erwinia amylovora_. Phytopathology 62:1201-1207.

Sutton, M. D., and W. Bell. 1954. The use of aureomycin as a treatment of swede seed for the control of black rot (_Xanthomonas campestris_). Plant Dis. Rep. 38:547-552.

Ulrychová, M., G. Vanek, M. Jokeš, Z. Klobáska, and O. Králík. 1975. Association of rickettsia-like organisms with infectious necrosis of grapevines and remission of symptoms after penicillin treatment. Phytopathol. Z. 82:254-265.

U.S. Environmental Protection Agency. 1978. Tolerances and exemptions from tolerances for pesticide chemicals in or on raw agricultural commodities. Oxytetracycline. Fed. Regist. 43(154):35309.

Whiffin, A. J. 1950. The activity *in vitro* of cycloheximide (actidione) against fungi pathogenic to plants. Mycologia 42:253-258.

APPENDIX C
GENETICS OF ANTIMICROBIAL RESISTANCE

George A. Jacoby[1] and K. Brooks Low[2]

NATURE OF ANTIBIOTIC RESISTANCE

Resistance to an antibacterial agent may be either natural or acquired. Some bacterial species are by nature uniformly resistant, some uniformly susceptible, and some include both susceptible and resistant strains. Natural resistance is reflected by gaps in the spectrum of activity of an antibiotic. Thus, broad spectrum drugs such as tetracyclines are effective against many bacterial species while narrow spectrum agents such as polymyxins are active against a restricted group of organisms.

Natural resistance (sometimes termed nonsusceptibility) to a particular antibiotic may be caused by a species' impermeability to an agent or by its lack of a target site, which is present in susceptible species.

Acquired resistance develops by mutation or by infection with resistance (R) plasmids. A single mutation may produce a high level of resistance to an antibiotic, such as streptomycin. For other drugs serial passage through gradually increasing concentrations of an antibiotic is required, and the resulting resistant strain generally carries multiple mutations, each providing a small increment in resistance. Resistance resulting from mutation is usually specific for the selecting agent or closely related drugs. It is inherited, but is rarely, if ever, spread to other bacteria. While some resistant mutants retain parental growth and virulence, other mutants are partially crippled. Mutants of this type are likely to be unstable and to revert or be lost due to a disadvantageous growth rate when antibiotic selection is withdrawn. In contrast, acquisition of an R plasmid generally confers resistance to clinically achievable levels of an antibiotic in a single step. A plasmid may carry resistance to one or to many chemically unrelated drugs. Furthermore, plasmids are transmissible by conjugation, transduction, or transformation to other bacteria and can thus disperse their resistance genes. They generally do not have deleterious effects on cell growth or virulence and may in fact carry

[1]Infectious Disease Unit, Massachusetts General Hospital, Boston, Mass.

[2]Radiobiology Laboratories, Yale University School of Medicine, New Haven, Conn.

genes contributing to virulence as well as to antibiotic resistance. Consequently, while study of mutational resistance to antibiotics has revealed much about normal cellular physiology and the actions of antibacterial agents, the major mechanism for resistance in clinical isolates of bacteria is plasmid carriage.

Bacteria with either natural or acquired resistance will be selectively favored in humans, animals, or environments in which antibiotics are used. How commonly this occurs depends on the particular antibiotic and on the genetic potential for development of resistance.

CHROMOSOMALLY DETERMINED RESISTANCE

Chromosomal mutations conferring resistance to antibiotics occur as spontaneous, random, and relatively rare alterations in the DNA composition of bacteria at frequencies of 10^{-6} to 10^{-10} per cell generation. Table 1 lists some well-studied examples of mutational resistance. Further details can be found in reviews by Benveniste and Davis (1973) and Davies and Smith (1978).

The biochemical basis of resistance usually involves one of four mechanisms:

- the target site is altered so that binding of the antibiotic is reduced or eliminated,
- there is a block in the transport of the drug into the cell,
- the antibiotic is detoxified or inactivated, or
- the inhibited step in a metabolic pathway is by-passed.

Resistance to the aminoglycosides kasugamycin, neamine, streptomycin, or spectinomycin can result from alteration of the amino acid in a specific protein of the 30S ribosomal subunit (Funatsu and Wittmann, 1972; Funatsu *et al.*, 1972; Yaguchi *et al.*, 1976; Yoshikawa *et al.*, 1975). Coresistance to neomycin and kanamycin probably involves the same mechanism but is less well characterized (Apirion and Schlessinger, 1968). Ribosomal mutants with broad resistance to aminoglycosides, including gentamicin, kanamycin, neomycin, and tobramycin, also occur, but additional nonribosomal mutations are required to achieve a high level of resistance (Buckel *et al.*, 1977).

TABLE 1

Mechanisms of Mutational Resistance to Antibiotics

Drug	Target	Mechanism of resistance
Aminoglycosides	Ribosome. Inhibition of protein synthesis	Altered ribosomal proteins (kasugamycin, S2[a]; neamine, S17; streptomycin, S12; spectinomycin, S5) Altered ribosomal protein (gentamicin, kanamycin, neomycin, tobramycin, and others, L6[a]) Altered 16S RNA methylation (kasugamycin) Altered drug transport
Erythromycin	Ribosome. Inhibition of protein synthesis	Altered ribosomal proteins (L4, L22) Altered assembly of ribosomal subunits
Nalidixic acid	DNA gyrase	Altered subunit of DNA gyrase (nalidixic or oxolinic acid) Altered drug transport
Novobiocin	DNA gyrase	Altered subunit of DNA gyrase (coumermycin A_1, novobiocin)
Penicillins	Cell wall biosynthesis	Altered penicillin-binding proteins Increased synthesis of chromosomal beta-lactamase Altered cell envelope
Rifampin	RNA polymerase	Altered beta subunit of RNA polymerase
Sulfonamide	Folic acid biosynthesis	Altered dihydropteroate synthase
Trimethoprim	Folic acid biosynthesis	Thymine auxotrophy sparing folic acid requirement

[a] Altered ribosomal protein: S = 30S subunit protein; L = 50S subunit protein.

Some kasugamycin-resistant mutants have altered 16S RNA methylation (Helser *et al.*, 1972).

Lower levels of resistance to aminoglycoside antibiotics can also be attributed to mutations in components of the system by which oxidative energy is coupled to drug transport (Kanner and Gutnick, 1972, Săsărman *et al.*, 1968). Some aminoglycoside transport mutants are broadly resistant to many other related drugs (Thorbjarnardóttir *et al.*, 1978). Resistance to rifampin develops as a result of an alteration in the beta subunit of its target site, RNA polymerase (Tocchini-Valentini *et al.*, 1968). *Escherichia coli* mutants that are resistant to erythromycin can be selected with alterations in specific ribosomal proteins or in the assembly of the two ribosomal subunits (Pardo and Rosset, 1977; Wittmann *et al.*, 1973). Penicillin-resistant mutants can result from alterations of penicillin-binding proteins (Spratt, 1978; Suzuki *et al.*, 1978) by increased synthesis of a chromosomally determined beta-lactamase, which is normally produced at low levels (Eriksson-Grennberg *et al.*, 1965) or by changes in the cell envelope (Nordstrom *et al.*, 1970).

Mutants that are resistant either to nalidixic acid or to novobiocin can result from alterations in components of DNA gyrase activity (Gellert *et al.*, 1977; Higgins *et al.*, 1978). Resistance to nalidixic acid can also be caused by altered drug permeability (Bourguignon *et al.*, 1973). Finally, resistance to sulfonamide can develop from decreased binding by dihydropteroate synthase (Ortiz, 1970), and resistance to trimethoprim can result from mutation to auxotrophy for thymine, thus sparing this important end-product of folic acid activity (Stacey and Simson, 1965).

Considering the variety of mechanisms that cause mutational resistance of bacteria to antibiotics, it is perhaps surprising that the genetic mechanism is not more common in clinical isolates. Mutational resistance is clinically important for nalidixic acid (Ronald *et al.*, 1966), streptomycin (Finland, 1955), rifampin (Eickhoff, 1971), and trimethoprim (Maskell *et al.*, 1976) and may be responsible for broadly aminoglycoside-resistant clinical isolates (Bryan *et al.*, 1976), but for most drugs plasmids provide the major source of resistance to antibiotics.

PLASMIDS

Plasmids are extrachromosomal genetic elements composed of circular double-stranded DNA. They vary from a molecular weight of approximately 1 million to over 300 million (Hansen and Olsen, 1978). Hence, they range from one-thousandth to one-tenth the size of the bacterial chromosome and can accommodate from a few to perhaps 500 genes.

Essential genes are concerned with plasmid replication and the partitioning of plasmid DNA to daughter cells at the time of bacterial division. Also in this category are genes that determine the number of plasmid copies per cell chromosome and the plasmid incompatibility behavior. In addition to these requirements, plasmids may carry other genes.

Many plasmids are infectious or conjugative and possess the genetic machinery for assuring their transmission on contact among bacterial cells by conjugation, a complex process that, for one well-studied plasmid, requires at least 17 genes (Miki *et al.*, 1978). Plasmids with a molecular weight less than approximately 20 million lack room for this equipment and are generally transfer-deficient (Tra^-) although some Tra^- plasmids can be transferred ("mobilized") by another conjugative plasmid that is present in the same cell (Clowes, 1972).

A third category of plasmid genes is involved with interactions with other replicons and includes genes that inhibit the propagation of certain bacteriophages or the transfer functions of other plasmids.

Finally, plasmids carry genes that effect the host cell's interaction with the environment. Antibiotic resistance genes are the most familiar, but as shown in Table 2 this category also includes genes determining resistance to metallic compounds (Summers and Silver, 1978) including arsenicals used as feed additives, genes for resistance to physical and chemical agents that damage DNA (Lehrbach *et al.*, 1977), genes for specialized metabolic pathways such as sugar fermentation (Smith *et al.*, 1978) or other catabolic functions (Wheelis, 1975), genes determining bacteriocin production and resistance, and genes involved in pathogenicity such as toxin production or colonization by adherence to mammalian cells.

Plasmids can be detected by physical or genetic techniques. Traditionally, plasmid DNA has most often been isolated by centrifuging a cell lysate in a cesium chloride density gradient

TABLE 2

Plasmid-Determined Properties Other Than Antibiotic Resistance [a]

Property	Plasmid carrier: Gram-negative bacteria	Plasmid carrier: Gram-positive bacteria
Resistance to metallic compounds		
Antimony		+
Arsenic	+	+
Bismuth		+
Boron	+	
Cadmium		+
Chromium	+	+
Cobalt	+	
Lead		+
Mercury	+	+
Nickel	+	
Silver	+	
Tellurium	+	
Zinc		+
Resistance to agents that damage DNA		
Alkylating agents	+	
γ-Irradiation	+	
Ultraviolet irradiation	+	
Metabolic functions		
Catabolism of camphor, naphthalene, nicotine, octane, salicylate, or toluene	+	
Citrate utilization	+	
Fermentation of lactose, raffinose, or sucrose	+	+
Hemolysin production	+	+
Hydrogen sulfide production	+	
Nuclease production	+	
Protease production		+
Urease production		+
Bacteriocin production and resistance	+	+

TABLE 2 CONTINUED

Property	Plasmid carrier Gram-negative bacteria	Gram-positive bacteria
Toxin production		
Enterotoxin	+	+
Exfoliative toxin		+
Other factors affecting virulence		
Colonization factors K88, K99, and others	+	
Colicin V	+	
Vir plasmid	+	

[a] From Jacoby and Swartz, in press, with permission.

containing an intercalating dye such as ethidium bromide that binds differentially to plasmid and chromosomal DNA to allow their separation (Helinski and Clewell, 1971). Recently, agarose gel electrophoresis has been adapted to allow simpler and more rapid visualization of extrachromosomal DNA (Meyers *et al.*, 1976). The presence of many plasmids can be demonstrated physically and their molecular weights identified within a day by modifications of this technique (Eckhardt, 1978). Conjugative plasmids can be detected by testing for transfer of the property they determine to a suitable recipient by mating. Transmission of nonconjugative plasmids can be accomplished by transduction with bacteriophage, transformation with purified plasmid DNA, or mobilization with another plasmid. Finally, certain agents, "curing" compounds, or physical techniques promote the loss of plasmids or select against plasmid-containing cells. Consequently, they can be used to provide presumptive evidence for the presence of a plasmid-determined characteristic.

Further physical and genetic characterization of plasmids is generally necessary to identify and assess the spread of plasmids in epidemiological investigations. Basic physical characteristics are plasmid size, DNA composition as expressed by percent guanine plus cytosine, and the fragmentation pattern produced by restriction endonucleases, which are enzymes that recognize specific DNA sequences as cleavage sites (Roberts, 1976). After endonuclease treatment, the fragments that are produced are separated by agarose gel electrophoresis to produce a characteristic pattern for a particular plasmid that is usually, but not always, independent of the host (Causey and Brown, 1978).

Incompatibility behavior is often used to classify plasmids further. Compatible plasmids can coexist in the same host cell while incompatible plasmids cannot and tend to displace each other. By this test plasmids found in enterobacteria can be divided into more than 30 groups (Chabbert *et al.*, 1972; Datta, 1975; Grindley *et al.*, 1973; Jacob *et al.*, 1977; see Table 3). Similar incompatibility schemes allow *Pseudomonas* plasmids to be classified into 11 or more groups (Jacoby and Matthew, 1979) and *Staphylococcus* plasmids to be assigned to at least seven groups (Novick *et al.*, 1977).

Although only a few genes are involved in incompatibility specificity (Palchaudhuri and Maas, 1977), plasmids belonging to the same incompatibility (Inc) group usually share much greater DNA homology than do plasmids of different Inc groups, thereby reflecting other similarities in gene function (Falkow *et al.*,

TABLE 3

Incompatibility Groups for Enteric Plasmids [a]

Incompatibility group designation	Synonyms [b]	Donor-specific phage susceptibility	Examples [c]
A			RA4
B	IncO, Com10		R16, ColIa-K9
C	IncA-C, Com6		R57b, P*lac*
D		fd	R711b
FI		fd, MS2, others	F, R386, ColV, Ent
FII		fd, MS2, others	R1, ColB2, Ent
FIII		fd, others	ColB-K98, MIP240 (Hly), Vir
FIV		fd, MS2, others	R124
FV		fd	F_o*lac*
FVI		MS2	Hly-P212
G		MS2	Rms149
H1			R27
H2	IncS		TP116, pWR23
H3			MIP233
I1	IncIα, Iβ, Com1	If1	R64, ColIb-P9
I2		If1	TP114, MIP241 (Hly)
I3	Incγ	If1	R621a, ColIb-IM1420
I4	IncIδ	If1	R721
J			R391
K			R387

ABLE 3 CONTINUED

ncompatibility roup	Synonyms	Donor-specific phage susceptibility	Examples
L			R946b
M	IncL, Com7		RIP69
N	Com2	Ike, PRD1	R46
P	Com4	PRR1, PRD1, Ike, others	RP1
Q			R300B
T		PilE/R1	Rts1
V			R753
W		PRD1	R388
X			R6K
Y			Phage P1
9	Com9		RIP71

---

[a]From Jacoby and Swartz, in press, with permission. Based on the compilation of Jacob *et al.* (1977), R. W. Hedges (Royal Postgraduate Medical School, London, personal communication, 1979), and other sources.

[b]Abbreviations: Inc, incompatibility; Com, compatibility.

[c]Abbreviations: Col, colicinogenic plasmid; Ent, enterotoxigenic plasmid; F, fertility plasmid; Hly, hemolysin-producing plasmid; R, resistance plasmid; Vir, the Vir plasmid. Some of the plasmids listed are metabolic plasmids carrying genes for sugar utilization, e.g., *Plac*, F_0*lac*, pWR23, and MIP233.

1974; Grindley et al., 1973). Plasmids that are transmissible to E. coli have also been broadly divided into those that inhibit the fertility factor (Fi^+) and those that do not (Fi^-) (Meynell et al., 1968). Bacteriophage interactions can also be used for plasmid classification. Certain phages, termed donor-specific or male phages (see Table 3), adsorb specifically to surface structures, such as thread-like pili, which are part of the conjugation apparatus for transfer-positive (Tra^+) plasmids. Other plasmids characteristically interfere with the propagation of certain phages so that both phage susceptibility and resistance can be used for plasmid classification.

PLASMID TRANSFER

In the laboratory Tra^+ plasmids vary in their transfer frequencies from barely detectable values of 10^{-7} to 10^{-8} to virtually 100% efficiency. Typical average values are 10^{-3} to 10^{-5} per donor. The transfer mechanism of some plasmids is naturally repressed, but is relieved from repression when the plasmid enters a new host (Meynell et al., 1968). Other plasmids transfer much more efficiently on solid rather than in liquid media. For some plasmids transfer is sensitive to temperature, occurring much more readily at 22°C than at 37°C (Rodriguez-Lemoine et al., 1975). Such plasmids have been responsible for outbreaks of resistant typhoid fever but could have been overlooked had mating experiments been performed at the conventional temperature (Smith et al, 1978).

In-vivo transfer of plasmids appears to be even less efficient than under laboratory conditions, although it has been observed in the gut of both humans and laboratory animals (Smith, 1969, 1970). A number of factors have been incriminated. Anderson (1974) found that strains containing R plasmids survive less well in the human intestine than do their R^- counterparts. The anaerobic environment also reduces the fertility of some plasmids (Burman, 1977) as does the presence of bile salts (Wiedemann, 1972) and the metabolic activity of other gut bacteria, especially Bacteroides (Anderson, 1975). Finally, smooth colony types are less efficient as plasmid recipients than are the rough variants used for laboratory experiments (Jarolmen and Kemp, 1969). After a volunteer drank a suspension containing 10^9 donor organisms, Smith (1969) found that few ingested R^+ Escherichia coli strains were able to colonize the intestine, that transfer to other E. coli occurred rarely, and that these strains persisted for only a few days. In similar studies with even larger inocula, Anderson et al. (1973a,b) were unable to detect transfer of R plasmids unless specific antibiotics were also administered, but under these conditions they found that plasmid transfer occurred at high frequency and that R^+ organisms could persist for several months. Similar results were obtained by Burton *et al.* (1974) who could only detect transfer of a plasmid determining resistance to tetracycline (among other antibiotics) when 1 g of tetracycline was given daily for 9 days. However, high-level shedding of resistant bacteria persisted from 2 to 43 days in the absence of continued administration of tetracycline. Since plasmid-containing strains, like those sensitive to antibiotics, have variable but finite persistence in the gut flora, continuous administration of antibiotics is more likely to promote plasmid carriage than would intermittent use (Linton *et al.*, 1975).

PLASMID HOST RANGE

An important biological limitation to transfer is plasmid host range, which correlates with plasmid Inc specificity. Transfer of intact plasmids between Gram-positive and Gram-negative bacteria has not been accomplished (Mahler and Halvorson, 1977), and transmission of plasmids between facultative and strict Gram-negative anaerobes has proven difficult to demonstrate (Burt and Woods, 1976; Del Bene *et al.*, 1976). Many plasmids transfer efficiently to closely related bacteria, for example, among *E. coli*, *Salmonella*, and *Shigella* (Datta and Hedges, 1972). Some, such as certain plasmids found in *P. aeruginosa*, transfer only to other *Pseudomonas* species (Shahrabadi *et al.*, 1975). Hence, it is important to use a related organism as a recipient when testing for transmission of a potentially plasmid-determined characteristic.

Other plasmids are much more promiscuous. Members of the IncP group have been transferred to virtually every Gram-negative host tested as recipient. Not surprisingly, P-type plasmids have been found in a variety of natural hosts. Other plasmid Inc groups tend to be associated more often with particular bacterial species, but the number of plasmids examined for host specificity is still small. The question of whether R plasmids of human and animal origin differ has been examined by Anderson *et al.* (1975). They found a high degree of DNA homology between plasmids of the same Inc group independent of their origin, suggesting a common pool of R factors in humans and animals.

PLASMID DISTRIBUTION

Plasmids have been found in practically all bacteria that have been carefully investigated. Not all are R plasmids. Indeed, some have no established function and are termed cryptic plasmids.

Table 4 lists the antibiotic resistances that have been found on plasmids in particular pathogenic organisms. Gram-negative pathogens have been studied most intensively. R plasmids have been observed in Enterobacteriaceae including *Enterobacter*, *Escherichia*, *Klebsiella*, *Proteus*, *Providencia*, *Salmonella*, *Serratia*, and *Shigella* and in other Gram-negative pathogens including *Acinetobacter*, *Bordetella*, *Haemophilus*, *Neisseria gonorrhoeae*, *Pasteurella*, *Pseudomonas*, *Vibrio*, and *Yersinia*. Among the Gram-positive pathogens, plasmids determining resistance are well known in *Staphylococcus aureus* and *S. epidermidis* and have also been found in streptococci of groups A, B, and D. Some streptococcal plasmids are even conjugative (Jacob and Hobbs, 1974). Plasmids have been found in *S. pneumoniae* as well (Young and Mayer, 1979) but have not yet been associated with antibiotic resistance. Recently, R plasmids have also been found in anaerobes including *Clostridium perfringens* (Brefort *et al.*, 1977) and *Bacteroides fragilis* (Mancini and Behme, 1977; Privitera *et al.*, 1979; Tally *et al.*, 1979). Evidently, plasmids provide a general mechanism for carrying a potentially advantageous but dispensable function in some members of a population in a form that can be spread to other bacteria under selective conditions (Clowes, 1972).

PLASMID PREVALENCE

Studies of primitive societies little exposed to antibiotics and of bacterial isolates from the preantibiotic era indicate that R plasmids preexisted contemporary antibiotic usage. Maré (1968) found resistant Gram-negative bacteria in 10% of over 500 fecal specimens from African bushmen and wild animals, but none of the bacteria could transfer their resistance patterns. In contrast, Gardner *et al.* (1969) reported the existence of R factors in 2 of 40 stool specimens from humans in a remote section of the Solomon Islands, and Davis and Anandan (1970) found six R^+ strains of *E. coli* in 4 of 128 stool specimens from natives living in North Borneo. These low frequencies provide a reasonable estimate of plasmid prevalence in the absence of obvious antibiotic selection.

TABLE 4

Detection of Plasmid-Determined Antibiotic Resistance in Pathogens[a]

Organism	Antibiotic[b] Beta-lactam	Cm	Gm	Km	MLS	Sm	Su	Tc	Tm	Tp
Gram-negative										
Enterobacteriaceae	+	+	+	+		+	+	+	+	+
Haemophilus influenzae	+	+		+				+		
Neisseria gonorrhoeae	+									
Pseudomonas aeruginosa	+	+	+	+		+	+	+	+	
Gram-positive										
Staphylococcus aureus	+	+	+	+	+	+		+	+	
Staphylococcus epidermidis	+	+		+				+	+	
Streptococcus										
Group A					+					
Group B		+			+			+		
Group D		+		+	+	+		+		
Anaerobes										
Clostridium perfringens		+			+			+		
Bacteroides fragilis	+	+			+			+		

[a] From Jacoby and Swartz, in press, with permission.

[b] Abbreviations: Beta-lactam, penicillin and cephalosporin; Cm, chloramphenicol; Gm, gentamicin; Km, kanamycin; MLS, macrolide (erythromycin), lincomycin, and streptogramin B-type antibiotics; Sm, streptomycin; Su, sulfonamide; Tc, tetracycline; Tm, tobramycin; Tp, trimethoprim.

The incidence of R factors in intestinal bacteria of healthy people in industrial societies is much higher. For example, Linton *et al.* (1972) reported that 53% of 193 healthy adults and children in Bristol, England, who had not received antibiotics or had not been recently hospitalized, carried antibiotic-resistant coliform bacteria in their feces. Transmissible R plasmids could be demonstrated in 61% of the resistant strains.

Antibiotic usage exerts a strong selective pressure favoring R plasmid carriage. Smith (1971) found sensitive *E. coli* in the fecal flora of 59% of pigs, 73% of chickens, and 90% of calves that had not been fed antibiotics, but in less than 2% of pigs and chickens that had been fed tetracycline. Datta *et al.* (1971) reported that 30% of the women admitted to hospitals in England excreted resistant *E. coli* but that 18 of 18 given tetracycline had resistant *E. coli* in their stools and that 66% of these strains contained transmissible R plasmids. Many studies have shown a higher frequency of antibiotic-resistant bacteria among hospitalized patients than among people outside the hospital. There is a higher incidence of antibiotic resistance in coliforms from hospital sewers than from domestic sewers, and multiple resistance is more common (Linton *et al.*, 1974).

The incidence of plasmids in hospital isolates is very high. For example, using agarose gel electrophoresis Laufs and Kleimann (1978) found plasmid DNA in 76% of *E. coli*, 31% of *Proteus*, 95% of *Klebsiella pneumoniae*, 24% of *Pseudomonas aeruginosa*, 40% of *Staphylococcus aureus*, and 36% of group D streptococci from clinical sources. Multiple plasmids were often present, and 45% of the plasmid-containing enteric strains could transfer antibiotic resistance to an *E. coli* recipient. In some cases, the presence of multiple plasmids leads to higher levels of antibiotic resistance than is observed with a single plasmid (Pinney and Smith, 1974).

In some pathogenic strains multiple resistance is becoming more common. In Japan, where plasmid-determined resistance to chloramphenicol, streptomycin, sulfonamide, and tetracycline appeared in *Shigella* during the 1950's, this pattern of quadruple resistance has remained by far the most common (Tanaka *et al.*, 1975). In Great Britain, on the other hand, plasmid-determined resistance to streptomycin and sulfonamide appeared in *Salmonella typhimurium* in 1963. As antibiotic usage, especially in animal feed, increased, resistance to tetracycline, ampicillin, and kanamycin as well as to streptomycin and sulfonamide became the predominant pattern (Anderson, 1968). In this case the strains acquired additional plasmids. In the last decade, the introduction of newer aminoglycosides has been followed by the appearance and spread of plasmid-determined resistance to amikacin, gentamicin, and tobramycin. In some cases, multiple resistance seems to be acquired as new resistance genes are incorporated into existing plasmids (Smith *et al.*, 1975).

PLASMID-DETERMINED ANTIBIOTIC RESISTANCE

Plasmids determine antibiotic resistance by the same general biochemical strategies discussed previously, but the mechanisms are usually different from those produced by chromosomal mutations. Some specific plasmid-determined mechanisms of resistance, which are listed in Table 5, have been reviewed by Davies and Smith (1978). Penicillins and cephalosporins are hydrolyzed by beta-lactamases, of which 11 types produced by plasmids of Gram-negative bacteria can be differentiated (Matthew, 1979). Chloramphenicol is also detoxified, but by acetylation. The aminoglycosides are attacked by a variety of enzymes that attach acetyl, nucleotidyl (adenylyl), or phosphate groups to key hydroxyl or amino moieties on the antibiotic. Modification of aminoglycoside occurs at a faster rate than the uptake of aminoglycoside so that no active drug is available to block protein synthesis. Tetracycline resistance is not due to drug degradation or modification but rather to a combination of diminished tetracycline uptake and an intracellular inhibition of tetracycline activity (Levy and McMurry, 1978).

Plasmid effects on antibiotic uptake have also been suggested for chloramphenicol, kanamycin, and penicillin. Plasmid-determined resistance to the MLS group of drugs (macrolide, lincosamide, and streptogramin B-type antibiotics) involves methylation of adenine residues in 23S RNA of the larger ribosomal subunit so that binding of these drugs to their target is prevented. Resistance to three drugs used in animal feed, oleandomycin, tylosin, and virginiamycin, develops in this way. Finally, resistance to sulfonamides and trimethoprim involves plasmid-determined folic acid biosynthetic enzymes that bypass the metabolic block produced by these chemotherapeutic agents. It is noteworthy that whenever antibiotic degradation is not involved, the drug can remain to exert a continued selective pressure for resistant organisms.

For a few antibiotics plasmid-determined resistance has not yet been found. Specifically, this mechanism of resistance is not known to occur for bacitracin, bambermycin, colistin, monensin, nalidixic

TABLE 5

Mechanisms of Plasmid-Determined Antibiotic Resistance[a]

Drug	Mechanism of resistance
Aminoglycosides[b]	
Amikacin	6'-N-Acetyltransferase
Gentamicin	3-N- and 6'-N-Acetyltransferases 2"-O-Adenylyltransferase
Kanamycin	6'-N-Acetyltransferase 4'-O-Adenylyltransferase 3'-O-Phosphotransferase
Streptomycin	3"-O-Adenylyltransferase 3"-O-Phosphotransferase
Spectinomycin	3"-O-Adenylyltransferase
Tobramycin	3-N- and 6'-N-Acetyltransferase 2"-O-Adenylyltransferase
Beta-lactams	
Penicillins	Various beta-lactamases (TEM-1, TEM-2, OXA-1, OXA-2, OXA-3, PSE-1, PSE-2, PSE-3, PSE-4, HMS-1, SHV-1)
Chloramphenicol	3-O-Acetyltransferase
Erythromycin	Methylation of 23S RNA
Lincomycin	Methylation of 23S RNA
Sulfonamide	Substitute dihydropteroate synthase
Tetracycline	Diminished uptake Inhibition of intracellular action
Trimethoprim	Substitute dihydrofolate reductase

[a]From Jacoby and Swartz, in press, with permission.

[b]Additional modifying enzymes for aminoglycosides found in Gram-positive bacteria are reviewed by Davies and Smith (1978).

acid, nitrofuran, novobiocin, polymyxin, rifampin, or vancomycin, although resistance to each of these agents can occur intrinsically or by chromosomal mutation.

PLASMID STRUCTURE AND REARRANGEMENTS

For some plasmid systems the resistance and transfer genes occur on separate molecules, each of which is capable of independent replication. Transfer of such an aggregate or multimolecular plasmid is achieved by mobilization of the Tra^- R-plasmid by its Tra^+ partner. In other plasmids the resistance genes and transfer functions are combined in a single molecule which may or may not be able to dissociate into separate replicons (Clowes, 1972). In a cointegrate plasmid the resistance genes are often clustered together on the R-determinant segment of the plasmid, while the genes for transfer and other basic plasmid functions are clustered on the resistance transfer factor (RTF) segment. These two segments may be linked by specific repeated segments of DNA known as insertion sequences since the insertion of such a DNA segment into a structural gene results in its inactivation.

Interactions between paired insertion sequences allow plasmids with this structure to dissociate into two component replicons. The resistance genes may also transpose to another replicon as a unit or duplicate to higher degrees of multiplicity in the presence of an antibiotic to amplify the level of resistance (Ptashne and Cohen, 1975; Rownd *et al.*, 1975; Yagi and Clewell, 1976). Individual resistance genes or groups of genes may also be located between repeated segments of DNA, which allow them to be transposed to another replicon such as another plasmid, a phage genome, or the bacterial chromosome. Such a transposable genetic element has been termed a transposon (Hedges and Jacob, 1974).

Transposons, some of which are listed in Table 6, comprise virtually all types of plasmid-determined antibiotic resistance, including resistance to beta-lactam antibiotics, chloramphenicol, erythromycin, gentamicin, kanamycin, streptomycin, sulfonamide, tetracycline, and trimethoprim. Plasmids must thus be thought of as assemblages of potentially transposable resistance genes. Transposition is not a common event. It generally occurs at frequencies of 10^{-3} or less, even under the most favorable conditions (Kleckner, 1977). However, where the selection pressure is high, the results of transposition events can be dramatic. Multiresistant R plasmids have evolved in this way (Rubens *et al.*, 1979). Furthermore, a resistance gene that becomes prevalent in one group

TABLE 6

Selected Drug-Resistance Transposons[a]

Transposon	Drug resistance	Molecular weight (x 10^6)
Tn1	Ampicillin	3.2
Tn4	Ampicillin, streptomycin, sulfonamide	13.6
Tn5	Kanamycin	3.5
Tn7	Streptomycin, trimethoprim	8.5
Tn9	Chloramphenicol	1.7
Tn10	Tetracycline	6.2
Tn551	Erythromycin, lincomycin	3.5
Tn1696	Chloramphenicol, gentamicin, streptomycin, sulfonamide	9.1

[a] From Jacoby and Swartz, in press, with permission.

of organisms, such as the transposon responsible for ampicillin resistance in enteric bacteria (Matthew and Hedges, 1976), seems to have crossed genetic boundaries to appear in unrelated pathogens and to have caused resistance to penicillin in gonococci (Elwell *et al*., 1977) and to ampicillin in *Haemophilus influenzae* (Elwell *et al*., 1975) by inserting into plasmids that are indigenous to these organisms.

Thus, when one takes into account all the known modes of alteration and transfer of genes in bacteria, it is clear that there is a broad spectrum of factors that can influence the activities and spread of genetic determinants leading to antibiotic resistance. These factors are:

Mutation: creation or loss of enzymatic activity by changes in DNA base sequence (see Table 1)

Derepression: increase in production of enzyme causing resistance in response to an external stimulus (Franklin, 1967)

Amplification: tandem multiplication of R-determinants per plasmid or increased number of plasmid copies per cell (Uhlin and Nordström, 1977)

Multiple plasmids: total level of antibiotic resistance sometimes higher than that due to individual plasmids

Genetic rearrangements:

> *Transposition*: insertion of R-determinants from one region of DNA into a new location
>
> *Fusion*: recombination between two plasmids to produce a composite plasmid
>
> *Disassociation*: separation of a plasmid into its component replicons
>
> *Microevolution*: small deletions, insertions, or duplications (Timmis *et al*., 1978)

Gene transfer (reviewed by Low and Porter, 1978):

> *Conjugation*: transfer through cell-to-cell connection of either plasmid or chromosomal DNA

Hormone-stimulated conjugation: intercellular signalling leading to cell aggregation and high frequency transfer (Dunny *et al.* 1979)

Transduction: infection by viral particles that carry drug resistance gene(s) from previous host cell

Transformation: uptake of naked DNA from surrounding medium

Loss of function:

Genetic deletion

Insertional inactivation

Plasmid loss or curing

PLASMIDS AND VIRULENCE

Other genes of importance for bacterial infection are also carried on plasmids. Production of enterotoxin in both *Staphylococcus aureus* (Shalita *et al.*, 1977) and *E. coli* (Smith and Linggood, 1971b) may be determined by plasmids. Two types of *E. coli* enterotoxin are produced: a small, heat-stable polypeptide and a larger, heat-labile protein toxin that has a structure and mechanism of action similar to that of cholera toxin (Dallas and Falkow, 1979). The production of toxin alone is not sufficient for *E. coli* to cause disease in animals. Enteropathogenic strains also carry a plasmid that codes for a surface antigen that facilitates adherence to the gut wall (Smith and Linggood, 1971a). Species-specific antigens have been described for pig strains (the K88 antigen), calf and lamb strains (the K99 antigen), and strains of human origin (Evans *et al.*, 1975; McNeish *et al.*, 1975). Commonly, enterotoxin-producing *E. coli* also carry R plasmids, and transfer of resistance often results in concurrent transfer of enterotoxin production (Echeverria *et al.*, 1978). Genes for antibiotic resistance and enterotoxin production can even be linked on the same plasmid (Gyles *et al.*, 1977), and there is evidence that the genes for toxin production are transposable (So *et al.*, 1979).

Whether plasmid carriage has other effects on virulence has long been debated. Watanabe (1971) initially found smooth R^+ strains of *Salmonella typhimurium* less virulent for mice than their R^- parents, but he was unable to repeat the observation.

Smith (1972) found that a few R plasmids caused a marked reduction in virulence of *S. typhimurium* for chicks, but that most had only a slight or no effect. The high prevalence of plasmids in hospital isolates of a variety of pathogenic bacteria suggests that most R^+ strains are fully virulent. In particular, Brumfitt *et al.* (1971) found that the incidence of resistant fecal *E. coli* was the same in women with or without urinary tract infection, that those women with resistant organisms in the urine carried the same organism in the stool, and that R plasmid carriage neither hindered nor facilitated infection of the urinary tract by intestinal *E. coli*.

E. coli that cause extraintestinal infections in humans are not likely to be toxigenic or invasive (Wachsmuth *et al.*, 1975). Whether they have other virulence properties is a subject of active current investigation. Smith (1974) found that an *E. coli* strain causing bacteremia in a lamb carried a virulence plasmid (Vir) that determined an exotoxin, which was lethal to other animals when intravenously injected. Only one of 190 *E. coli* isolates had the same property and it also came from a lamb with bacteremia.

In the same study, Smith (1974) also found an *E. coli* strain isolated from an outbreak of bacteremia in chickens that could transfer increased animal lethality to other *E. coli*. Increased survival in blood and peritoneal fluids rather than toxin production was associated with this virulence factor, which proved to be identical with the Col V plasmid (Smith and Huggins, 1976). The prevalence of Col V is high in invasive *E. coli* strains from animals and humans. The production of colicin per se is not essential for enhanced virulence (Quackenbush and Falkow, 1979). Rather, increased virulence correlates with serum resistance and, hence, with decreased sensitivity to host defense mechansims that depend on antibody and complement (Binns *et al.*, 1979). Col V plasmids can carry antibiotic resistance genes. Therefore, as in the case of enterotoxin production, factors that increase the prevalence of R plasmids can also increase the prevalence of virulence factors.

ATTACK ON R FACTOR REPLICATION OR TRANSFER

A wide variety of physical and chemical agents, including some antibiotics and at least one drug used in animal feed, bambermycin, can block plasmid transfer or enhance loss *in vitro* (Brinton, 1971). Conjugation, which is probably the predominant mode of plasmid transfer in nature, requires several conditions. The formation of sex pili, which is essential for mating pair formation, requires a certain temperature range. For the well studied F factor, this range is approximately 30° C to 43° C. The recipient cell surface must also contain certain components such as outer membrane proteins, the lack of which results in conjugative deficiency (Skurray *et al.*, 1974). In the laboratory, plasmid transfer can be blocked by the addition of a small amount of sodium dodecylsulfate (Yokota and Akiba, 1961), which presumably disrupts either the recipient or donor cell surface. Rifampin (Mándi and Béládi, 1974), levallorphan (Löser *et al.*, 1971), phenylethyl alcohol (Brinton, 1971), donor-specific phages, or the concomitant presence of an Fi^+ plasmid prevent formation or function of sex pili as do mutations in the plasmid genes that confer transmissibility (*tra* genes). Nalidixic acid also blocks DNA transfer during conjugation (Hane, 1971), presumably by its action on DNA gyrase.

In many studies these agents have been tested against only a limited number of plasmids. Consequently, whether their effects apply to all plasmids is not known. Their effectiveness in blocking transfer *in vivo* has not been studied. It is possible that mutants resistant to their action could develop. Further studies are needed to determine the potential value of this approach.

APPLICATIONS AND FUTURE PROSPECTS

The variety of mechanisms that bacteria have evolved to deal with antibiotics is impressive, and there is no assurance that new ones will not appear. Plasmids provide microorganisms with a remarkably versatile system for packaging resistance genes, toxin determinants, and other virulence factors in a form that can be both transmitted from cell to cell and transposed from plasmid to plasmid. While there appears to be a natural barrier to the transfer of plasmids between Gram-negative and Gram-positive organisms, there is considerable potential for the flow of genetic information within each group. Antibiotic usage leads to antibiotic-resistant organisms in both animals and humans. Studies not reviewed here leave little doubt that resistant organisms from animals are, on occasion, a cause of human disease. Even if certain organisms lack the ability to infect both humans and animals, resistance plasmids that can be carried by bacteria from animals or humans share no such specificity. Hence, antibiotic resistance arising in animals from subtherapeutic antibiotic usage is undoubtedly a potential cause of resistance of bacteria to antimicrobials used to treat infections in humans.

The relative importance of an animal reservoir of resistant pathogens is, however, not known. One could assume that selection of resistant bacteria should be proportional to antibiotic usage for animals or humans. Therefore, since approximately 36% of U.S. antibiotic production in 1974 was devoted to animal feeds or other nonmedicinal uses (Food and Drug Administration, 1978), one might assume that a similar percentage of the total selection pressure for resistant bacteria arose from the use of antibiotics in animal feeds.

In one attempt to study the issue directly, Richmond and Linton (1980) conducted a survey of tetracycline usage in the Avon area near Bristol, England. They found that most tetracycline was prescribed by general practitioners in their offices rather than by physicians in hospitals. From earlier studies of the effect of the antibiotic on fecal flora, they calculated that 0.75% of Avon's population would be expected to excrete tetracycline-resistant organisms because of tetracycline therapy. "On the basis of the data reported here," they concluded, "there hardly seems a need to postulate a veterinary source for the resistant coliforms encountered in the human population." However, the observed frequency of tetracycline-resistant coliforms in Bristol sewage in 1974 was 3% (Linton *et al.*, 1974). It can be argued that the use of other antibiotics to treat humans and the linkage of other antibiotic resistance genes to tetracycline resistance on plasmids account for the discrepancy between 0.75% and 3% or, alternatively, that only 25% of the observed tetracycline resistance can be attributed to the use of antibiotics in humans. Further surveys of this sort are needed.

Inasmuch as some antibiotics suited for use in animal feed do not select for transmissible resistance to drugs used in humans, studies sould be conducted to document the potential economic and therapeutic benefits of their subtherapeutic use.

More extensive epidemiological studies of nosocomial infection caused by plasmids in bacteria are also desirable. Many investigators have documented the prevalence of antibiotic resistance in hospital pathogens. Combining detailed classification of resistant organisms and molecular and genetic characterization of the plasmids they contain should help elucidate the relative roles of cross-infection by resistant organisms as opposed to spread of resistance by particular plasmids. The epidemiology of plasmids in resistant Gram-positive pathogens has been particularly neglected.

Finally, while the search continues for better antibiotics and combinations that are effective against plasmid-containing strains, attention should also be directed to a search for naturally occurring agents that might directly attack R factor replication or maintenance.

REFERENCES

Anderson, E. S. 1968. The ecology of transferable drug resistance in the enterobacteria. Annu. Rev. Microbiol. 22:131-180.

Anderson, E. S., G. O. Humphreys, and G. A. Willshaw. 1975. The molecular relatedness of R factors in enterobacteria of human and animal origin. J. Gen. Microbiol. 91:376-382.

Anderson, J. D. 1974. The effect of R-factor carriage on the survival of Escherichia coli in the human intestine. J. Med. Microbiol. 7:85-90.

Anderson, J. D. 1975. Factors that may prevent transfer of antibiotic resistance between gram-negative bacteria in the gut. J. Med. Microbiol. 8:83-88.

Anderson, J. D., W. A. Gillespie, and M. H. Richmond. 1973a. Chemotherapy and antibiotic-resistance transfer between enterobacteria in the human gastro-intestinal tract. J. Med. Microbiol. 6:461-473.

Anderson, J. D., L. C. Ingram, M. H. Richmond, and B. Wiedemann. 1973b. Studies on the nature of plasmids arising from conjugation in the human gastro-intestinal tract. J. Med. Microbiol. 6:475-486.

Apirion, D., and D. Schlessinger. 1968. Coresistance to neomycin and kanamycin by mutations in an Escherichia coli locus that affects ribosomes. J. Bacteriol. 96:768-776.

Benveniste, R., and J. Davis. 1973. Mechanisms of antibiotic resistance in bacteria. Annu. Rev. Biochem. 42:471-506.

Binns, M. M., D. L. Davies, and K. G. Hardy. 1979. Cloned fragments of the plasmid ColV,I-K94 specifying virulence and serum resistance. Nature 279:778-781.

Bourguignon, G. J., M. Levitt, and R. Sternglanz. 1973. Studies on the mechanism of action of nalidixic acid. Antimicrob. Agents Chemother. 4:479-486.

Brefort, G., M. Magot, H. Ionesco, and M. Sebald. 1977. Characterization and transferability of Clostridium perfringens plasmids. Plasmid 1:52-66.

Brinton, C. C., Jr. 1971. The properties of sex pili, the viral nature of "conjugal" genetic transfer systems, and some possible approaches to the control of bacterial drug resistance. Crit. Rev. Microbiol. 1:105-160.

Brumfitt, W., D. S. Reeves, M. C. Faiers, and N. Datta. 1971. Antibiotic-resistant *Escherichia coli* causing urinary-tract infection in general practice: Relation to faecal flora. Lancet 1:315-317.

Bryan, L. E., R. Haraphongse, and H. M. Van Den Elzen. 1976. Gentamicin resistance in clinical-isolates of *Pseudomonas aeruginosa* associated with diminished gentamicin accumulation and no detectable enzymatic modification. J. Antibiot. (Tokyo) 29:743-753.

Buckel, P., A. Buchberger, A. Böck, and H. G. Wittmann. 1977. Alteration of ribosomal protein L6 in mutants of *Escherichia coli* resistant to gentamicin. Mol. Gen. Genet. 158:47-54.

Burman, L. G. 1977. Expression of R-plasmid functions during anaerobic growth of an *Escherichia coli* K-12 host. J. Bacteriol. 131:69-75.

Burt, S. J., and D. R. Woods. 1976. R factor transfer to obligate anaerobes from *Escherichia coli*. J. Gen. Microbiol. 93:405-409.

Burton, G. C., D. C. Hirsh, D. C. Blenden, and J. L. Zeigler. 1974. The effects of tetracycline on the establishment of *Escherichia coli* of animal origin, and *in vivo* transfer of antibiotic resistance, in the intestinal tract of man. Pp. 241-253 in F. A. Skinner and J. G. Carr, eds. The Society for Applied Bacteriology Symposium Series No. 3. The Normal Microbial Flora of Man. Academic Press, London and New York.

Causey, S. C., and L. R. Brown. 1978. Transconjugant analysis: Limitations on the use of sequence-specific endonucleases for plasmid identification. J. Bacteriol. 135:1070-1079.

Chabbert, Y. A., M. R. Scavizzi, J. L. Witchitz, G. R. Gerbaud, and D. H. Bouanchaud. 1972. Incompatibility groups and the classification of *fi*⁻ resistance factors. J. Bacteriol. 112:666-675.

Clowes, R. C. 1972. Molecular structure of bacterial plasmids. Bacteriol. Rev. 36:361-405.

Dallas, W. S., and S. Falkow. 1979. The molecular nature of heat-labile enterotoxin (LT) of Escherichia coli. Nature 277: 406-407.

Datta, N. 1975. Epidemiology and classification of plasmids. Pp. 9-15 in D. Schlessinger, ed. Microbiology--1974. American Society for Microbiology, Washington, D.C.

Datta, N., and R. W. Hedges. 1972. Host ranges of R factors. J. Gen. Microbiol. 70:453-460.

Datta, N., W. Brumfitt, M. C. Faiers, F. Ørskov, D. S. Reeves, and I. Ørskov. 1971. R factors in Escherichia coli in faeces after oral chemotherapy in general practice. Lancet 1:312-315.

Davies, J., and D. I. Smith. 1978. Plasmid-determined resistance to antimicrobial agents. Annu. Rev. Microbiol. 32:469-518.

Davis, C. E., and J. Anandan. 1970. The evolution of R factor. A study of a "preantibiotic" community in Borneo. N. Engl. J. Med. 282:117-122.

Del Bene, V. E., M. Rogers, and W. E. Farrar, Jr. 1976. Attempted transfer of antibiotic resistance between Bacteroides and Escherichia coli. J. Gen. Microbiol. 92:384-390.

Dunny, G. M., R. A. Craig, R. L. Carron, and D. B. Clewell. 1979. Plasmid transfer in Streptococcus faecalis: Production of multiple sex pheromones by recipients. Plasmid 2:454-465.

Echeverria, P., C. V. Ulyangco, M. T. Ho, L. Verhaert, S. Komalarini, F. Ørskov, and I. Ørskov. 1978. Antimicrobial resistance and enterotoxin production among isolates of Escherichia coli in the Far East. Lancet 2:589-592.

Eckhardt, T. 1978. A rapid method for the identification of plasmid desoxyribonucleic acid in bacteria. Plasmid 1:584-588.

Eickhoff, T. C. 1971. In-vitro and in-vivo studies of resistance to rifampin in meningococci. J. Infect. Dis. 123:414-420.

Elwell, L. P., J. De Graaff, D. Seibert, and S. Falkow. 1975. Plasmid-linked ampicillin resistance in *Haemophilus influenzae* type *b*. Infect. Immun. 12:404-410.

Elwell, L. P., M. Roberts, L. W. Mayer, and S. Falkow. 1977. Plasmid-mediated beta-lactamase production in *Neisseria gonorrhoeae*. Antimicrob. Agents Chemother. 11:528-533.

Eriksson-Grennberg, K. G., H. G. Boman, J. A. Torbjörn Jansson, and S. Thorén. 1965. Resistance of *Escherichia coli* to penicillins. I. Genetic study of some ampicillin-resistant mutants. J. Bacteriol. 90:54-62.

Evans, D. G., R. P. Silver, D. J. Evans, Jr., D. G. Chase, and S. L. Gorbach. 1975. Plasmid-controlled colonization factor associated with virulence in *Escherichia coli* enterotoxigenic for humans. Infect. Immun. 12:656-667.

Falkow, S., P. Guerry, R. W. Hedges, and N. Datta. 1974. Polynucleotide sequence relationships among plasmids of the I compatibility complex. J. Gen. Microbiol. 85:65-76.

Finland, M. 1955. Emergence of antibiotic-resistant bacteria. N. Engl. J. Med. 253:909-922, 969-979, 1019-1028.

Food and Drug Administration. 1978. Draft Environmental Impact Statement--Subtherapeutic Antibacterial Agents in Animal Feeds. Bureau of Veterinary Medicine, Food and Drug Administration, Department of Health, Education, and Welfare, Rockville, Md. [371 + xviii] pp.

Franklin, T. J. 1967. Resistance of *Escherichia coli* to tetracyclines. Changes in permeability to tetracyclines in *Escherichia coli* bearing transferable resistance factors. G. B. Med. J. 105: 371-378.

Funatsu, G., and H. G. Wittmann. 1972. Ribosomal proteins. XXXIII. Location of amino-acid replacements in protein S12 isolated from *Escherichia coli* mutants resistant to streptomycin. J. Mol. Biol. 68:547-550.

Funatsu, G., K. Nierhaus, and B. Wittmann-Liebold. 1972. Ribosomal proteins. XXII. Studies on the altered protein S5 from a spectinomycin-resistant mutant of *Escherichia coli*. J. Mol. Biol. 64:201-209.

Gardner, P., D. H. Smith, H. Beer, and R. C. Moellering, Jr. 1969. Recovery of resistance (R) factors from a drug-free community. Lancet 2:774-776.

Gellert, M., K. Mizuuchi, M. H. O'Dea, T. Itoh, and J. I. Tomizawa. 1977. Nalidixic acid resistance: A second genetic character involved in DNA gyrase activity. Proc. Nat. Acad. Sci. (USA) 74:4772-4776.

Grindley, N. D. F., J. N. Grindley, and E. S. Anderson. 1972. R factor compatibility groups. Mol. Gen. Genet. 119:287-297.

Grindley, N. D. F., G. O. Humphreys, and E. S. Anderson. 1973. Molecular studies of R factor compatibility groups. J. Bacteriol. 115:387-398.

Gyles, C. L., S. Palchaudhuri, and W. K. Maas. 1977. Naturally occurring plasmid carrying genes for enterotoxin production and drug resistance. Science 198:198-199.

Hane, M. W. 1971. Some effects of nalidixic acid on conjugation in *Escherichia coli* K-12. J. Bacteriol. 105:46-56.

Hansen, J. B., and R. H. Olsen. 1978. Isolation of large bacterial plasmids and characterization of the P2 incompatibility group plasmids pMG1 and pMG5. J. Bacteriol. 135:227-238.

Hedges, R. W., and A. E. Jacob. 1974. Transposition of ampicillin resistance from RP4 to other replicons. Mol. Gen. Genet. 132: 31-40.

Helinski, D. R., and D. B. Clewell. 1971. Circular DNA. Annu. Rev. Biochem. 40:899-942.

Helser, T. L., J. E. Davies, and J. E. Dahlberg. 1972. Mechanism of kasugamycin resistance in *Escherichia coli*. Nature (London) New Biol. 235:6-9.

Higgins, N. P., C. L. Peebles, A. Sugino, and N. R. Cozzarelli. 1978. Purification of subunits of *Escherichia coli* DNA gyrase and reconstitution of enzymatic activity. Proc. Nat. Acad. Sci. (USA) 75:1773-1777.

Jacob, A. E., and S. J. Hobbs. 1974. Conjugal transfer of plasmid-borne multiple antibiotic resistance in *Streptococcus faecalis* var. *zymogenes*. J. Bacteriol. 117:360-372.

Jacob, A. E., J. A. Shapiro, L. Yamamoto, D. I. Smith, S. N. Cohen, and D. Berg. 1977. Table: Plasmids studied in Escherichia coli and other enteric bacteria. Pp. 607-638 in A. I. Bukhari, J. A. Shapiro, and S. L. Adhya, eds. DNA Insertion Elements, Plasmids, and Episomes. Cold Spring Harbor Laboratory, N.Y.

Jacoby, G. A., and M. Matthew. 1979. The distribution of β-lactamase genes on plasmids found in Pseudomonas. Plasmid 2:41-47.

Jacoby, G. A., and M. N. Swartz. In press. Plasmids: Microbiological and clinical importance in L. Weinstein and B. N. Fields, eds. Seminars in Infectious Diseases, Vol. III. Thieme-Stratton, Inc. N.Y.

Jarolmen, H., and G. Kemp. 1969. Association of increased recipient ability for R factors and reduced virulence among variants of Salmonella choleraesuis var. kunzendorf. J. Bacteriol. 97:962-963.

Kanner, B. I., and D. L. Cutnick. 1972. Use of neomycin in the isolation of mutants blocked in energy conservation in Escherichia coli. J. Bacteriol. 111:287-289.

Kleckner, N. 1977. Translocatable elements in procaryotes. Cell 11:11-23.

Laufs, R., and F. Kleimann. 1978. [In German; English summary.] Antibiotika-Resistenzfaktoren und andere Plasmide in Bakterienisolaten von hospitalisierten Patienten. Zentralbl. Bakteriol. Parasitenkd. Infektionskr. Hyg., I. Abt. Orig. Reihe A 240:503-516.

Lehrbach, P., A. H. C. Kung, B. T. O. Lee, and G. A. Jacoby. 1977. Plasmid modification of radiation and chemical-mutagen sensitivity in Pseudomonas aeruginosa. J. Gen. Microbiol. 98:167-176.

Levy, S. B., and L. McMurry. 1978. Probing the expression of plasmid-mediated tetracycline resistance in Escherichia coli. Pp. 177-180 in D. Schlessinger, ed. Microbiology--1978. American Society for Microbiology, Washington, D.C.

Linton, A. H., K. Howe, and A. D. Osborne. 1975. The effects of feeding tetracycline, nitrovin and quindoxin on the drug-resistance of Coli-aerogenes bacteria from calves and pigs. J. Appl. Bacteriol. 38:255-275.

Linton, K. B., P. A. Lee, M. H. Richmond, W. A. Gillespie, A. J. Rowland, and V. N. Baker. 1972. Antibiotic resistance and transmissible R-factors in the intestinal coliform flora of healthy adults and children in an urban and a rural community. J. Hyg., Camb. 70:99-104.

Linton, K. B., M. H. Richmond, R. Bevan, and W. A. Gillespie. 1974. Antibiotic resistance and R factors in coliform bacilli isolated from hospital and domestic sewage. J. Med. Microbiol. 7:91-103.

Löser, R., P. L. Boquet, R. Röschenthaler, and C. E. N. Saclay. 1971. Inhibition of R-factor transfer by levallorphan. Biochem. Biophys. Res. Commun. 45:204-211.

Low, K. B., and D. D. Porter. 1978. Modes of gene transfer and recombination in bacteria. Annu. Rev. Genet. 12:249-287.

Mahler, I., and H. O. Halvorson. 1977. Transformation of *Escherichia coli* and *Bacillus subtilis* with a hybrid plasmid molecule. J. Bacteriol. 131:374-377.

Mancini, C., and R. J. Behme. 1977. Transfer of multiple antibiotic resistance from *Bacteroides fragilis* to *Escherichia coli*. J. Infect. Dis. 136:597-600.

Mándi, Y., and I. Béládi. 1974. Effect of rifamycin and its derivatives on the transfer of R factor in *Escherichia coli*. Acta Microbiol. Acad. Sci. Hung. 21:385-389.

Maré, I. J. 1968. Incidence of R factors among gram negative bacteria in drug-free human and animal communities. Nature 220: 1046-1047.

Maskell, R., R. H. Payne, and O. A. Okubadejo. 1976. Thymine-requiring bacteria associated with co-trimoxazole therapy. Lancet 1:834-835.

Matthew, M. 1979. Plasmid-mediated β-lactamases of gram-negative bacteria: Properties and distribution. J. Antimicrob. Chemother. 5:349-358.

Matthew, M., and R. W. Hedges. 1976. Analytical isoelectric focusing of R factor-determined β-lactamases: Correlation with plasmid compatibility. J. Bacteriol. 125:713-718.

McNeish, A. S., J. Fleming, P. Turner, and N. Evans. 1975. Mucosal adherence of human enteropathogenic *Escherichia coli*. Lancet 2:946-948.

Meyers, J. A., D. Sanchez, L. P. Elwell, and S. Falkow. 1976. Simple agarose gel electrophoretic method for the identification and characterization of plasmid deoxyribonucleic acid. J. Bacteriol. 127:1529-1537.

Meynell, E., G. G. Meynell, and N. Datta. 1968. Phylogenetic relationships of drug-resistance factors and other transmissible bacterial plasmids. Bacteriol. Rev. 32:55-83.

Miki, T., T. Horiuchi, and N. S. Willetts. 1978. Identification and characterization of four new *tra* cistrons on the *E. coli* K12 sex factor F. Plasmid 1:316-323.

Nordström, K., L. G. Burman, and K. G. Eriksson-Grennberg. 1970. Resistance of *Escherichia coli* to penicillins. VIII. Physiology of a class II ampicillin-resistant mutant. J. Bacteriol. 101:659-668.

Novick, R. P., S. Cohen, L. Yamamoto, and J. A. Shapiro. 1977. Table: Plasmids of *Staphylococcus aureus*. Pp. 657-662 in A. I. Bukhari, J. A. Shapiro, and S. L. Adhya, eds. DNA Insertion Elements, Plasmids, and Episomes. Cold Spring Harbor Laboratory, N.Y.

Ortiz, P. J. 1970. Dihydrofolate and dihydropteroate synthesis by partially purified enzymes from wild-type and sulfonamide-resistant pneumococcus. Biochemistry 9:355-361.

Palchaudhuri, S., and W. K. Maas. 1977. Physical mapping of a DNA sequence common to plasmids of incompatibility group FI. Proc. Nat. Acad. Sci. (USA) 74:1190-1194.

Pardo, D., and R. Rosset. 1977. A new ribosomal mutation which affects the two ribosomal subunits in *Escherichia coli*. Mol. Gen. Genet. 153:199-204.

Pinney, R. J., and J. T. Smith. 1974. Antibiotic resistance levels of bacteria harbouring more than one R factor. Chemotherapy 20:296-302.

Privitera, G., A. Dublanchet, and M. Sebald. 1979. Transfer of multiple antibiotic resistance between subspecies of Bacteroides fragilis. J. Infect. Dis. 139:97-101.

Ptashne, K., and S. N. Cohen. 1975. Occurrence of insertion sequence (IS) regions on plasmid deoxyribonucleic acid as direct and inverted nucleotide sequence duplications. J. Bacteriol. 122:776-781.

Quackenbush, R. L., and S. Falkow. 1979. Relationship between colicin V activity and virulence in Escherichia coli. Infect. Immun. 24:562-564.

Richmond, M. H., and K. B. Linton. 1980. The use of tetracycline in the community and its possible relation to the excretion of tetracycline-resistant bacteria. J. Antimicrob. Chemother. 6: 33-41.

Roberts, R. J. 1976. Restriction endonucleases. CRC Crit. Rev. Biochem. 4:123-164.

Rodriguez-Lemoine, V., A. E. Jacob, R. W. Hedges, and N. Datta. 1975. Thermosensitive production of their transfer systems by group S plasmids. J. Gen. Microbiol. 86:111-114.

Ronald, A. R., M. Turck, and R. G. Petersdorf. 1966. A critical evaluation of nalidixic acid in urinary-tract infections. N. Engl. J. Med. 275:1081-1089.

Rownd, R. H., D. Perlman, and N. Goto. 1975. Structure and replication of R-factor deoxyribonucleic acid in Proteus mirabilis. Pp. 76-94 in D. Schlessinger, ed. Microbiology--1974. American Society for Microbiology, Washington, D.C.

Rubens, C. E., W. F. McNeill, and W. E. Farrar, Jr. 1979. Transposable plasmid deoxyribonucleic acid sequence in Pseudomonas aeruginosa which mediates resistance to gentamicin and four other antimicrobial agents. J. Bacteriol. 139:877-882.

Săsărman, A., M. Surdeanu, G. Szégli, T. Horodniceanu, V. Greceanu, and A. Dumitrescu. 1968. Hemin-deficient mutants of Escherichia coli K-12. J. Bacteriol. 96:570-572.

Shahrabadi, M. S., L. E. Bryan, and H. M. Van Den Elzen. 1975. Further properties of P-2 R-factors of Pseudomonas aeruginosa and their relationship to other plasmid groups. Can. J. Microbiol. 21:592-605.

Shalita, Z., I. Hertman, and S. Sarid. 1977. Isolation and characterization of a plasmid involved with enterotoxin B production in Staphylococcus aureus. J. Bacteriol. 129:317-325.

Skurray, R. A., R. E. W. Hancock, and P. Reeves. 1974. Con$^-$ mutants: Class of mutants in Escherichia coli K-12 lacking a major cell wall protein and defective in conjugation and adsorption of a bacteriophage. J. Bacteriol. 119:726-735.

Smith, D. I., R. Gomez Lus, M. C. Rubio Calvo, N. Datta, A. E. Jacob, and R. W. Hedges. 1975. Third type of plasmid conferring gentamicin resistance in Pseudomonas aeruginosa. Antimicrob. Agents Chemother. 8:227-230.

Smith, H. W. 1969. Transfer of antibiotic resistance from animal and human strains of Escherichia coli to resident E. coli in the alimentary tract of man. Lancet 1:1174-1176.

Smith, H. W. 1970. The transfer of antibiotic resistance between strains of enterobacteria in chicken, calves and pigs. J. Med. Microbiol. 3:165-180.

Smith, H. W. 1971. The effect of the use of antibacterial drugs on the emergence of drug-resistant bacteria in animals. Adv. Vet. Comp. Med. 15:67-100.

Smith, H. W. 1972. The effect on virulence of transferring R factors to Salmonella typhimurium in vivo. J. Med. Microbiol. 5:451-458.

Smith, H. W. 1974. A search for transmissible pathogenic characters in invasive strains of Escherichia coli: The discovery of a plasmid-controlled toxin and a plasmid-controlled lethal character closely associated, or identical, with colicine V. J. Gen. Microbiol. 83:95-111.

Smith, H. W., and M. B. Huggins. 1976. Further observation on the association of the colicine V plasmid of Escherichia coli with pathogenicity and with survival in the alimentary tract. J. Gen. Microbiol. 92:335-350.

Smith, H. W., and M. A. Linggood. 1971a. Observations on the pathogenic properties of the K88, Hly and Ent plasmids of Escherichia coli with particular reference to porcine diarrhoea. J. Med. Microbiol. 4:467-485.

Smith, H. W., and M. A. Linggood. 1971b. The transmissible nature of enterotoxin production in a human enteropathogenic strain of Escherichia coli. J. Med. Microbiol. 4:301-305.

Smith, H. W., Z. Parsell, and P. Green. 1978. Thermosensitive antibiotic resistance plasmids in enterobacteria. J. Gen. Microbiol. 109:37-47.

So, M., F. Heffron, and B. J. McCarthy. 1979. The E. coli gene encoding heat stable toxin is a bacterial transposon flanked by inverted repeats of IS1. Nature 277:453-456.

Spratt, B. G. 1978. Escherichia coli resistant to β-lactam antibiotics through a decrease in the affinity of a target for lethality. Nature 274:713-715.

Stacey, K. A., and E. Simson. 1965. Improved method for the isolation of thymine-requiring mutants of Escherichia coli. J. Bacteriol. 90:554-555.

Summers, A. O., and S. Silver. 1978. Microbial transformations of metals. Annu. Rev. Microbiol. 32:637-672.

Suzuki, H., Y. Nishimura, and Y. Hirota. 1978. On the process of cellular division in Escherichia coli: A series of mutants of E. coli altered in the penicillin-binding proteins. Proc. Nat. Acad. Sci. (USA) 75:664-668.

Tally, F. P., D. R. Syndman, S. L. Gorbach, and M. H. Malamy. 1979. Plasmid-mediated, transferable resistance to clindamycin and erythromycin in Bacteroides fragilis. J. Infect. Dis. 139:83-88.

Tanaka, T., M. Tsunoda, and S. Mitsuhashi. 1975. Drug resistance in Shigella strains isolated in Japan from 1965 to 1973. Pp. 187-199 in S. Mitsuhashi and H. Hashimoto, eds. Microbial Drug Resistance. University Park Press, Baltimore, Md.

Thorbjarnardóttir, S. H., R. A. Magnúsdóttir, G. Eggertsson, S. A. Kagan, and Ó. S. Andrésson. 1978. Mutations determining generalized resistance to aminoglycoside antibiotics in Escherichia coli. Mol. Gen. Genet. 161:89-98.

Timmis, K. N., F. Cabello, I. Andrés, A. Nordheim, H. J. Burkhardt, and S. N. Cohen. 1978. Instability of plasmid DNA sequences: Macro and micro evolution of the antibiotic resistance plasmid R6-5. Mol. Gen. Genet. 167:11-19.

Tocchini-Valentini, G. P., P. Marino, and A. J. Colvill. 1968. Mutant of *E. coli* containing an altered DNA-dependent RNA polymerase. Nature 220:275-276.

Uhlin, B. E., and K. Nordström. 1977. R plasmid gene dosage effects in *Escherichia coli* K-12: Copy mutants of the R plasmid R1*drd*-19. Plasmid 1:1-7.

Wachsmuth, I. K., W. E. Stamm, and J. E. McGowan, Jr. 1975. Prevalence of toxigenic and invasive strains of *Escherichia coli* in a hospital population. J. Infect. Dis. 132:601-603.

Watanabe, T. 1971. Transferable antibiotic resistance in Enterobacteriaceae: Relationship to the problems of treatment and control of coliform enteritis. Ann. N. Y. Acad. Sci. 176: 371-384.

Wheelis, M. L. 1975. The genetics of dissimilatory pathways in *Pseudomonas*. Annu. Rev. Microbiol. 29:505-524.

Wiedemann, B. 1972. Resistance transfer *in vivo* and its inhibition. Pp. 75-90 in V. Krčméry, L. Rosival, and T. Watanabe, eds. Bacterial Plasmids and Antibiotic Resistance. First International Symposium. Infectious Antibiotic Resistance. Castle of Smolenice, Czechoslovakia, 1971. Springer-Verlag, N.Y.

Wittmann, H. G., G. Stöffler, D. Apirion, L. Rosen, K. Tanaka, M. Tamaki, R. Takata, S. Dekio, E. Otaka, and S. Osawa. 1973. Biochemical and genetic studies on two different types of erythromycin resistant mutants of *Escherichia coli* with altered ribosomal proteins. Mol. Gen. Genet. 127:175-189.

Yagi, Y., and D. B. Clewell. 1976. Plasmid-determined tetracycline resistance in *Streptococcus faecalis*: Tandomly repeated resistance determinants in amplified forms of pAM$_{\alpha}$1 DNA. J. Mol. Biol. 102:583-600.

Yaguchi, M., H. G. Wittmann, T. Cabezón, M. DeWilde, R. Villarroel, A. Herzog, and A. Bollen. 1976. Alteration of ribosomal protein S17 by mutation linked to neamine resistance in *Escherichia* coli. II. Localization of the amino acid replacement in protein S17 from a neaA mutant. J. Mol. Biol. 104:617-620.

Yokota, T., and T. Akiba. 1961. Studies on the mechanism of transfer of drug-resistance in bacteria. VII. Inhibition of transfer of the resistance-factor from E. coli to Shigella flexneri by some chemicals. [In Japanese] Med. Biol. (Tokyo) 58:188-191 (cited in Watanabe, T. 1963. P. 90 in Infective heredity of multiple drug resistance in bacteria. Bacteriol. Rev. 27: 87-115).

Yoshikawa, M., A. Okuyama, and N. Tanaka. 1975. A third kasugamycin resistance locus, ksgC, affecting ribosomal protein S2 in Escherichia coli K-12. J. Bacteriol. 122:796-797.

Young, F. E., and L. Mayer. 1979. Genetic determinants of microbial resistance to antibiotics. Rev. Infect. Dis. 1:55-62.

APPENDIX D

IMPACT OF ANTIMICROBIALS ON THE MICROBIAL ECOLOGY OF THE GUT

Dwayne C. Savage[1]

Much evidence has been published on the influence of antibiotics on population levels and antimicrobial resistance in *Escherichia coli*. *E. coli* and some of its close relatives, such as salmonellae, are pervasive pathogens. Possibly because *E. coli* is easy to culture and manipulate *in vitro*, it has also become the major bacterial tool of molecular biologists. Thus, there is great interest concerning its resistance to antimicrobial agents. As documented below, it can be recognized as a member of the "normal gut floras" of many species of animals. It is usually a minority member of such floras.

Studies of the antimicrobial resistance of *E. coli* have been reported in depth (see, for example, Food and Drug Administration, 1978). However, the findings of these studies may be inadequate to demonstrate how predominant flora may interact with antimicrobial drugs. Consequently, I have chosen to minimize discussion of *E. coli* and to emphasize findings and concepts concerning the types of bacteria that predominate in the "normal gut flora."

"NORMAL" GUT FLORA

The Gastrointestinal Ecosystem

In my opinion, the term "normal gut flora" is confusing and probably obsolete (Savage, 1977). The confusion begins with the word "gut," which usually means "intestine." Much evidence supports the hypothesis that most higher animals, including cattle, swine, and chickens (possibly even humans), have "gastrointestinal microbiota" composed of indigenous microbes colonizing specific habitats located throughout the gastrointestinal tract, not just in the gut. Some of this evidence is presented later in this paper.

The words "normal flora" also are confusing. "Normal flora" is usually used collectively to describe various microbial species found by cultures or microscopy to be on the skin and mucous membranes and in certain body cavities of both healthy and sick animals. The term is also used as a synonym for "indigenous microbiota" meaning, collectively, those autochthonous microbial resi-

[1]Department of Microbiology, University of Illinois, Urbana.

dents of habitats on certain body surfaces or in particular body cavities of normal animals. These definitions do not necessarily describe the same microorganisms. The first suggests that all microbial types found on or in, or cultured from, certain surfaces or cavities are normal residents of habitats in those sites. However, much recent evidence supports the concept that many microbial types that can be isolated at any given time from an open ecosystem such as the gastrointestinal tract cannot be identified as indigenous to the system and must be regarded as transients.

Transients can be transported to a habitat in a gastrointestinal ecosystem in food and other materials (including feces in coprophagous animals such as chickens and pigs) or even by passing down from habitats above the one being sampled. Certain transients, some of which may be pathogens, may temporarily colonize niches in habitats in perturbed ecosystems. Systems may be perturbed by antimicrobial drugs (as shall be amplified), by starvation or other forms of malnutrition, and perhaps by certain environmental conditions such as hyperbaric atmospheres and circumstances generating fear and other stresses. Such conditions influence the factors that regulate the population levels and localization of indigenous microorganisms in the ecosystem (Savage, 1977). These factors are discussed later in this paper.

Anatomy of the Gastrointestinal Tract

As already noted, microbial habitats can be found in various locations in the gastrointestinal tracts of animals of different species. The gastrointestinal tracts of mammals and birds have five major sections: esophagus, stomach, small intestine, cecum, and large intestine. Depending upon the animal species, any of these sections may be further compartmentalized or divided into subsections. In mammals, there are three basic variations on this overall theme: the ruminant, cecal, and "straight tube" systems. In the ruminant, the stomach is ramified into compartments (Hungate, 1966). In mammals with a cecum, the cecum is a blind pouch extending laterally from the distal end of the small intestine and the proximal end of the large bowel (McBee, 1977). In chickens, the "stomach" consists of a storage compartment (crop), proventriculus, and gizzard (Fuller and Turvey, 1971); two ceca are present (Bauchop, 1977; McBee, 1977). Depending upon the species of animal, any or all of these areas may contain habitats for indigenous microorganisms. Such habitats may include the contents of the lumen, the epithelial surface, or even pits in the mucosa called Crypts of Lieberkühn.

The epithelial and cryptal habitats may be particularly important. In mammals and birds, the esophagus is lined with a stratified squamous epithelium that may or may not be keratinized (Savage, 1977). Some "gastric" compartments, such as the crop in chickens (Fuller and Turvey, 1971), part of the stomach in rodents (Savage, 1977), and the rumens of cattle and sheep (McCowan *et al.*, 1978), are lined with a stratified squamous epithelium that is usually keratinized. In chickens and mammals that have been examined (including humans) gastric compartments not lined with a squamous epithelium and the small and large intestines (including the cecum) are lined with a single layer of columnar cells. In the small intestine, the mucosa is organized so that the epithelium covers finger- or leaf-shaped villi that protrude into the lumen. Villi are not found in the stomach or large intestine, although the mucosa in both areas may fold when the lumen is empty. Columnar epithelium also lines the Crypts of Lieberkühn, which are located at the bases of the villi in the small bowel and are spaced periodically in the mucosa of the stomach and large bowel (Savage, 1977). Depending upon the animal species, crypts and epithelial surfaces may provide habitats for microbial communities throughout the gastrointestinal tract.

Evidence that epithelial, cryptal, and luminal habitats exist for indigenous microorganisms in all areas of the gastrointestinal tract has been provided primarily by studies of laboratory rodents (Savage, 1977). The indigenous microbiotas of most mammalian and avian species have not been defined as well as they have for rodents. Nevertheless, some evidence on the microbiotas of calves, swine, and chickens supports a hypothesis that the concepts discussed above apply to those species as they do to laboratory rodents. In the discussion to follow, that point is amplified for swine and chickens, and some information on humans is included to provide perspective. The calf is treated separately because it is an ungulate with an enormous complex biota in its rumen. However, the biota in the rumen is similar to that in the large intestines of monogastric animals such as humans, pigs, and chickens.

The Microbiota of the Stomach

Microorganisms of many types have been isolated from the contents of the stomachs of humans and swine (Savage, 1977) and from the crops of chickens (Fuller and Turvey, 1971). Most of the types isolated should probably be regarded as transients since the stomachs of most animals undoubtedly empty more rapidly than microorganisms can multiply. Thus, microbes in the lumen pass out of the stomach with the contents (Savage, 1977). Nevertheless, certain types may be regarded as autochthonous to habitats in the area. *Lactobacillus* spp. at high population levels (10^9 organisms per gram of mucosa) can be cultured from and observed microscopically on the squamous epithelium of the crops of chickens (Fuller and Turvey, 1971). Likewise, *Lactobacillus* spp. and *Candida* spp. can be cultured at comparable population levels from the squamous epithelium in the pars oesophagia of swine (Fuller *et al*., 1978; Savage, 1977). Although such organisms are usually found in the stomachs of humans as well (Savage, 1977), much more research is needed to test the hypothesis that humans have an indigenous gastric microbiota.

The Microbiota of the Small Intestine

The small intestines of humans and chickens (and undoubtedly also swine and calves) also yield many microbial species (Dickman *et al*., 1976; Savage, 1977). Most of the organisms are probably transients, especially in the upper two-thirds of the bowel where peristalsis moves luminal content much more rapidly than microbes can multiply (Savage, 1977). Microbes of types found in the large bowel (see below) may be identified, occasionally at high population levels, in cultures from the lower third of the gastrointestinal tract, where the content moves somewhat sluggishly and may not move at all for a time. Such organisms may be indigenous to the region or may be contaminants from the large bowel that have crossed the ileo-cecal valve into the area. Neither of these hypotheses can be set aside on the basis of evidence that is available at this time.

In chickens, however, microbes seen adhering to the epithelium of the small intestine (Fuller and Turvey, 1971) may be indigenous to that area (Savage, 1977). These organisms are filamentous prokaryotes with Gram-negative ultrastructure (Savage, 1977). Their population levels are unknown (they have not been cultured *in vitro*), but are probably quite high. Similar organisms are recognized as indigenous inhabitants of the epithelial surfaces of the small bowels of laboratory rodents (Savage, 1977).

The Microbiota of the Large Intestine

The large bowels of humans and the ceca and colons of swine and chickens contain enormous populations of microorganisms (more than 1×10^{11} microbes per gram dry weight of content). The contents of those regions move sluggishly and allow ample time for microbial multiplication (Savage, 1977). The populations are composed primarily of Gram-positive and Gram-negative bacteria that cannot multiply in atmospheres containing oxygen (Table 1). Indeed, many of the species are intolerant of oxygen and are killed by exposure to it or to growth media or diluting fluids with oxidation-reduction potentials above certain negative levels. Human feces yield up to 400 species in as many as 40 microbial genera (Drasar and Hill, 1974; Holdeman *et al.*, 1976; Moore and Holdeman, 1974). The vast majority of the species are oxygen-intolerant anaerobic bacteria. More than 99% of the total microbial population obligately gains its energy through anaerobic processes. In the gastrointestinal ecosystem of humans, facultative bacteria (i.e., able to use both aerobic and anaerobic processes to generate energy) such as *E. coli* are usually outnumbered by the anaerobes by as much as 1,000 to 1. The systems of swine and chickens are undoubtedly similar (Table 1).

Some of the microbial species in the ecosystems adhere to or colonize secretions in the epithelium of the ceca or colons (Savage, 1977). In swine, spirochetes and a variety of other microbial species have been found in epithelial habitats (Allison *et al.*, 1979; Savage, 1977). In chickens, both Gram-positive and Gram-negative bacteria can be observed on the colonic surface (Fuller and Turvey, 1971). In humans, bacteria have been seen microscopically on the surface, but have not been characterized well (Savage, 1977). Since many such microbial species have not been cultured *in vitro* (Savage, 1977), they are not listed in Table 1. Nevertheless, they cannot be ignored as components of the ecosystem.

The Microbiota of the Rumen

The biota in the rumen of the adult bovine animal is also highly complex, consisting of protozoa and bacteria at enormous population levels (total levels greater than 1×10^{11} organisms per gram dry weight of content) (Bauchop, 1977; Hungate, 1966). Most of the bacterial species in the rumen belong to anaerobic genera. Some of them are similar to those found in the large bowels of monogastric animals (Table 1), but others are undoubtedly unique to the ecosystem of the rumen (Hungate, 1966). The population levels of facultative

TABLE 1

Principal Bacterial Genera Reported to be Present in the Feces or Content of the Large Bowels of Swine, Chickens, or Humans[a]

Predominant Genera[b]

Swine	Chickens	Humans
Eubacterium	Eubacterium	Eubacterium
Peptostreptococcus	Bacteroides	Bacteroides
Clostridium	Fusobacterium	Fusobacterium
Lactobacillus	Peptostreptococcus	Peptostreptococcus
Propionibacterium	Bifidobacterium	Ruminococcus
Streptococcus	Gemminger	Coprococcus
Peptococcus	Clostridium	Bifidobacterium
Megasphaera	Lactobacillus	Gemminger
	Propionibacterium	Clostridium
		Lactobacillus

Minor Genera[c]

Swine	Chickens	Humans
Bacteroides	Staphylococcus	Acidaminococcus
Bifidobacterium	Streptococcus	Staphylococcus
Treponema	Escherichia	Propionibacterium
Veillonella		Peptococcus
Escherichia		Desulfomonas
		Succinivibrio
		Streptococcus
		Escherichia

[a]Swine: Fuller *et al.*, 1978; Hackman and Wilkins, 1975; Kinyon and Harris, 1979; Kolacz *et al.*, 1971; Morishita and Ogata, 1970; Ogata and Morishita, 1969; Russell, 1979; Terada *et al.*, 1976.
Chickens: Barnes and Impey, 1968, 1970; Fuller and Turvey, 1971; Gilliland *et al.*, 1975; Ochi *et al.*, 1964; Salanitro *et al.*, 1974, 1977, 1978; Timms, 1968.
Humans: Akama and Otani, 1970; Dickman *et al.*, 1976; Drasar and Hill, 1974; Gilliland *et al.*, 1975; Holdeman *et al.*, 1976; Mitsuoka, 1969; Mitsuoka and Ohno, 1977; Moore and Holdeman, 1974.

[b]Population levels of many species exceed 1×10^9 organisms per gram of content. Most exceed 1×10^{10} organisms per gram.

[c]Population levels less than 1×10^9 organisms per gram of content. Many species have levels of less than 1×10^8 organisms per gram.

organisms such as *E. coli* are usually nonexistant or quite low. Certain bacterial types, including some facultative ones, are believed to adhere to the epithelium of the rumen (McCowan *et al.*, 1978). The biota of the remainder of the bovine intestinal tract has not been characterized.

Summary

There is no doubt that all mammalian and avian species have microbial floras that are indigenous to their gastrointestinal tracts. In humans, calves, swine, and chickens, climax floras, such as might be found in a healthy adult, contain primarily anaerobic bacteria in most habitats of the tract. Under normal conditions those anaerobes vastly outnumber facultative microbes such as *E. coli*. In fact, in normal, unperturbed systems the anaerobes undoubtedly function to restrict the population levels of *E. coli* and its relatives. Unfortunately, as noted earlier, information on the anaerobes with pertinence to this report is far less well developed than it is for *E. coli*. This problem complicates the answers to most of the questions raised in the following paragraphs.

ANTIBIOTIC-RESISTANT STRAINS IN "NORMAL FLORA"

Investigators interested in *E. coli*, primarily as a potential pathogen, have provided considerable data on antibiotic-resistant strains in "normal flora." Strains of *E. coli* with resistance to numerous antibiotics, many carrying transferable plasmids coding for such resistance, can be isolated from calves, swine, and poultry being fed (Table 2) or treated (Table 3) with antimicrobial drugs. Such strains can also be isolated from animals ostensibly not fed or treated with the drugs, but with much less frequency than from animals receiving them (Franklin and Glatthard, 1977; Petrocheilou *et al.*, 1976) (Tables 1, 2). Most investigators do not provide reassurance, however, that these controls have not been in contact with antibiotics, for example, through association with parental animals treated with drugs.

Reliable information of the type available for *E. coli* is virtually unavailable for the bacterial species predominating in the gastrointestinal ecosystem. Anaerobic bacteria of many genera can develop resistance to antimicrobial drugs. This has been demonstrated for organisms from the rumen (Fulghum *et al.*, 1968; Wang *et al.*, 1969), from feces of humans (Anderson and Sykes, 1973; Burt and

TABLE 2

Some Reports Containing Evidence that Resistant Strains of *Escherichia coli* can be Isolated More Frequently from Animals Fed Diets Containing Certain Antibiotics than from Animals Fed Drug-Free Diets[a]

Animal	Antibiotic[b]	Reference
Swine	Tetracyclines	Fuller et al., 1960 Smith, 1968 Mercer et al., 1971 Siegel et al., 1974 Linton et al., 1975 Ahart et al., 1978 Langlois et al., 1978
	Penicillin	Fuller et al., 1960 Mercer et al., 1971 Siegel et al., 1974
	Virginiamycin	Langlois et al., 1978
	A mixture of chlortetracycline, penicillin, and sulfamethazine	Mercer et al., 1971
	A mixture of virginiamycin, tylosin, Furoxone, and sulfaguanidine	Pohl et al., 1977
Calves	Tetracyclines	Edwards, 1962 Loken et al., 1971 Siegel et al., 1974 Linton et al., 1975 Ahart et al., 1978
	Penicillin	Siegel et al., 1974
Chickens	Tetracycline	Smith, 1968
Turkeys	Tetracycline	Baldwin et al., 1976

[a]Isolated resistant strains of E. coli were resistant to one or more antimicrobial drugs, often not only to the drug used in the feed but also to one or more other compounds.

[b]Present at subtherapeutic levels in the feed.

TABLE 3

Some Reports Containing Evidence that Resistant Strains of *Escherichia coli* can be Isolated More Frequently from Animals being Treated with Certain Antibiotics than from Untreated Animals[a]

Animal	Antibiotic[b]	Reference
Swine	Many different types	Larsen and Nielsen, 1975
Cows	Penicillin plus dihydrostreptomycin	Rollins *et al.*, 1974
Chickens	Tetracyclines	Chopra *et al.*, 1963 Howe *et al.*, 1976
Humans	Tetracyclines	Schmidt *et al.*, 1973 Hirsh *et al.*, 1973 Bartlett *et al.*, 1975 Møller *et al.*, 1977

[a] Isolated resistant strains of *E. coli* were resistant to one or more antimicrobial drugs, often not only to the drug used in treatment but also to one or more other compounds.

[b] Used prophylactically or to treat a particular disease.

Woods, 1975; Finegold, 1970, 1977) and swine (Rood *et al.*, 1978), and from the ceca of chickens (Barnes and Goldberg, 1962). Moreover, investigators have demonstrated that plasmids code for resistance to several antibiotics in certain species of *Streptococcus* (Malke, 1979; Van Embden *et al.*, 1977), *Lactobacillus* (Klaenhammer *et al.*, 1979), and *Bacteroides* (Guiney and Davis, 1978; Onderdonk *et al.*, 1979; Welch *et al.*, 1979), and in *Clostridium perfringens* (Sebald and Bréfort, 1975), all bacterial species recognized to be members of the large bowel flora of mammals and birds (Table 1). Plasmids coding for resistance can be transferred *in vitro* from donor to recipient strains of *Clostridium perfringens* (Sebald and Bréfort, 1975). Such plasmids may also transfer from donor to recipient strains of *Bacteroides in vitro* (Welch *et al.*, 1979) and *in vivo* in formerly germfree rodents (Onderdonk *et al.*, 1979) and from donor *Bacteroides* to *E. coli in vitro* (Mancini and Behme, 1977). Strong evidence supports findings that there is a conjugative transfer of an R plasmid from a strain of *Bacteroides ochraceus* isolated from the human mouth to a strain of *E. coli* (Guiney and Davis, 1978). Burt and Woods (1976) reported that "R-factor" plasmids from *E. coli* can be transferred *in vitro* to strains of *B. fragilis*, other species of *Bacteroides*, and some species of *Fusobacterium*, if the recipient strains are heated before being exposed to the donor.

Most such information has been gained in studies conducted within the last 4 or 5 years. Indeed, many recent reports on the transmissibility of plasmids in anaerobes appear only as abstracts in the literature. Much of the work concerns anaerobic bacteria as pathogens rather than as members of the indigenous microbiota. However, these efforts provide good indications of gene transmission among the anaerobic members of the gastrointestinal ecosystem. Unfortunately, little of the evidence has been gained in such a way that the proportion of antibiotic-resistant strains in "normal" flora can be determined.

CHANGES INDUCED BY SUBTHERAPEUTIC LEVELS OF ANTIBIOTICS IN FEED

The Proportion of Resistant Strains in Gastrointestinal Microbiota

As suggested above, reliable information on the proportion of resistant strains in gastrointestinal microbiota is almost nonexistent for the major components of the indigenous biota. Ample evidence supports observations that strains of *E. coli* with resistance to penicillins, tetracyclines, and other antibiotics can be isolated much more frequently from animals fed subtherapeutic doses of tetracycline and penicillin in their diets (Table 2) than from animals eating diets free of the drugs. Indeed, after animals have consumed the diets containing drugs for just a few days, more than 90% of the *E. coli* strains isolated are resistant to the drugs used in the diets and to other compounds. By contrast, less than 10% of the strains isolated from animals not fed the drugs are resistant to antibiotics. Some efforts have been made to develop such information for certain other types of bacteria that can be cultured from the gastrointestinal tracts of animals. For example, dietary chlortetracycline was found to induce resistant strains of *Streptococcus faecalis* that predominate over sensitive strains in ceca of chickens (Elliott and Barnes, 1959). One such resistant strain predominated in the animals 5 months after the antibiotic had been removed from the diet.

Similarly, 90% of the strains of lactobacilli or streptococci isolated from the feces of swine were commonly resistant to penicillin or to chlortetracycline if isolated from animals fed diets containing that drug. By contrast, more than 90% of the same strains isolated from animals not fed the drugs were sensitive to them (Fuller *et al.*, 1960). Some other studies (Ahart *et al.*, 1978) in which "anaerobes" were isolated and found to be resistant to antibiotics cannot be evaluated. The methods used by those investigators provide no clues to the types of bacteria involved.

Potential Pathogens in the Gastrointestinal Microbiota

Virtually no information is available on the influence of antimicrobial drugs on the relative proportions and absolute numbers of potential pathogens in the indigenous biotas except for *E. coli* and its relatives. Actually, "pathogen" is difficult to define in reference to the biota. In swine, *Treponema hyodysenteriae* can cause dysentery only when acting with other anaerobic components of the indigenous biota, none of which are known to be pathogens (Kinyon and Harris, 1979). Likewise, many other indigenous species have the capacity to cause disease under the right circumstances. In several species of animal, including pigs and chickens, *Clostridium perfringens* can cause diarrheal disease under certain conditions (Finegold, 1977; Rood *et al.*, 1978). In humans and other animals, certain *Bacteroides* spp. induce abscesses in normally sterile tissues, often in association with facultative bacterial species (Finegold, 1977). Many other species of anaerobic bacteria can cause disease under certain conditions (Finegold, 1977). Most of them are normally present in the gastrointestinal tracts of animals at extremely high population levels. Thus, the question of whether or not antibiotics tend to increase the relative proportions and absolute numbers of potential pathogens is moot.

Flora of Areas of the Body Other Than the Skin

Information pertaining to the effects of antibiotics on flora at sites other than the skin is sparse. Strains of bacteria with resistance to antibiotics have been isolated from the vaginal secretions of cows (Panangala and Barnum, 1978). However, these studies were conducted with cows that had been treated with antibiotics but not necessarily given feed containing subtherapeutic doses of the drugs. Moreover, there was no evidence that the bacteria were members of the indigenous flora of the bovine vagina.

Virtually nothing of which I am aware has been published on the composition of the skin flora of chickens and mammals other than humans (McBride *et al.*, 1977). The skin and noses of pigs and chickens fed diets containing tetracyclines yield abnormally high proportions of strains of *Staphylococcus aureus* with resistance to the drug (Smith and Crabb, 1960). However, *S. aureus* may or may not be a member of the indigenous skin and nasal biota of such animals.

Persistence of Changes when Selection Pressure is Removed

The duration of resistance when selection pressure is removed cannot be determined satisfactorily for most species found in the gastrointestinal tract. *E. coli* strains bearing drug resistance plasmids may persist in the biotas of animals for months after the selection pressure is removed (Hartley and Richmond, 1975; Smith, 1975). Similarly, as already noted, *Streptococcus* strains with resistance to chlortetracycline may persist in the ceca of chickens for months after the drug is removed from their diets (Elliott and Barnes, 1969). Whether or not such findings apply to the majority components of the biota is not known.

CHANGES IN FLORA RESULTING FROM THE THERAPEUTIC USE OF ANTIBIOTICS

There are few definitive data concerning changes in the anaerobic components of flora resulting from the therapeutic use of antibiotics. Evidence does substantiate that therapeutic doses of certain antibiotics enable resistant strains of *E. coli* to proliferate in the gastrointestinal tracts of several species of animals (Table 3) and to transfer plasmids coding for such resistance in the gastrointestinal tracts of humans (Anderson *et al.*, 1973). Likewise, many streptococcal strains isolated from the mouths and blood of humans treated with penicillin and some other antibiotics may be resistant to the drugs used (Phillips *et al.*, 1976). Moreover, there is no doubt that antimicrobial therapy allows strains of other types of pathogenic anaerobic bacteria to grow in and be isolated from lesions of diseases in humans (Finegold, 1977). Strains of such organisms may persist for a time in the human gut (Finegold, 1977); however, there are no data pertaining to the development and persistance of resistance in the major components of the indigenous biota of the gastrointestinal tract.

CHANGES IN FLORA RESULTING FROM LEVELS OF ANTIBIOTICS USED TO PROMOTE GROWTH

There is no reliable information pertaining to the action of antibiotics used as growth promoters on the major components of the indigenous microbiota *in vivo*. As discussed above, both penicillin and tetracycline can induce resistance in anaerobes of many species.

FACTORS AFFECTING ABILITY TO COLONIZE

Many factors influence the population levels and localization of microorganisms in the gastrointestinal ecosystem (Tables 4 and 5). Some of the forces are exerted by the host, its environment, and diet (the allogenic factors). Some are exerted by the microorganisms themselves (the autogenic factors). The microbiota can alter the forces generated by the host, making them either more or less effective in controlling the biota. Thus, the processes influencing a microbe's ability to colonize a niche in a habitat in the gastrointestinal tract are enormously complex. It is known, however, that the strictly anaerobic bacteria are the most important components of the biota involved in stabilizing established communities in adult animals.

The processes involved in maintaining such stability undoubtedly work most effectively in adult animals with unperturbed indigenous biotas. Most importantly, these processes prevent transient microbial species from colonizing niches in the system (Savage, 1977). Such transients (many of which may be potential microbial

TABLE 4

Some Allogenic Factors Known to Influence the Composition of the Indigenous Microbiota in Certain Regions of the Gastrointestinal Tract[a]

Factor	Possible Region of Influence	Normal Features that Influence Composition of Microbiota
Temperature	Stomach Small intestine Large intestine	Body temperature (37°C)
pH	Stomach Small intestine Large intestine	Acidic Neutral to alkaline Neutral to alkaline
Stasis	Stomach Small intestine Large intestine (including cecum)	Periodic Periodic in lower part of region Prolonged (residence time) especially in cecum
Oxygen	Large intestine[b]	Concentration low, if present at all
Oxidation-reduction potential	Large intestine[b]	Low potential, especially when microbes are present
Enzymes	Small intestine[b]	Pancreatic enzymes present
Bile acids	Stomach Small intestine Large intestine	Low concentration Conjugated bile acids present Deconjugated bile acids present
Epithelial turnover	All regions of tract	Sloughing of cells necessitates replacement of attached cells but the cells may provide microbial nutrients
Urea	Large intestine[b]	Can be carbon and nitrogen source for certain microbial species

TABLE 4
(Continued)

Factor	Possible Region of Influence	Normal Features that Influence Composition of Microbiota
Mucin	All regions of tract	Mucin contributes to the viscosity of the environment and may act as a microbial nutrient
Diet	All regions of tract	The diet provides microbial nutrients and affects the nature of habitats in the tract
Drugs	All regions of tract	Influence is characteristic of the drug(s)
Phagocytic cells	Crypts of Leiberkühn	Microbiota may be phagocytosed (selectively)
Antibodies	All regions of tract	Precise effect on biota not known Antibody protein may be utilize nutritionally by microorganisms

[a] Adapted from Savage, 1977; see also Booth et al., 1977, and Gibbons and van Houte, 1975.

[b] Evidence is insufficient to suggest that the factor may operate in other regions.

TABLE 5

Some Autogenic Factors Known to Influence the Composition of the Indigenous Microbiota in Certain Regions of the Gastrointestinal Tract[a]

Factor	Possible Region of Influence	Normal Features that Influence Composition of Microbiota
Volatile fatty acids	Any habitat	Effect dependent upon oxidation-reduction potential
Bacteriocins	Any habitat	Effects uncertain
Nutritional competition	Any habitat	Effects uncertain
Hydrogen sulfide	Probably in large intestine[b]	May depress population levels of some facultative species of bacteria
Adherence to epithelium	Any habitat	Allows microorganisms to colonize areas of the tract where peristaltic rate moves contents more rapidly than bacteria can multiply

[a] Adapted from Savage, 1977; see also Booth *et al.*, 1977, and Gibbons and van Houte, 1975.

[b] Evidence is insufficient to suggest that the factor may operate in other regions.

pathogens constantly enter the system via food, water, and other ingesta. They usually do not persist long in the unperturbed system, but may colonize a niche in a perturbed system.

As mentioned above, a system may be perturbed by antimicrobial drugs (Decuypere *et al.*, 1973; Dubos *et al.*, 1963; Savage and Dubos, 1968; Savage and McAllister, 1971; Van der Waaij and Berghuis, 1974), starvation and other forms of nutritional stress (Savage, 1977), and even by some less drastic changes in an animal's lifestyle (Holdeman *et al.*, 1976). In infants, in whom the climax gastrointestinal microbiota characteristic of the adult has not yet been established, the biota may also be regarded as perturbed. During this developmental period of animals, the population levels of *E. coli* may be quite high (Savage, 1977). Once the anaerobic components of the biota are established, however, the levels drop to the normally low levels of adults. As long as the communities of anaerobes remain intact in adult animals, the population levels of *E. coli* remain low. If the communities of anaerobes are perturbed (e.g., by antimicrobial drugs), the levels of *E. coli* may rise dramatically. Such evidence has been considered strong support for the hypothesis that the anaerobes control the levels of *E. coli* in the ecosystems (Morishita and Mitsuoka, 1976). However, the mechanisms of such control are not well understood. *In vitro*, anaerobes may also inhibit R-factor transfer among strains of *E. coli* (Anderson, 1975).

Because antimicrobial drugs perturb the gastrointestinal ecosystem, they must upset the balance of forces that regulate the biota. The precise factors that are perturbed, especially those affected by subtherapeutic doses of drugs, can only be conjectured. No doubt exists, however, that subtherapeutic doses of both penicillin and tetracycline in animal feeds somehow tip the balance towards resistant strains in the biota of the animal fed the diets. Interestingly, when certain antibiotics are administered, some microbial strains may not themselves have to be resistant to the drugs to survive because resistance in another organism may enable them to do so (Hackman and Wilkins, 1975).

Humans associating with animals fed subtherapeutic doses of antibiotics may temporarily carry resistant strains of *E. coli* that are present in the animals. Such bacterial strains may transfer from animals to humans, however, whether or not the animals are fed antibiotics (Hirsh and Wiger, 1977, 1978; Hirsh *et al.*, 1974; Linton *et al.*, 1977).

When antibiotics are removed from an ecosystem, the maintenance of resistance may become an undue physiological burden for some strains. Thus, they may fail to compete with unhandicapped strains of the same species and eventually decline in prevalence and disappear from the system (Anderson, 1974). At this time, however, this hypothesis can be neither supported nor rejected by evidence provided by studies of the major components of the indigenous microbiota--the strictly anaerobic bacteria (Finegold, 1970).

SUMMARY

Antibacterial drugs such as penicillin and the tetracyclines, when incorporated as growth promotants into the feed of animals, provide a selective environment in the gastrointestinal tract favoring the proliferation of resistant strains of *Escherichia coli*, *Streptococcus* spp., and at least some of the major (strictly anaerobic) bacterial components of the indigenous microbiota. As with *E. coli*, some strains of strict anaerobes carry genetic information for resistance on plasmids. For a few such bacterial species, the plasmids can be transferred to recipient strains of the same species. Certain strains of *Bacteroides* may even be able to transfer their plasmids to recipient strains of *E. coli* and vice versa.

Such information provides limited evidence that the mechanisms of antibiotic resistance in some strains of anaerobic bacteria in the gastrointestinal ecosystem are similar to the mechanisms of such resistance in *E. coli*. However, it does not reveal anything about the proportion of resistant anaerobic strains that reside in animals receiving drugs in feed. Most importantly, perhaps, it reveals nothing about whether or not such resistance is transferred between microbial species in the gastrointestinal tract and whether or not resistance is maintained in the tract of an animal not being fed or treated with drugs. Information pertaining to these questions is insufficient for the major components of the biota, especially as they interact with each other and their host. Microorganisms in the gastrointestinal ecosystem interact biochemically and genetically with each other and biochemically with their animal host. Such interactions are complex mechanistically and not well understood. Much more evidence is needed before the impact of antibiotics on the system can be understood.

REFERENCES

Ahart, J. G., G. C. Burton, and D. C. Blenden. 1978. The influence of antimicrobial agents on the percentage of tetracycline-resistant bacteria in faeces of humans and animals. J. Appl. Bacteriol. 44:183-190.

Akama, K., and S. Otani. 1970. Clostridium perfringens as the flora in the intestine of healthy persons. Jpn. J. Med. Sci. Biol. 23:161-175.

Allison, M. J., I. M. Robinson, J. A. Bucklin, and G. D. Booth. 1979. Comparison of bacterial populations of the pig cecum and colon based upon enumeration with specific energy sources. Appl. Environ. Microbiol. 37:1142-1151.

Anderson, J. D. 1974. The effect of R-factor carriage on the survival of Escherichia coli in the human intestine. J. Med. Microbiol. 7:85-90.

Anderson, J. D. 1975. Factors that may prevent transfer of antibiotic resistance between gram-negative bacteria in the gut. J. Med. Microbiol. 8:83-88.

Anderson, J. D., and R. B. Sykes. 1973. Characterisation of a β-lactamase obtained from a strain of Bacteroides fragilis resistant to β-lactam antibiotics. J. Med. Microbiol. 6:201-206.

Anderson, J. D., W. A. Gillespie, and M. H. Richmond. 1973. Chemotherapy and antibiotic-resistance transfer between enterobacteria in the human gastro-intestinal tract. J. Med. Microbiol. 6:461-473.

Baldwin, B. B., M. C. Bromel, D. W. Aird, R. L. Johnson, and J. L. Sell. 1976. Effect of dietary oxytetracycline on microorganisms in turkey feces. Poult. Sci. 55:2147-2154.

Barnes, E. M., and H. S. Goldberg. 1962. The isolation of anaerobic gram-negative bacteria from poultry reared with and without antibiotic supplements. J. Appl. Bacteriol. 25:94-106.

Barnes, E. M., and C. S. Impey. 1968. Anaerobic gram negative non-sporing bacteria from the caeca of poultry. J. Appl. Bacteriol. 31:530-541.

Barnes, E. M., and C. S. Impey. 1970. The isolation and properties of the predominant anaerobic bacteria in the caeca of chickens and turkeys. Br. Poult. Sci. 11:467-481.

Bartlett, J. G., L. A. Bustetter, S. L. Gorbach, and A. B. Onderdonk. 1975. Comparative effect of tetracycline and doxycycline on the occurrence of resistant *Escherichia coli* in the fecal flora. Antimicrob. Agents Chemother. 7:55-57.

Bauchop, T. 1977. Foregut fermentation. Pp. 223-250 in R. T. J. Clarke and T. Bauchop, eds. Microbial Ecology of the Gut. Academic Press, London, New York, and San Francisco.

Booth, S. J., J. L. Johnson, and T. D. Wilkins. 1977. Bacteriocin production by strains of *Bacteroides* isolated from human feces and the role of these strains in the bacterial ecology of the colon. Antimicrob. Agents Chemother. 11:718-724.

Burt, S. J., and D. R. Woods. 1975. Studies on multiple antibiotic resistance in obligate anaerobes. S. Afr. Med. J. 49:1804-1806.

Burt, S. J., and D. R. Woods. 1976. R factor transfer to obligate anaerobes from *Escherichia coli*. J. Gen. Microbiol. 93:405-409.

Chopra, S. L., A. C. Blackwood, and D. G. Dale. 1963. The effect of chlortetracycline medication on the coliform microflora of newly hatched chicks. Can. J. Comp. Med. Vet. Sci. 27:74-76.

Decuypere, J., H. K. Henderickx, and I. Vervaeke. 1973. Influence of nutritional doses of Virginiamycin and Spiramycin on the quantitative and topographical composition of the gastrointestinal flora of artificially reared piglets. Zentralbl. Bakteriol. Parasitenkd. Infektionskr. Hyg., I. Abt. Orig. Reihe A 223:348-355.

Dickman, M. D., A. R. Chappelka, and R. W. Schaedler. 1976. The microbial ecology of the upper small bowel. Am. J. Gastroenterol. 65:57-62.

Drasar, B. S., and M. J. Hill. 1974. Human Intestinal Flora. Academic Press, London, New York, and San Francisco. 263 pp.

Dubos, R., R. W. Schaedler, and M. Stephens. 1963. The effect of antibacterial drugs on the fecal flora of mice. J. Exp. Med. 117:231-243.

Edwards, S. J. 1962. Effect of antibiotics on the growth rate and intestinal flora (Escherichia coli) of calves. J. Comp. Pathol. 72:420-432.

Elliott, S. D., and E. M. Barnes. 1959. Changes in serological type and antibiotic resistance of Lancefield group D streptococci in chickens receiving dietary chlortetracycline. J. Gen. Microbiol. 20:426-433.

Finegold, S. M. 1970. Interaction of antimicrobial therapy and intestinal flora. Am. J. Clin. Nutr. 23:1466-1471.

Finegold, S. M. 1977. Antimicrobial agent susceptibility of anaerobic bacteria. Pp. 513-533 in Anaerobic Bacteria in Human Disease. Academic Press, New York, San Francisco, and London.

Food and Drug Administration. 1978. Draft Environmental Impact Statement--Subtherapeutic Antibacterial Agents in Animal Feeds. Bureau of Veterinary Medicine, Food and Drug Administration, Department of Health, Education, and Welfare, Rockville, Md. [371 + xviii] pp.

Franklin, A., and V. Glatthard. 1977. [In German; English summary.] R-Faktor-determinierte Antibiotika-Resistenz bei coli-Stämmen isoliert von Ferkeln in Schweden. Zentralbl. Bakteriol. Parasitenkd. Infektionskr. Hyg., I Abt. Orig. Reihe A 238:208-215.

Fulghum, R. S., B. B. Baldwin, and P. P. Williams. 1968. Antibiotic susceptibility of anaerobic ruminal bacteria. Appl. Microbiol. 16:301-307.

Fuller, R., and A. Turvey. 1971. Bacteria associated with the intestinal wall of the fowl (Gallus domesticus). J. Appl. Bacteriol. 34:617-622.

Fuller, R., L. G. M. Newland, C. A. E. Briggs, R. Braude, and K. G. Mitchell. 1960. The normal intestinal flora of the pig. IV. The effect of dietary supplements of penicillin, chlortetracycline or copper sulphate on the faecal flora. J. Appl. Bacteriol. 23:195-205.

Fuller, R., P. A. Barrow, and B. E. Brooker. 1978. Bacteria associated with the gastric epithelium of neonatal pigs. Appl. Environ. Microbiol. 35:582-591.

Gibbons, R. J., and J. van Houte. 1975. Bacterial adherence in oral microbial ecology. Annu. Rev. Microbiol. 29:19-44.

Gilliland, S. E., M. L. Speck, and C. G. Morgan. 1975. Detection of Lactobacillus acidophilus in feces of humans, pigs, and chickens. Appl. Microbiol. 30:541-545.

Guiney, D. G., Jr., and C. E. Davis. 1978. Identification of a conjugative R plasmid in Bacteroides ochraceus capable of transfer to Escherichia coli. Nature 274:181-182.

Hackman, A. S., and T. D. Wilkins. 1975. In vivo protection of Fusobacterium necrophorum from penicillin by Bacteroides fragilis. Antimicrob. Agents Chemother. 7:698-703.

Hartley, C. L., and M. H. Richmond. 1975. Antibiotic resistance and survival of E. coli in the alimentary tract. Br. Med. J. 4:71-74.

Hirsh, D. C., and N. Wiger. 1977. Effect of tetracycline upon transfer of an R plasmid from calves to human beings. Am. J. Vet. Res. 38:1137-1139.

Hirsh, D. C., and N. Wiger. 1978. The effect of tetracycline upon the spread of bacterial resistance from calves to man. J. Anim. Sci. 46:1437-1446.

Hirsh, D. C., G. C. Burton, and D. C. Blenden. 1973. Effect of oral tetracycline on the occurrence of tetracycline-resistant strains of Escherichia coli in the intestinal tract of humans. Antimicrob. Agents Chemother. 4:69-71.

Hirsh, D. C., G. C. Burton, and D. C. Blenden. 1974. The effect of tetracycline upon establishment of Escherichia coli of bovine origin in the enteric tract of man. J. Appl. Bacteriol. 37:327-333.

Holdeman, L. V., I. J. Good, and W. E. C. Moore. 1976. Human fecal flora: Variation in bacterial composition within individuals and a possible effect of emotional stress. Appl. Environ. Microbiol. 31:359-375.

Howe, K., A. H. Linton, and A. D. Osborne. 1976. The effect of tetracycline on the coliform gut flora of broiler chickens with special reference to antibiotic resistance and O-serotypes of Escherichia coli. J. Appl. Bacteriol. 41:453-464.

Hungate, R. E. 1966. The Rumen and Its Microbes. Academic Press, New York and London. 533 pp.

Kinyon, J. M., and D. L. Harris. 1979. Treponema innocens, a new species of intestinal bacteria, and emended description of the type strain of Treponema hyodysenteriae Harris et al. Int. J. Syst. Bacteriol. 29:102-109.

Klaenhammer, T. R., L. F. Scott, S. M. Sutherland, and M. L. Speck. 1979. Plasmid DNA isolation from Lactobacillus acidophilus and Lactobacillus bulgaricus. P. 132 in Abstracts of the 79th Annual Meeting of the American Society for Microbiology, Los Angeles, Calif., 4-8 May. American Society for Microbiology, Washington, D.C.

Kolacz, J. W., R. B. Wescott, and A. R. Dommert. 1971. Influence of age and rations on fecal microflora of hormel miniature swine. Am. J. Vet. Res. 32:597-602.

Langlois, B. E., G. L. Cromwell, and V. W. Hays. 1978. Influence of type of antibiotic and length of antibiotic feeding period on performance and persistence of antibiotic resistant enteric bacteria in growing-finishing swine. J. Am. Sci. 46:1383-1396.

Larsen, J. L., and N. C. Nielsen. 1975. [In Norwegian; English summary.] Indflydelse af restriktiv antibiotika-anvendelse pa Escherichia coli floraens resistensforhold i svine besaetninger. Nord. Veterinaermed. 27:353-364.

Linton, A. H., K. Howe, and A. D. Osborne. 1975. The effects of feeding tetracycline, nitrovin and quindoxin on the drug-resistance of coli-aerogenes bacteria from calves and pigs. J. Appl. Bacteriol. 38:255-275.

Linton, A. H., K. Howe, P. M. Bennett, M. H. Richmond, and E. J. Whiteside. 1977. The colonization of the human gut by antibiotic resistant Escherichia coli from chickens. J. Appl. Bacteriol. 43:465-469.

Loken, K. I., L. W. Wagner, and C. L. Henke. 1971. Transmissible drug resistance in Enterobacteriaceae isolated from calves given antibiotics. Am. J. Vet. Res. 32:1207-1212.

Malke, H. 1979. Conjugal transfer of plasmids determining resistance to macrolides, lincosamides and streptogramin-B type antibiotics among group A, B, D and H streptococci. Fed. Eur. Microbiol. Lett. 5:335-338.

Mancini, C., and R. J. Behme. 1977. Transfer of multiple antibiotic resistance from Bacteroides fragilis to Escherichia coli. J. Infect. Dis. 136:597-600.

McBee, R. H. 1977. Fermentation in the hindgut. Pp. 185-222 in R. T. J. Clarke and T. Bauchop, eds. Microbial Ecology of the Gut. Academic Press, London, New York, and San Francisco.

McBride, M. E., W. C. Duncan, and J. M. Knox. 1977. The environment and the microbial ecology of human skin. Appl. Environ. Microbiol. 33:603-608.

McCowan, R. P., K. J. Cheng, C. B. M. Bailey, and J. W. Costerton. 1978. Adhesion of bacteria to epithelial cell surfaces within the reticulo-rumen of cattle. Appl. Environ. Microbiol. 35: 149-155.

Mercer, H. D., D. Pocurull, S. Gaines, S. Wilson, and J. V. Bennett. 1971. Characteristics of antimicrobial resistance of Escherichia coli from animals: Relationship to veterinary and management uses of antimicrobial agents. Appl. Microbiol. 22:700-705.

Mitsuoka, T. 1969. [In German; English summary.] Vergleichende Untersuchungen über die Laktobazillen aus den Faeces von Menschen, Schweinen und Hühnern. Zentralbl. Bakteriol. Parasitenkd. Infektionskr. Hyg., I Abt. Orig. 210:32-51.

Mitsuoka, T., and K. Ohno. 1977. [In German; English summary.] Die Faekalflora bei Menschen. V. Mitteilung: Die Schwankungen in der Zusammensetzung der Faekalflora gesunder Erwachsener. Zentralbl. Bakteriol. Parasitenkd. Infektionskr. Hyg., I. Abt. Orig. Reihe A 238:228-236.

Møller, J. K., A. Leth Bak, A. Stenderup, H. Zachariae, and H. Afzelius. 1977. Changing patterns of plasmid-mediated drug resistance during tetracycline therapy. Antimicrob. Agents Chemother. 11:388-391.

Moore, W. E. C., and L. V. Holdeman. 1974. Human fecal flora: The normal flora of 20 Japanese-Hawaiians. Appl. Microbiol. 27:961-979.

Morishita, Y., and T. Mitsuoka. 1976. Microorganisms responsible for controlling the populations of *Escherichia coli* and enterococcus and the consistency of cecal contents in the chicken. Jpn. J. Microbiol. 20:197-202.

Morishita, Y., and M. Ogata. 1970. Studies on the alimentary flora of pig. V. Influence of starvation on the microbial flora. Jpn. J. Vet. Sci. 32:19-24.

Ochi, Y., T. Mitsuoka, and T. Sega. 1964. [In German; English summary.] Untersuchungen über die Darmflora des Huhnes. III. Mitteilung: Die Entwicklung der Darmflora von Küken bis zum Huhn. Zentralbl. Bakteriol. Parasitenkd. Infektionskr. Hyg., Orig. 193:80-95.

Ogata, M., and Y. Morishita. 1969. Studies on the alimentary flora of pigs. IV. The alimentary flora of pigs infected with hog cholera. Jpn. J. Vet. Sci. 31:71-82.

Onderdonk, A. B., D. R. Snydman, M. H. Malamy, and F. P. Tally. 1979. Colonization of germfree mice with *Bacteroides* and transfer of antibiotic resistance *in vivo*. P. 19 in Abstracts of the 79th Annual Meeting of the American Society for Microbiology, Los Angeles, Calif., 4-8 May, and the 79th Annual Meeting of the U.S.-Japan Intersociety Microbiology Congress, Honolulu, Ha., 8-11 May. American Society for Microbiology, Washington, D.C.

Panangala, V. S., and D. A. Barnum. 1978. Antibiotic resistance patterns of organisms isolated from cervico-vaginal mucus of cows. Can. Vet. J. 19:113-118.

Petrocheilou, V., J. Grinsted, and M. H. Richmond. 1976. R-plasmid transfer *in vivo* in the absence of antibiotic selection pressure. Antimicrob. Agents Chemother. 10:753-761.

Phillips, I., C. Warren, J. M. Harrison, P. Sharples, L. C. Ball, and M. T. Parker. 1976. Antibiotic susceptibilities of streptococci from the mouth and blood of patients treated with penicillin or lincomycin and clindamycin. Med. Microbiol. 9:393-404.

Pohl, P., J. Thomas, G. Van Robaeys, and J. Moury. 1977. [In French; English summary.] Résistance de flores colibacillaires en présence et en l'absence d'antibiotique étude dans l'intestin du porc. Annu. Méd. Vét. 121:345-349.

Rollins, L. D., D. W. Pocurull, H. D. Mercer, R. P. Natzke, and D. S. Postle. 1974. Use of antibiotics in a dairy herd and their effect on resistance determinants in enteric and environmental Escherichia coli. J. Dairy Sci. 57:944-950.

Rood, J. I., E. A. Maher, E. B. Somers, E. Campos, and C. L. Duncan. 1978. Isolation and characterization of multiply antibiotic-resistant Clostridium perfringens strains from porcine feces. Antimicrob. Agents Chemother. 13:871-880.

Russell, E. G. 1979. Types and distribution of anaerobic bacteria in the large intestine of pigs. Appl. Environ. Microbiol. 37: 187-193.

Salanitro, J. P., I. G. Blake, and P. A. Muirhead. 1974. Studies on the cecal microflora of commercial broiler chickens. Appl. Microbiol. 28:439-447.

Salanitro, J. P., I. G. Blake, and P. A. Muirhead. 1977. Isolation and identification of fecal bacteria from adult swine. Appl. Environ. Microbiol. 33:79-84.

Salanitro, J. P., I. G. Blake, P. A. Muirhead, M. Maglio, and J. R. Goodman. 1978. Bacteria isolated from the duodenum, ileum, and cecum of young chicks. Appl. Environ. Microbiol. 35:782-790.

Savage, D. C. 1977. Microbial ecology of the gastrointestinal tract. Annu. Rev. Microbiol. 31:107-133.

Savage, D. C., and R. Dubos. 1968. Alterations in the mouse cecum and its flora produced by antibacterial drugs. J. Exp. Med. 128:97-110.

Savage, D. C., and J. S. McAllister. 1971. Cecal enlargement and microbial flora in suckling mice given antibacterial drugs. Infect. Immun. 3:342-349.

Schmidt, H., E. From, and G. Heydenreich. 1973. Bacteriological examination of rectal specimens during long-term oxytetracycline treatment for acne vulgaris. Acta Dermatol. Venereol. 53:153-156.

Sebald, M., and G. Bréfort. 1975. Bactériologie transfert du plasmide tetracycline-chloramphénicol chez Clostridium perfringens. C. R. Acad. Sci., Paris 281:317-319.

Siegel, D., W. G. Huber, and F. Enloe. 1974. Continuous non-therapeutic use of antibacterial drugs in feed and drug resistance of the gram-negative enteric florae of food-producing animals. Antimicrob. Agents Chemother. 6:697-701.

Smith, H. W. 1968. Anti-microbial drugs in animal feeds. Nature 218:728-731.

Smith, H. W. 1975. Persistence of tetracycline resistance in pig E. coli. Nature 258:628-630.

Smith, H. W., and W. E. Crabb. 1960. The effect of diets containing tetracyclines and penicillin on the Staphylococcus aureus flora of the nose and skin of pigs and chickens and their human attendants. J. Pathol. Bacteriol. 79:243-249.

Terada, A., K. Uchida, and T. Mitsuoka. 1976. [In German; English summary.] Die Bacteroidaceenflora in den Faeces von Schweinen. Zentralbl. Bakteriol. Parasitenkd. Infektionskr. Hyg., I Abt. Orig. Reihe A 234:362-370.

Timms, L. 1968. Observations on the bacterial flora of the alimentary tract in three age groups of normal chickens. Br. Vet. J. 124:470-477.

van der Waaij, D., and J. M. Berghuis. 1974. Determination of the colonization resistance of the digestive tract of individual mice. J. Hyg., Camb. 72:379-387.

Van Embden, J. D. A., H. W. B. Engel, and B. Van Klingeren. 1977. Drug resistance in group D streptococci of clinical and nonclinical origin: Prevalence, transferability, and plasmid properties. Antimicrob. Agents Chemother. 11:925-932.

Wang, C. L., B. B. Baldwin, R. S. Fulghum, and P. P. Williams. 1969. Quantitative antibiotic sensitivities of ruminal bacteria. Appl. Microbiol. 18:677-679.

Welch, R. A., K. R. Jones, and F. L. Macrina. 1979. Plasmid-mediated conjugational transfer of lincosamide-macrolide resistance in *Bacteroides*. Plasmid 2:261-268.

APPENDIX E

ANTIMICROBIAL RESIDUES AND RESISTANT ORGANISMS: THEIR OCCURRENCE, SIGNIFICANCE, AND STABILITY

Stanley E. Katz[1]

The occurrence of antibiotic residues in animal tissue and animal products resulting from the subtherapeutic, prophylactic, or therapeutic use of antibiotics is a function of the antibiotic, the method of application, the level of treatment, and, most importantly, adherance to withdrawal periods. Because of the extreme variability in both the use of drugs and adherence to withdrawal periods, it is inevitable that residues would occur in a small but significant percent of animal products found in the marketplace.

RESIDUE LEVELS FROM SUBTHERAPEUTIC ANTIBIOTIC USE

Huber (1971) reported the results of a 1969 survey of animals slaughtered in Illinois, Wisconsin, Iowa, and Indiana. In 27% of the swine slaughtered, there was evidence of recent treatment with antibacterial substances, of which 10% were penicillin. Because of the lack of visible evidence of injection, these residues most likely were the result of improper withdrawal times or levels of usage. There was a 9% rate of positive findings in beef cattle, 2% of which were attributed to penicillin. In veal, 7% of 17% of the samples in which antibiotics were found resulted from penicillin. Some 21% of market lambs were positive for antibacterial residues. Of these, 4% were positive for penicillin. The presence of antimicrobial residues was found in 26% of the chickens, 6% of which were positive for penicillin activity. The incidence of antibiotic residues in milk during the early 1950's was approximately 11%, dropping to 0.5% at the time of Huber's report.

Mussman (1975) reviewed the inspection and sampling procedures used in the U.S. Department of Agriculture (USDA) program to monitor levels of residues in conformance with Food and Drug Administration (FDA) regulations and analyzed the data contained in the USDA *Biological Residue Report* for 1973 (USDA, 1974). The USDA figures indicated that 5.3% of 529 carcass samples examined for residues of streptomycin, tetracycline, erythromycin, neomycin, oxytetracycline, and chlortetracycline were positive; only 17 of

[1]Department of Biochemistry and Microbiology, Cook College - New Jersey Agricultural Experiment Station, Rutgers University, The State University of New Jersey, New Brunswick, N.J.

5,301 samples, or 0.32%, were positive for penicillin; and 12 samples of 728, or 1.6%, were positive for sulfonamides. Non-specific antimicrobial activity was found in 154 (2.9%) of 5,301 samples.

Table 1 summarizes the U.S. Department of Agriculture sampling program for 1976-1978. Violations exist when residue levels exceed established tolerances or when residues are found when no residue is permitted.

If the results of the USDA sampling program are at all representative, there is no doubt that violative residues occur in almost all animals used for food and that residues that are not in violation occur in even higher percentages. The rates of antibiotic and sulfonamide residue violations are lowest among poultry and cattle, and the highest rates occur in swine and in veal calves.

The levels of residues that can be expected from feeding subtherapeutic quantities of antibiotics vary with the degree of absorption from the intestinal tract. Because of very poor absorption from the intestine, residues resulting from the consumption of such antibiotics as streptomycin, neomycin, bacitracin, and the bambermycins rarely, if ever, occur. Residues from the subtherapeutic feeding of chlortetracycline (CTC) and oxytetracycline (OTC) occur regularly and have been also reported for penicillin. In chickens, the continuous feeding of 50 to 200 g of CTC per ton of feed resulted in residue levels ranging from 0.036 to 0.11 μg CTC/g muscle tissue and from 0.058 to 0.199 μg CTC/g liver tissue (Katz _et al._, 1972). These residues disappeared after 1 day of withdrawal from the medicated feed.

Messersmith _et al._ (1967) reported residue levels of 0.08 μg CTC/g muscle and 0.46 μg CTC/g liver resulting from feeding 100 g CTC/ton to swine. After a 5-day withdrawal, no detectable levels could be measured in muscle and fat, but trace levels were detected in the liver and kidney. Gale _et al._ (1967) reported from 0.04 to 0.08 μg CTC/g muscle and from 0.24 to 0.46 μg CTC/g liver from the continuous feeding of 100 g/ton. After a 5-day withdrawal period, there were no measurable levels in muscle, and only trace levels could be found in the liver. OTC residues occurring in poultry muscle from the continuous feeding of 25 to 200 g/ton were approximately 1/1,000 of the feeding level. This is similar to levels resulting from the feeding of CTC. Measurable tissue residues of CTC disappeared after a 1-day withdrawal period (Katz _et al._, 1972). Cooking destroyed all residues of both OTC and CTC in the muscle (Katz _et al._, 1972, 1973; Meredith _et al._, 1965). The only CTC residues surviving cooking were found in the liver.

TABLE 1

Violative Actions for Antibiotics and Sulfonamides[a]

Species	Antibiotic Samples	Viola-tions	%	Sulfonamide Samples	Viola-tions	%
1976:						
Cattle	545	7	1.3	476	4	0.
Calves	1,378	118	8.6	327	12	3.
Sheep and goats	70	5	7.1	100	1	1.
Swine	247	4	1.6	1,493	141	9.
Chickens	155	1	0.6	331	1	0.
Turkeys	258	0	0.0	648	16	2.
Geese and ducks	160	1	0.6	265	0	0.
1977:						
Cattle	1,739	22	1.3	175	4	2.
Calves	1,120	46	4.1	166	5	3.
Sheep and goats	176	2	1.1	12	0	0.
Swine	449	6	1.3	9,461	1,242	13.
Chickens	366	0	0.0	1	0	0.
Turkeys	450	3	0.7	445	4	0.
Geese and ducks	161	1	0.6	206	1	0.
1978:						
Cattle	1,769	46	2.6	243	2	0.
Calves	1,409	94	6.7	214	6	2.
Sheep and goats	210	5	2.4	40	6	15.
Swine	1,399	76	5.4	6,687	648	9.
Chickens	470	8	1.7	119	1	0.
Turkeys	447	15	3.3	443	19	4.
Geese and ducks	175	2	1.1	148	0	0.

[a]From U.S. Department of Agriculture, 1977-1979.

Residues of OTC and CTC in eggs were not completely destroyed by cooking. The lower temperatures and shorter times of cooking were responsible for the survival of the residues.

Filson *et al.* (1965) found CTC levels ranging from 0.072 μg/ml in the serum of old birds to 0.330 μg/ml in the serum of young birds that had received 200 g of the antibiotic per ton of feed. They reported no muscle deposition levels, but it is generally assumed that muscle residue levels usually correspond to serum levels.

Another potential source of tetracycline residues, especially if the kidneys are used as the indicator organ, would be tetracyclines released from deposition in the bones. Brüggemann *et al.* (1966) noted that the bones of all domestic animals fed tetracycline contain measureable amounts of the antibiotic. After the feeding of the tetracycline ceases, levels in the bones decrease, indicating mobilization and excretion.

After feeding pigs 100 μg procaine penicillin per gram of feed, Loftsgaard *et al.* (1968) found residues of 2 μg/ml urine and levels in muscle no higher than 0.005 μg/g. Kidney levels ranged from 0.003 to 0.24 μg/g, and liver levels were 0.012 μg/g. After feeding the unmedicated basal ration for 24 hours, the investigators found no measurable antibiotic activity. However, residues from intramuscular injections of procaine penicillin disappeared by day 6. After injections of benzathine penicillin G, activity was detected in the urine and kidney for as long as 14 days.

The feeding of procaine penicillin to broilers and laying hens did not result in any penicillin activity in the blood, muscle, liver, and kidney tissue of broilers or in the eggs of hens fed 100 g/ton. Approximately 98% of the penicillin activity was destroyed in the upper portion of the intestinal tract, and little or no activity reached the small intestine (Katz *et al.*, 1974; Messersmith *et al.*, 1967). One of the major degradation products was penicilloic acid.

McCracken (1977) reported that intramuscular injections of 3 mg penicillin and OTC per kilogram of body weight yielded muscle residue levels less than 0.04 μg/g and 0.20 μg/g, respectively. Surprisingly, no residues in muscle were found after an intramuscular injection of neomycin at 100 mg/kg.

These few reports indicate that OTC and CTC residues can and do appear as a result of subtherapeutic and therapeutic oral feeding. Residues attributed to the feeding of penicillin were variable, but tended to be very low or at the level of detectability of the methodology used. Most of the analytical methods used for penicillin were capable of detecting levels of 0.0125 μg/g or less.

FATE OF ANTIBIOTIC RESIDUES

Residues of the tetracyclines in the muscle tissue of animals will not survive normal food preparation procedures. No residues will enter the diet of humans unless the muscle tissue is eaten raw or very rare. Cooking degrades CTC to isochlortetracycline (Shirk *et al.*, 1957), and OTC is thought to be converted to α- and β-apooxytetracyclines (Katz *et al.*, 1973). The literature contains no data to indicate that either of these compounds has any biological significance.

Tetracycline residues remain only in products that are subjected to a minimum amount of cooking. Even in chickens soaked in CTC solutions to increase shelf life, which resulted in tissue levels of 3 μg/g or greater (Broquist *et al.*, 1956), no residues could be measured after cooking (Kohler *et al.*, 1955). However, if residues do survive cooking, the potential for biological action remains. After feeding raw chicken meat containing an average of 2.6 μg/g CTC to dogs, Rollins *et al.* (1975) found an increase in the number of resistant coliforms shed by the dogs.

The metabolic fate of tetracycline has been studied by several investigators. Kelly and Buyske (1960) found that tetracycline was metabolically unaltered in the rat and, for the most part, in the dog. Eisner and Wulf (1963) reported that epichlortetracycline and demethylchlortetracycline were metabolic products of CTC. The formation of isochlortetracycline in the intestinal tract of poultry was observed by Shirk *et al.* (1957). Katz and Fassbender (1967) reported that epichlortetracycline and an unknown highly fluorescent compound was formed in feeds, but that isochlortetracycline was not. These authors suggested that an equilibrium was established between CTC and its epimer followed by a breakdown of either the CTC or its epimer into unidentified products.

There is no apparent significance to the presence of tetracycline residues if the product is adequately cooked, unless some unknown compound forms in the animals fed the antibiotics or the breakdown products of tetracyclines stimulate the development of resistance in enteric organisms or the transfer of resistance determinants between R^+ *Escherichia coli* and recipient *E. coli* or salmonellae. In Great Britain, the data indicate that the destruction of CTC and OTC residues during cooking renders the meat adequately safe for consumption by humans (Brander, 1970).

ALLERGIC RESPONSE

The situation is somewhat different with penicillin residues. Huber (1971) reported that 10% of the general population is sensitive to penicillin. McGovern *et al.* (1970) stated that from 1% to 10% of the population of North America and Western Europe may be allergic to it. Parker (1963) and Levine and Ovary (1961) suggested that degradation products from acid and alkaline breakdowns could be responsible for hypersensitivity reactions. Altman and Tompkins (1978) reported that penicillin degrades, forming benzyl penicilloic acid, a major determinant of hypersensitivity, and some minor determinants. These degradation products are haptens that can become antigens when they conjugate to endogenous protein *in vivo*. Katz *et al.* (1974) found that penicilloic acid formed in the intestinal tract of chickens that had been fed growth promotional and prophylactic levels of penicillin.

Weinstein (1975) estimated that 66% of a dose of penicillin passed into the intestine of humans where it was inactivated. Such inactivation would undoubtedly lead to the formation of penicilloic acid and the possible adsorption and deposition of this compound into muscle tissue.

The use of injectables and the residues resulting from them can always be a source of unwanted and potentially dangerous residues. Perhaps the only truly documented death resulting from residues of penicillin occurred when a butcher consumed fresh pork that contained 0.31 μg/g penicillin (Tscheyschner, 1972).

As early as 1956 it was known that penicillin residues could survive pasteurization at 60°C and 71°C, but not at 121°C (Shahani *et al.*, 1956). Katz *et al.* (1978) reported that penicillin residues in meat could survive all but the most rigorous cooking. These investigators measured only penicillin activity and provided no information concerning the degradation products.

Breakdown Products

The literature does not provide much information regarding the significance of breakdown products in relation to potential hypersensitivity reactions from eating products containing residues and breakdown products of penicillin. Warrington *et al.* (1978) found that both the major and minor degradation products of benzyl penicillin were useful reagents in determining hypersensitivity. Hypersensitivity of one-fifth of the patients that they tested would have been missed if only the major product had been tested. Borrie and Barrett (1961) reported the case history of a woman who had relapses of allergy when she consumed dairy products. The problem disappeared when the patient received no commercial dairy products or milk known to be free from penicillin.

Batchelor *et al.* (1967) reported that a penicilloylated polymer with a high molecular weight produced immunological responses in the guinea pig.

Ferrando (1975) reported that 40 units of benzyl penicillin was sufficient to trigger allergic responses in very sensitive individuals. He noted that some investigators have suggested that from 2 to 3 units of penicillin would trigger anaphylactic reactions in sensitive people. From his own calculations and from the opinions expressed by allergists in France and elsewhere in Europe, he believes that the risk is "more theoretical than real."

The significance to human health of the residues of penicillin and its breakdown products cannot be determined by reviewing the literature. However, it is known that the breakdown products of penicillin do have biological significance ranging from their ability to sensitize individuals to their action as selecting agents for the development of antibiotic resistance in *E. coli*. Since up to 10% of the population is potentially sensitive to penicillin and its breakdown products, the risk is too great to be ignored. Oral feeding of subtherapeutic doses of penicillin should be avoided, and injections should be carefully controlled.

ROUTES OF ADMINISTRATION

Residues of other antibiotics resulting from injections can be a more serious problem than residues attributed to feeding because of the higher concentrations that can be deposited and/or sequestered in the tissue. As was noted previously, the only documented fatality from hypersensitivity to penicillin was caused by a penicillin residue that resulted from an injection of the antibiotic. Gaines *et al.* (1978) pointed out that dihydrostreptomycin residues of 2 and 10 μg/g, which were observed in bovine kidneys after intramuscular injection or intramammary infusion, caused a significant increase in resistance in the enteric bacteria of animals. Residues of dihydrostreptomycin, unlike those of tetracycline, are known to be refractory to thermal decomposition (Inglis and Katz, 1978) and are strong selectors of resistant organisms (Huber, 1971). Wilson (1958) reported that streptomycin readily sensitized from 2% to 3% of the nurses who handled it.

Residues of neomycin have been found in serum and urine up to 144 hours after administration of an intramuscular injection. Residues of this antibiotic have been reported to be relatively stable in cooked eggs (Katz and Levine, 1978) and in cooked muscle tissue of animals (Katz and Levine, 1980, unpublished data).

Residues arising from injectables are a more serious problem because of the high levels in which they accumulate. Therefore, every effort must be made to minimize the use of injectables in animals going to market.

THE ROLE OF RESIDUES IN THE DEVELOPMENT OF RESISTANCE

It is doubtful that antibiotic residues or their degradation products will provide any selective pressure on enteric bacteria contaminating the carcasses of animals. Residue levels are usually low, contact time in relation to the number of generations relatively short, the nutritional requirements too variable and usually insufficient for sustained growth, and the temperature of storage too low for growth. The selection process requires the inhibition of susceptible strains, thereby allowing the more resistant strains to grow. The transfer of resistant determinants between strains of *E. coli* would be of low frequency, or nonexistent, for all the aforementioned reasons. The resistant organisms contaminating the carcasses come from the environment of the slaughterhouse itself--not from the residues that may be present.

THE EFFECT OF REGULATION ON RESIDUES

Enforcement of FDA regulations controlling tolerances for antibiotic residues is a function of the perceived seriousness of the problem and the amount of money that regulatory agencies budget for this purpose. It is both impossible and impractical to design a program to insure that every animal going to slaughter and every gallon of milk is free of residues. The USDA sampling program, which results in the *Biological Residue Reports* (e.g., USDA, 1977-1979) is the first line of information allowing regulatory officials to define a problem and marshall efforts to solve it. Practices that can result in residues, such as ignoring withdrawal times, the use of antibiotics beyond the period of effective growth promotion, the subtle sales approach used by the drug companies suggesting that continuous usage could be an "insurance policy" protecting against carcass condemnations, should be modified.

There is no doubt that strict adherence to proper usage and adherence to withdrawal periods, which are both stimulated by increased regulatory activity, will minimize the residue problem. This regulatory approach was successful in lowering the incidence of residues in milk from 11% to 0.5% (Huber, 1971) and appears to be having similar success with the sulfonamide residues in swine. Only through monitoring and changes in agricultural practice can the problem be minimized. State Agricultural Experiment Stations, through their research and extension arms, should provide the farmer with the knowledge to develop proper agricultural practices. The pharmaceutical industry should sell farmers only effective drugs and stipulate adamantly the requirements for their use. Considering the size and complexity of the enforcement problem and the limits of the laboratory and inspection staffs, regulatory efforts are reasonable.

EXCRETION OF ANTIBIOTICS

Antibiotics that are not absorbed, not metabolized or are free or bound in a conjugated form are excreted in the feces and urine. Antibiotics such as streptomycin, which are not readily absorbed, are excreted in their active form (Huber, 1971). Neomycin, like streptomycin, is poorly absorbed in the gut and is excreted unchanged in the feces (Weinstein, 1975). Bacitracin is poorly absorbed from the intestinal tract, but a large percentage of the dose is destroyed in the intestinal tract (Scudi *et al.*, 1947).

Many different antimicrobials are absorbed in varying amounts from the intestinal tract. Those that are most easily absorbed, such as the tetracyclines, are excreted in both urine and feces. Huber (1977) estimated that from 10% to 25% of an oral dose of the tetracyclines is excreted in the feces. Elmund *et al.* (1971) observed that 75% of the CTC ingested by yearling steers was excreted. Alderson *et al.* (1975) reported that 21% of the OTC fed to sheep was recovered from the feces. In the accumulated feces of feedlots, the level of tetracyclines extracted was 75% of that fed (Elmund *et al.*, 1971). Webb and Fontenot (1975) reported that the litter of broilers contained levels of OTC ranging from 5.5 to 29.1 $\mu g/g$

(average, 10.9 μg/g); CTC ranging from 0.8 to 26.3 μg/g (average, 12.5 μg/g); penicillin ranging from 0 to 25 μg/g (average 12.5 μg/g); bacitracin levels ranging from 0.16 to 36.0 μg/g (average, 12.3 μg/g); and arsenic residues ranging from 1.1 to 59.7 μg/g (average 40.4 μg/g). They found no residues of neomycin.

Arsenicals are excreted unchanged and can be recovered from feces at a level of 0.1 μg/g after 12 days of ingesting the compound in doses of 90 g/ton (Overby and Frost, 1960). Morrison (1969) reported a rather constant level of arsenic in soil after 20 years of fertilization with poultry litter. This finding may be related to metabolism and microbial conversions. Arsenicals, such as 3-nitro-4-hydroxyphenylarsonic acid, are partially reduced to the 3-amino product. Moreover, arsanilic acid residues can be metabolized to arsenate in soils (Woolson, 1977).

PERSISTENCE OF ANTIMICROBIALS IN SOILS

In agricultural areas, residues of antimicrobials can be leached from soils and pastures into streams. Van Dijck and Van de Voorde (1976) reported that 12 of 41 water samples showed inhibitory activity against *Staphylococcus aureus*, but believed that the low activity in the water samples posed no hazard. Unfortunately, they made no attempt to correlate this inhibition with the types of antimicrobials used in the area.

There is a paucity of definitive information on the degradation of antibiotics and antimicrobials in the environment. Although Jefferys (1952) observed that penicillin is readily inactivated in garden soils, the FDA (1978) reported that no information was available on the *time* required for the inactivation in soils or in wastes from animals. Streptomycin forms such strong complexes with clays that it can be irreversibly inactivated at low levels (Pinck *et al.*, 1961). Soulides *et al.* (1961) observed that bioactive streptomycin can be desorbed, and Pramer and Starkey (1951, 1972) reported that it could be microbiologically decomposed in soil.

The FDA (1978) summarized the information on the stability of tetracyclines in the environment. In soils, where as much as 5 tons of waste from cattle feedlots was applied per acre as a fertilizer, no measurable CTC activity could be detected. Rumsey *et al.* (1975) reported that measurable levels of CTC were not found in most run-off water from pastures on which wastes containing that antibiotic had been spread. Little pertinent information has been reported for OTC. Metcalf (1976) reported that sulfamethazine was biodegradable in a 33-day terrestrial-aquatic model ecosystem, but he provided no data on the stability of the compound in soils and in mixtures of feces and soil.

From the data available it is difficult to make an accurate assessment of the persistence of antibiotics in the environment.

We know that antibiotics degrade in soils, but must learn how quickly they do and what effects they have on the bacterial populations in the soil. Antibiotics are added to the soil in a mixture of feces, urine, and bedding that probably does not exceed 50 tons per acre. Therefore, this mixture accounts for no more than 5% of the top 15-cm layer of soil. Based on the average amount of antibiotics in broiler litter ($\sim$12.5 μg/g) (Webb and Fontenot, 1975), the level of antibiotic in the soil would be approximately 0.6 μg/g. Because of the absorptive reactions, the low concentrations of antibiotics, and the variety of organisms available to act upon the antibiotic molecules, it is doubtful that the antibiotics will persist for any great length of time in the soil.

Will low levels of antibiotics added to the soil cause the development of antibiotic-resistant populations? There is no general answer. It is doubtful that penicillin will survive sufficiently long in soil to act as a selective agent (Jefferys, 1952). Jefferys also reported that streptomycin was absorbed irreversibly into soil at relatively low concentrations and became inactivated. Hence, streptomycin would be an unlikely selective agent. The tetracyclines can survive microbial degradation in the gut of animals and be present in fresh manure at a concentration of 14 μg/g and at 0.34 μg/g in aged manure (Elmund *et al.*, 1971). The degradation of CTC in soil fertilized with cattle feedlot manure was indicated by a finding of no measurable CTC (Rumsey *et al.*, 1975). Although soluble, weakly absorbed, and potentially mobile in the soil, it is doubtful that the tetracyclines will be a strong selective agent.

SHEDDING OF RESISTANT ORGANISMS

Animals fed antibiotics shed antibiotic-resistant organisms (Smith, 1969; Smith and Crabb, 1957). The longer they are fed antibiotics, the greater the percentage of antibiotic-resistant organisms that will be shed. For the most part, the ubiquitous *E. coli* has been used as an indicator organism because it is representative of the Gram-negative enteric bacilli, but resistance in other genera is as common as in E. coli. Kelch and Lee (1978) noted that the antibiotic resistance pattern of Gram-negative bacteria of different genera correlated well with patterns found with E. coli, indicating that bacteria that share a common environment also share a common mode for developing resistance to antibiotics.

E. coli, in freshly voided feedlot manure, numbered 2.5 x 10^7 colony-forming units (CFU)/g (Thayer et al., 1974). This is as representative an estimation as any available. There is no exact number or even a totally representative value since numbers range from 10^5 to 10^8 CFU/g feces, depending on the species and age of the animals.

More than 200 species of bacteria are estimated to be present in the intestinal tracts of humans and other warm-blooded animals (Moore, 1969). In excess of 90% of the intestinal bacteria consist of the lactobacilli, enterococci, and the less oxygen-sensitive bacteroides. Smith and Crabb (1957, 1961) reported 10^{10} to 10^{11} total bacteria per gram of feces from several species of animals. E. coli comprise approximately 1% of the estimated total count, or 10^8 organisms per gram of feces.

Estimates of levels of resistance or of increases or decreases in resistance involve large numbers of organisms. To say that only 1% of the E. coli in feces are resistant is to lose sight of the fact that this involves 10^6 CFU/g. Even the 1% value represents a very large number of organisms.

Ahart et al. (1978) reported that 100% of the fecal samples from calves and pigs, 56% of the fecal samples from humans, 36% of the fecal samples from horses, 90% of the fecal samples from dogs, and 67% of the fecal samples from cats contained tetracycline-resistant coliforms. They concluded that the 1971 prohibition of the subtherapeutic use of tetracyclines in Great Britain resulted in little or no difference in the shedding of tetracycline-resistant strains of E. coli by pigs.

Smith (1970, 1975) summarized sensitivity testing data for tetracycline-resistant E. coli shed by pigs. He concluded that resistant populations may have decreased slightly but that the prohibition did not have any great impact during the study, which was conducted from 1971 to 1975. These observations underline the potential fallacy in assuming that ecological changes can be reversed simply by withdrawing the subtherapeutic use of antibiotics.

Once in the environment, soil, and/or water, organisms shed by animals tend to persist for extended periods. Throughout a 13-month observation period, Thayer *et al.* (1974) found surviving coliforms in a 4-year-old stockpile of feedlot manure. The estimated number of survivors was 2.5×10^7 CFU/g in fresh manure, 8.6×10^4 CFU/g in the top layer of accumulated manure, and 5.7×10^5 CFU/g in the middle layer.

Rankin and Taylor (1969) studied the potential disease hazards resulting from applying a slurry of cattle waste to a pasture. He found pathogens among the isolates, albeit in low frequency. These organisms survived from 11 to 12 weeks with no evidence of multiplication. Evans and Owens (1972) observed a 90% reduction in the numbers of organisms in pasture drainage water in 57 days. Tannock and Smith (1971) reported that salmonellae survived in contaminated waters for 12 weeks. Berkowitz *et al.* (1974) concluded that the application to soil of animal excreta containing large numbers of pathogens was not an acceptable practice because of the long survival time of pathogens in dried excreta.

SURVIVAL IN THE ENVIRONMENT

Cooke (1976a,b,c) noted a high incidence of resistance among coliforms isolated from sewage, freshwater, seawater, marine shellfish, freshwater mussels, and effluents. He reported that 48.7% of the total coliform isolates from tainted wells were resistant to one or more antibiotics, 67.5% of the isolates from the freshwater mussel had multiple antibiotic resistance, and 71.5% of the coliforms isolated from seawater were resistant. Because of these relatively high percentages of resistance, Cooke hypothesized that antibiotic-resistant bacteria may have a selective advantage for survival once these organisms are disseminated into natural waters.

Sewage treatment plants reduced the number of coliforms but did not remove the antibiotic-resistant strains from the effluent selectively or effectively. This observation was supported by Smith *et al.* (1974) who demonstrated that there were no significant changes in the ratios of presumptive fecal coliforms and fecal coliforms carrying R-factors between incoming sewage and effluents.

Grabow *et al.* (1975) found no difference in the survival of antibiotic-resistant and antibiotic-sensitive strains in distilled water, saline water, or in dialysis bags immersed in river water. Smith *et al.* (1974) noted that the survival of *E. coli* in seawater is not affected by the fact that they carry R factors.

Anderson (1974) found that the number of organisms carrying R factors declined faster in the gut than did sensitive strains and that they may be at an ecological disadvantage in nature in the absence of selection pressure from antibiotics. He suggested that the rapid decline in the resistant organisms resulted from an impaired vitality of the organisms rather than the loss of R factors from the cell.

Although there is a difference of opinion regarding whether resistant strains have a selective advantage for survival in the environment over nonresistant strains, the evidence in favor of their not having a selective advantage is more compelling. Anderson's observations of a decline in the number of antibiotic-resistant organisms in some populations, Grabow's comparison of survival in various waters, and Smith's observations all point to the fact that there are no easily measurable differences in survival rates in the environment between resistant and nonresistant *E. coli* strains. If anything, there might be a slight advantage to the antibiotic-sensitive *E. coli* because of the observations that resistant populations decline and are replaced by nonresistant strains over an extended period. However, there is one inescapable fact: because both antibiotic-resistant and sensitive strains survive for long periods in the environment, changes of populations will be slow.

The source of the relatively high incidence of antibiotic-resistant *E. coli* in sewage, effluents, and streams can never be established. Only where the sources of the organisms are easily discernible can a considered judgment be made.

Smith (1970) concluded that human beings rather than animals are the main source of antibiotic-resistant *E. coli*. He found that the incidence of antibiotic-resistant organisms was generally low in rivers and canals that flowed through rural areas and high in rivers that flowed through urban areas. In waters with the highest incidence of antibiotic-resistant organisms, inadequately treated sewage was the source. No antibiotic-resistant *E. coli* were found in a river before it entered predominantly urban areas.

Feary *et al.* (1972) concluded that the high incidence of resistance to streptomycin and tetracycline among coliforms isolated from waters near livestock feedlots were probably a direct result of the use of antibiotics in the feed. Hughes and Meynell (1974) indicated that there has been an increase in antibiotic-resistant coliforms in rivers since 1970. Popp (1974) reported that thorough treatment of sewage failed to remove salmonellae and that there were considerable numbers of the organisms in the water into which the treated sewage flowed. Morse and Duncan (1974) concluded that the aquatic environment was a favorable environment for the survival of salmonellae.

The above data seem to indicate that human beings rather than animals are the main source of antibiotic-resistant E. coli in the environment.

CONCLUSIONS

Several conclusions can be drawn from literature reviewed, namely:

(1) The incidence of antibiotic residues in animal products will continue at a relatively modest rate regardless of surveys and enforcement procedures. The current surveillance procedures are extremely effective in identifying problem areas, but no regulatory system can guarantee a "residue-free" food supply.

(2) Residues of oxytetracycline and chlortetracycline will usually not enter the human diet unless the foods containing these residues are subjected to minimal cooking times and temperatures. Hence, such residues should not be considered a serious factor in the development of resistance among intestinal microorganisms. The thermal degradation products of the tetracyclines are not known to have any biological effects.

(3) Penicillin residues and related breakdown products are not innocuous and have the potential of causing hypersensitivity reactions. Because approximately 10% of the population is potentially sensitive to penicillin and its breakdown products, the subtherapeutic feeding of penicillin should be avoided and the use of injectable forms carefully controlled.

(4) Antibiotic residues and/or their degradation products are doubtful agents for the selection of antibiotic-resistant organisms or as promoters of resistance transfer on the carcasses of animals. Resistant organisms result from contamination by intestinal contents during the handling of the carcasses.

(5) Although there is a paucity of definitive information, the available data indicate that antibiotics are not stable in the soil and should not act as a selective agent for the development of antibiotic resistance among microorganisms in the soil.

(6) Antibiotic-resistant microorganisms shed by animals persist for extended periods in the environment but do not appear to have any superior advantage for survival as compared to sensitive strains.

(7) Although animal agriculture contributes drug-resistant species to the environment, especially in rural areas, human beings rather than animals appear to be the main source of antibiotic-resistant organisms in the environment.

REFERENCES

Ahart, J. G., G. C. Burton, and D. C. Blenden. 1978. The influence of antimicrobial agents on the percentage of tetracycline-resistant bacteria in faeces of humans and animals. J. Appl. Bacteriol. 44:183-190.

Alderson, N. E., W. Knight, R. Robinson, J. Colaianne, and P. Bradley. 1975. Ovine absorption and excretion of oxytetracycline. J. Anim. Sci. 41:388-399 (Abstract).

Altman, L. C., and L. S. Tompkins. 1978. Toxic and allergic manifestations of antimicrobials. Postgrad. Med. 64:157-167.

Anderson, J. D. 1974. The effect of R-factor carriage on the survival of Escherichia coli in the human intestine. J. Med. Microbiol. 7:85-90.

Batchelor, F. R., J. M. Dewdney, J. G. Feinberg, and R. D. Weston. 1967. A penicilloyalted protein impurity as a source of allergy to benzyl-penicillin and 6-aminopenicillanic acid. Lancet 2:1175-1177.

Berkowitz, J. H., D. J. Kraft, and M. S. Finstein. 1974. Persistence of salmonellae in poultry excreta. J. Environ. Qual. 3: 158-160.

Borrie, P., and J. Barrett. 1961. Dermatitis caused by penicillin in bulked milk supplies. Br. Med. J. 2:1267.

Brander, G. C. 1970. Possible hazards to man from the use of drugs in and on animals. Br. Med. Bull. 26:217-221.

Broquist, H. P., A. R. Kohler, and W. H. Miller. 1956. Retardation of poultry spoilage by processing with chlortetracycline. Agric. Food Chem. 4:1030-1032.

Brüggemann, J., U. Lösch, M. Merkenschlager, and I. Offterdinger. 1966. [In German; English summary.] Ablagerung von Tetracyclin im Knocengewelbe von Tieren bei dem Zusatz von Tetracyclin zum Futter. Zentralbl. Veterinaermed. 13:59-74.

Cooke, M. D. 1976a. Antibiotic resistance among coliform and faecal coliform bacteria from natural waters and effluents. N. Z. J. Mar. Freshwater Res. 10:391-397.

Cooke, M. D. 1976b. Antibiotic resistance among coliform and fecal coliform bacteria isolated from the freshwater mussel _Hydridella menziesii_. Antimicrob. Agents Chemother. 9:885-888.

Cooke, M. D. 1976c. Antibiotic resistance among coliform and fecal coliform bacteria isolated from sewage, seawater, and marine shellfish. Antimicrob. Agents Chemother. 9:879-884.

Eisner, H. J., and R. J. Wulf. 1963. The metabolic fate of chlortetracycline and some comparisons with other tetracyclines. J. Pharmacol. Exp. Ther. 142:122-131.

Elmund, G. K., S. M. Morrison, D. W. Grant, and M. P. Nevins. 1971. Role of excreted chlortetracycline in modifying the decomposition process in feedlot waste. Bull. Environ. Contam. Toxicol. 6:129-132.

Evans, M. R., and J. D. Owens. 1972. Factors affecting the concentration of faecal bacteria in land-drainage water. J. Gen. Microbiol. 71:477-485.

Feary, T. W., A. B. Sturtevant, Jr., and J. Lankford. 1972. Antibiotic-resistant coliforms in fresh and salt water. Arch. Environ. Health 25:215-220.

Ferrando, R. 1975. Future of additives in animal feeding. World Rev. Nutr. Diet. 22:183-235.

Filson, D. R., H. H. Weiser, W. E. Meredith, and A. R. Winter. 1965. Absorption of chlortetracycline from the alimentary tract in white leghorn hens. Poult. Sci. 44:761-767.

Food and Drug Administration. 1978. Draft Environmental Impact Statement--Subtherapeutic Antibacterial Agents in Animal Feed. Bureau of Veterinary Medicine, Food and Drug Administration, Department of Health, Education, and Welfare, Rockville, Md. [371 + xviii] pp.

Gaines, S. A., L. D. Rollins, R. R. Silver, and M. Washington. 1978. Effect of low concentrations of dihydrostreptomycin on drug resistance in enteric bacteria. Antimicrob. Agents Chemother. 14:252-256.

Gale, G. O., A. Abbey, and A. L. Shor. 1967. Disappearance of chlortetracycline residues from edible tissues of animals fed rations containing the drug. I. Cattle and swine. Antimicrob. Agents Chemother. 7:749-756.

Grabow, W. O. K., O. W. Prozesky, and J. S. Burger. 1975. Behavior in a river and dam of coliform bacteria with transferable or non-transferable drug resistance. Water Res. 9:777-782.

Huber, W. G. 1971. The impact of antibiotic drugs and their residues. Adv. Vet. Sci. Comp. Med. 15:101-132.

Huber, W. G. 1977. Streptomycin, chloramphenicol, and other antibacterial agents. Pp. 940-971 in L. Meyer Jones, N. H. Booth, and L. E. McDonald, eds. Veterinary Pharmacology and Therapeutics. Fourth Edition. Iowa State University Press, Ames, Ia.

Hughes, C., and G. G. Meynell. 1974. High frequency of antibiotic-resistant enterobacteria in the River Stour, Kent. Lancet 2:451-453.

Inglis, J. M., and S. E. Katz. 1978. Determination of streptomycin residues in eggs and stability of residues after cooking. J. Assoc. Off. Anal. Chem. 61:1098-1102.

Jefferys, E. G. 1952. The stability of antibiotics in soils J. Gen. Microbiol. 7:295-312.

Katz, S. E., and C. A. Fassbender. 1967. Studies on the stability of chlortetracycline in mixed feeds: Epimerization of chlortetracycline. J. Assoc. Off. Anal. Chem. 50:821-827.

Katz, S. E., and P. R. Levine. 1978. Determination of neomycin residues in eggs and stability of residues after cooking. J. Assoc. Off. Anal. Chem. 61:1103-1106.

Katz, S. E., C. A. Fassbender, D. Dorfman, and J. J. Dowling, Jr. 1972. Chlortetracycline residues in broiler tissue and organs. J. Assoc. Off. Anal. Chem. 55:134-138.

Katz, S. E., C. A. Fassbender, and J. J. Dowling, Jr. 1973. Oxytetracycline residues in tissue, organs, and eggs of poultry fed supplemented rations. J. Assoc. Off. Anal. Chem. 56:77-81.

Katz, S. E., C. A. Fassbender, P. S. Dinnerstein, and J. J. Dowling, Jr. 1974. Effects of feeding penicillin to chickens. J. Assoc. Off. Anal. Chem. 57:522-526.

Katz, S. E., C. A. Fassbender, A. M. DePaolis, and J. D. Rosen. 1978. Improved microbiological assay for penicillin residues in tissues and stability of residues under cooking procedures. J. Assoc. Off. Anal. Chem. 61:564-568.

Kelch, W. J., and J. S. Lee. 1978. Antibiotic resistance patterns of gram-negative bacteria isolated from environmental sources. Appl. Environ. Microbiol. 36:450-456.

Kelly, R. G., and D. A. Buyske. 1960. Metabolism of tetracycline in the rat and the dog. J. Pharmacol. Exp. Ther. 130:144-149.

Kohler, A. R., W. H. Miller, and H. P. Broquist. 1955. Aureomycin chlortetracycline and the control of poultry spoilage. Food Technol. 9:151-154.

Levine, B. B., and Z. Ovary. 1961. Studies on the mechanism of formation of the penicillin antigen. III. The N-(D-α-Benzylpenicilloyl) group as an antigenic determinant responsible for hypersensitivity to penicillin G. J. Exp. Med. 114:875-904.

Loftsgaard, G., E. J. Briskey, N. Nes, and C. Olson. 1968. Residual penicillin in the tissues of pigs. Am. J. Vet. Res. 29: 1613-1618.

McCracken, A. 1977. Detection of antibiotic residues in slaughtered animals. Pp. 239-244 in M. Woodbine, ed. Antibiotics and Antibiosis in Agriculture with Special Reference to Synergism. Butterworths, Boston, Mass.

McGovern, J. P., C. E. Roberson, and G. T. Stewart. 1970. Incidence and manifestations of penicillin allergy. Pp. 3-22 in G. T. Stewart and J. P. McGovern, eds. Penicillin Allergy. Clinical and Immunologic Aspects. Charles C Thomas, Springfield, Ill.

Meredith, W. E., H. H. Weiser, and A. R. Winter. 1965. Chlortetracycline and oxytetracycline residues in poultry tissue and eggs. Appl. Microbiol. 13:86-88.

Messersmith, R. E., B. Sass, H. Berger, and G. O. Gale. 1967. Safety and tissue residue evaluations in swine fed rations containing chlortetracycline, sulfamethazine, and penicillin. J. Am. Vet. Med. Assoc. 151:719-724.

Metcalf, R. L. 1976. Evaluation of the Utility of the Model Ecosystem for Determining the Ecological Fate of Substances Subject to FDA Regulatory Authority. Final Report. Contract FDA 74-127. Food and Drug Administration, Rockville, Md. 133 pp.

Moore, W. E. C. 1969. Current research on the anaerobic flora of the gastrointestinal tract. Pp. 107-113 in The Use of Drugs in Animal Feeds. Proceedings of a Symposium. Publication No. 1679. National Academy of Sciences, Washington, D.C.

Morrison, J. L. 1969. Distribution of arsenic from poultry litter in broiler chickens, soil, and crops. J. Agric. Food Chem. 17:1288-1290.

Morse, E. V., and M. A. Duncan. 1974. Salmonellosis--an environmental health problem affecting animals and man. J. Am. Vet. Med. Assoc. 165:1015-1019.

Mussman, H. C. 1975. Drug and chemical residues in domestic animals. Fed. Proc. 34:197-201.

Overby, L. R., and D. V. Frost. 1960. Excretion studies in swine fed arsanilic acid. J. Anim. Sci. 19:140-145.

Pinck, L. A., D. A. Soulides, and F. E. Allison. 1961. Antibiotics in soils: II. Extent and mechanism of release. Soil Sci. 91:94-99.

Popp, L. 1974. [In German; English summary.] Salmonellen und naturliche Selbstreinigung der Gewasser. Zentralbl. Bakteriol. Parasitenkd. Infektionskr. Hyg., I. Abt. Orig. Reihe B 158: 432-445.

Pramer, D., and R. L. Starkey. 1951. Decomposition of streptomycin. Science 113:127.

Pramer, D., and R. L. Starkey. 1972. Decomposition of streptomycin in soil and by an isolated bacterium. Soil Sci. 114: 451-455.

Rankin, J. D., and R. J. Taylor. 1969. A study of some disease hazards which could be associated with the system of applying cattle slurry to pasture. Vet. Rec. 85:578-581.

Rollins, L. D., S. A. Gaines, D. W. Pocurull, and H. D. Mercer. 1975. Animal model for determining the no-effect level of an antimicrobial drug on drug resistance in lactose-fermenting enteric flora. Antimicrob. Agents Chemother. 7:661-665.

Rumsey, T. S., D. A. Dinius, and R. R. Oltjen. 1975. DES, antibiotic and ronnel in beef feedlot waste. J. Anim. Sci. 41:275 (Abstract).

Scudi, J. V., M. E. Clift, and R. A. Krueger. 1947. Some pharmacological characteristics of bacitracin. II. Absorption and excretion of bacitracin in the dog. Proc. Soc. Exp. Biol. Med. 65:9-13.

Shahani, K. M., I. A. Gould, H. H. Weiser, and W. Slatter. 1956. Stability of small concentrations of penicillin in milk as affected by heat treatment and storage. J. Dairy Sci. 39: 971-977.

Shirk, R. J., A. R. Whitehall, and L. R. Hines. 1957. A degradation product in cooked chlortetracycline-treated poultry. Pp. 843-848 in H. Welch, ed. Antibiotics Annual, 1956-1957. Medical Encyclopedia, Inc., N.Y.

Smith, H. W. 1969. The influence of antimicrobial drugs in animal feeds on the emergence of drug-resistant, disease-producing bacteria in animals. Pp. 304-317 in The Use of Drugs in Animal Feeds. Proceedings of a Symposium. Publication No. 1679. National Academy of Sciences, Washington, D.C.

Smith, H. W. 1970a. Effect of antibiotics on bacterial ecology in animals. Am. J. Clin. Nutr. 23:1472-1479.

Smith, H. W. 1970b. Incidence of river water of *Escherichia coli* containing R factors. Nature 228:1286-1288.

Smith, H. W. 1975. Persistence of tetracycline resistance in pig *E. coli*. Nature 258:628-630.

Smith, H. W., and W. E. Crabb. 1957. The effect of the continuous administration of diets containing low levels of tetracyclines on the incidence of drug-resistant Bacterium coli in the faeces of pigs and chickens: The sensitivity of the Bact. coli to other chemotherapeutic agents. Vet. Rec. 69:24-30.

Smith, H. W., and W. E. Crabb. 1961. The faecal bacterial flora of animals and man: Its development in the young. J. Pathol. Bacteriol. 82:53-66.

Smith, P. R., E. Farrell, and K. Dunican. 1974. Survival of R^+ Escherichia coli in sea water. Appl. Microbiol. 27:983-984.

Soulides, D. A., L. A. Pinck, and F. E. Allison. 1961. Antibiotics in soils. 3. Further studies on release of antibiotics from clays. Soil Sci. 92:90-93.

Stewart, G. T., and J. P. McGovern, eds. 1970. Penicillin allergy. Clinical and Immunologic Aspects. Charles C Thomas, Springfield, Ill. 196 pp.

Tannock, G. W., and J. M. B. Smith. 1971. Studies on the survival of Salmonella typhimurium and Salmonella bovismorbificans on pasture and in water. Aust. Vet. J. 47:557-559.

Thayer, D. W., P. Lewter, J. Barker, and J. J. J. Chen. 1974. Microbiological and chemical survey of beef cattle waste from a nonsurfaced feedlot. Bull Environ. Contam. Toxicol. 11: 26-32.

Tscheuschner, I. 1972. Anaphylaktische Reaktion auf Penicillin nach Genuss von Schweinefleisch. Z. Haut. Geschlechskr. 47: 591-592.

U.S. Department of Agriculture. 1974. Objective Phase Biological Residue Reports, January through December 1973. Data from Residue Monitoring Program, Food Safety and Quality Service, U.S. Department of Agriculture, Washington, D.C.

U.S. Department of Agriculture. 1977-1979. Objective Phase Biological Residue Reports, January through December, 1976-1978. Data from Residue Monitoring Program, Food Safety and Quality Service, U. S. Department of Agriculture, Washington, D.C.

Van Dijck, P. J., and H. Van de Voorde. 1976. [In Dutch; English summary.] Residu's van antimicrobiële stoffen in effluenten van landbouwbedrijven. Tijdschr. Diergeneeskd. 101:297-302.

Warrington, R. J., F. E. R. Simons, H. W. Ho, B. A. Gorski, and K. S. Tse. 1978. Diagnosis of penicillin allergy by skin testing: The Manitoba experience. Can. Med. Assoc. J. 118: 787-791.

Webb, K. E., Jr., and J. P. Fontenot. 1975. Medicinal drug residues in broiler litter and tissues from cattle fed litter. J. Anim. Sci. 41:1212-1217.

Weinstein, L. 1975. Section XIV, Chapters 55-61 in L. S. Goodman and A. Gilman, eds. The Pharmacological Basis of Therapeutics. Fifth Edition. MacMillan Publishing Co., Inc., N.Y.

Wilson, H. T. H. 1958. Streptomycin dermatitis in nurses. Br. Med. J. 1:1378-1382.

Woolson, E. A. 1977. Fate of arsenicals in different environmental substrates. Environ. Health Perspect. 19:73-81.

APPENDIX F

ZOONOTIC ASPECTS OF SUBTHERAPEUTIC ANTIMICROBIALS IN FEED

John F. Timoney[1]

BACTERIAL COLONIZATION OF HUMANS

The pathogenic bacteria found in animals and humans can be arranged into two groups based on their host specificity (Table 1). The first, and by far the largest, group contains host-adapted bacteria, most of which are uniquely adapted to specific hosts and rarely infect or colonize other hosts. This specificity may be an attribute of genus, species, serotype, phage-type, etc. The second, and much smaller, group of bacteria have limited or no host specificity and may colonize or infect a variety of hosts. Transfer of these bacteria between host species may occur at a perceptible rate, but this rate is difficult to quantitate because of overlapping reservoirs.

Only salmonellae in the second group, some serotypes of nonpathogenic *Escherichia coli*, and possibly some strains of *Staphylococcus aureus* may be involved in the transfer of antibiotic resistance genes between animals and human beings.

THE TRANSFER OF BACTERIA FROM ANIMALS TO HUMANS

To what extent do bacteria from poultry, pigs, or calves transfer to humans? Is the transfer greater in farm workers, rural inhabitants, and meat handlers than in others? Is food contamination the primary route of transfer? These questions are addressed in the following paragraphs. *E. coli* and *Salmonella* are used as models since these organisms appear to have the greatest potential as vehicles for plasmid transfer between the reservoirs in animals and humans.

E. coli

There remains substantial doubt as to whether strains of *E. coli* from farm animals (poultry, pigs, calves) contribute to the composition of flora in the human gut (Garrod, 1976; Siegel, 1976; Siegel *et al.*, 1974). Tools used for studying this issue have included serotyping (Bettelheim *et al.*, 1974; Howe and Linton, 1976), phage-typing (Siegel *et al.*, 1974), and a combination of

[1]Department of Microbiology, New York State College of Veterinary Medicine, Cornell University, Ithaca, N.Y.

TABLE 1

Representative Common Pathogenic Bacteria of Humans and Animals Grouped According to Presence or Absence of Host Adaptation[a]

Adapted to Host	
Actinobacillus lignieresii	(cattle)
Bordetella pertussis	(humans)
Brucella abortus	(cattle)
Brucella canis	(dog)
Brucella ovis	(sheep)
Campylobacter fetus (venerealis)	(cattle)
Clostridium perfringens Type A	(humans)
Clostridium perfringens Type B	(sheep)
Clostridium perfringens Type D	(sheep)
Corynebacterium diphtheriae	(humans)
Enteropathogenic *E. coli*: Specific serotypes for lambs, calves, infants, humans, piglets, and older pigs	
Erysipelothrix rhusiopathiae	(swine, turkeys)
Haemophilus influenzae	(humans)
Haemophilus suis	(pigs)
Moraxella bovis	(cattle)
Mycobacterium avium	(birds)
Neisseria gonorrhoeae	(humans)
Neisseria meningitidis	
Salmonella cholerae-suis	(pigs)
Salmonella pullorum	(poultry)
Salmonella typhi	(humans)
Shigella spp.	
Staphylococcus aureus--Most strains are adapted to specific hosts (Davidson, 1972; Gibbs *et al.*, 1978; Shimizu, 1977; Wang, 1978)	
Streptococcus equi	(horse)
Streptococcus pneumoniae	(humans)
Streptococcus pyogenes	(humans)
Treponema hyodysenteriae	(swine)
Treponema pallidum	(humans)

Not Adapted to Host
Bacillus anthracis
Some serotypes of nonpathogenic *E. coli*
Listeria monocytogenes
Pasteurella pseudotuberculosis
Salmonella typhimurium and many other serotypes
Staphylococcus aureus--A few strains may not be adapted to hosts (Live, 1972)
Klebsiella pneumoniae[b]
Proteus spp.[b]
Pseudomonas aeruginosa[b]
Serratia marcescens[b]
Yersinia enterocolitica

[a]From Bruner and Gillespie, 1973, and Dubos and Hirsch, 1965.
[b]No evidence exists that animals are a source of these organisms for humans.

serotyping and fermentation reactions (Guinée, 1963). Investigators have found a wide variety of *E. coli* strains in feces of humans and animals.

Serotypes and phage types in samples from humans and animals were substantially different. Only a small proportion of strains from animals and humans had the same serotype (Bettleheim *et al.*, 1974, 1976; Fein *et al.*, 1974) or phage-type (Fein *et al.*, 1974; Siegel *et al.*, 1974).

In the surveys cited above, a major proportion of the strains from animals could not be typed. In contrast, most of the strains from humans reacted in the typing system, thereby providing further evidence that the *E. coli* flora of humans and animals are essentially separate and discrete. Even when similar serotypes are found in humans and animals, there is substantial doubt as to their common identity since a large number of subtypes can be found within one serologic O group (Guinée, 1963).

Varying results were obtained from experiments in which volunteers were dosed with cultures of *E. coli* of animal origin. Smith (1969) dosed himself with a series of up to 1 billion *E. coli* strains of animal origin, but found that these strains persisted only briefly in his alimentary tract. Recently, Linton *et al.* (1977b) reported that one out of five volunteers who handled raw chicken meat subsequently exhibited intestinal colonization by *E. coli* strains from the meat. These strains persisted in the intestine for approximately 10 days. Cooke *et al.* (1972) observed that an antibiotic-sensitive *E. coli* of animal origin persisted for 120 days in a volunteer who received a large dose of organisms. Hirsh and Wiger (1978) reported a crossover of resistant *E. coli* from calves to their handlers.

There is also circumstantial evidence of brief colonization of the human intestine by *E. coli* of animal origin. Dorn *et al.* (1975) have shown that antibiotic resistance patterns of *E. coli* from farm families who killed and consumed their own animals for meat resembled those of their livestock. No such relationship was evident for families who did not process their own cattle or swine for meat. Wells and James (1973) found that resistance to more than three antibiotics was twice as common in *E. coli* from farm people who had direct contact with swine fed antibiotics than it was in their relatives who had only indirect contact with pigs. Both studies imply that the bacteria from the livestock had colonized the intestines of the humans long enough to pass on their resistance factors to the indigenous *E. coli*. However, Wiedemann and Knothe (1971) and Moorhouse (1971) were unable to prove that contact with livestock was related to the occurrence of antibiotic resistance in indigenous strains of *E. coli* in humans.

The conflicting nature of these results indicates that brief colonization of the intestines of humans by bacteria from animals and transfer of resistance to indigenous *E. coli* in humans occur only sporadically and that further study *is* required to elucidate the factors that facilitate this process.

The opportunity for resistant *E. coli* to transfer from meat or other animal products to humans, either by ingestion or indirectly by contact, is certainly available since many investigators, e.g., Kim and Stephens (1972), Lakhotia and Stephens (1973a, b), Linton *et al.* (1977a, c), and Walton and Lewis (1971), have shown that eggs and the carcasses of poultry, swine, and calves may be contaminated with antibiotic-resistant *E. coli*.

Furthermore, there is evidence that meat handling is an important factor in the transfer of resistant bacteria from animals to humans (Dorn *et al.*, 1975; Linton *et al.*, 1977b). Siegel (1976) observed that slaughterhouse personnel shared *E. coli* phage types more often than would normally be expected. He postulated that this was due to common exposure of these workers to contaminated meat.

In the United States and in Britain, meats and other foods of animal origin are usually cooked sufficiently to inactivate *E. coli*. Consequently, in those countries, colonization of humans by animal strains probably occurs mainly through contact with the contaminated product before cooking or via secondary contamination of other cooked items in the kitchen. The possible importance of handling in the transfer of *E. coli* is indicated by the findings of Linton *et al.* (1977b) and Dorn *et al.* (1975). However, since their observations are very limited, much more study of this subject is required.

Cooking routines vary greatly among different regions of the world. For example, in the Netherlands, many potentially contaminated meat items are eaten in a relatively uncooked condition. Such variations are seldom considered when comparing data on human salmonellosis in different countries.

Factors that are not related to the consumption of meat are also involved in the prevalence of antibiotic-resistant *E. coli* in the human intestine, but their mechanisms are not understood. The well-known study of Guinée *et al.* (1970), showing that vegetarians and babies were somewhat more likely to carry resistant *E. coli* than were meat-eaters, has not yet been explained. Other studies unrelated to the food of humans have shown that antibiotic-resistant bacteria may be very prevalent in ecosystems in which there is no obvious selection pressure from antibiotic usage (Cooke, 1976a, 1976b; Sizemore and Colwell, 1977; Timoney et al., 1978).

Salmonella spp.

It is an almost universally accepted dogma that human salmonellosis (with the exception of typhoid and paratyphoid) is a zoonosis (Christopher et al., 1974; Hook, 1971) and that animals are the immediate reservoir of Salmonella infections in humans. A logical extension of this dogma is that much of the antibiotic resistance in salmonellae in humans also derives from this reservoir in animals. There is extensive documentation that various food items derived from poultry, swine, and cattle have served as sources of Salmonella infection for man (National Academy of Sciences, 1969). Moreover, there have been detailed reports describing epidemics of specific clones of S. typhimurium that originated in calves and spread into the human population carrying with them R factors apparently acquired in the original host (Anderson, 1968; Threlfall et al., 1978a,b).

There is, however, a substantial and convincing body of evidence indicating that the role of animals as a source of Salmonella infection and associated R factors for humans is greatly exaggerated and that humans themselves are a major part of the Salmonella reservoir. This evidence is outlined in the succeeding paragraphs.

A major epidemic of Salmonella wien has been progressing in North Africa and Europe since 1969 (McConnell et al., 1979). Most of the strains involved are resistant to antibiotics and have not been found in animals. The largest epidemic of typhoid in history, which occurred in Mexico during the early 1970's, was also caused by a multiresistant strain (Gangarosa et al., 1972). Since S. typhi is found only in humans, animals were not implicated in the emergence of this resistant strain either. Both of these epidemics indicate that salmonellosis caused by multiresistant strains can occur in humans without involving an animal reservoir.

Salmonellosis in the United States is most common in infants less than 1 year old (Ryder et al., 1976). Because of the small proportion of meat in the diet consumed by these infants, there is a low probability that the infection was derived from animals via meats. Salmonellosis is also common among institutionalized children, where person-to-person transmission occurs (Aaron *et al.*, 1971; Schroeder *et al.*, 1968). Interestingly, dramatic outbreaks of salmonellosis attributed to ingestion of contaminated foods of animal origin involve mostly young and middle-aged adults (Hook, 1971), and there is minimal secondary lateral spread. The importance of lateral spread in the epidemiology of human salmonellosis is underscored by the proliferation of that disease among the urban poor (Cherubin *et al.*, 1969), where personal hygiene would be expected to be deficient.

Comparison of the 10 most frequently isolated serotypes from human and nonhuman sources reveals that about half of the serotypes are common to human and nonhuman sources and half are not (Mallory and Gangarosa, 1970; Ryder *et al.*, 1976). This implies that approximately half of the serotypes causing salmonellosis in humans during the surveys were probably not derived from nonhuman sources. Interestingly, a 2-year survey of *Salmonella* serotypes in the Gulf of Aarhus, Denmark, provides additional evidence for this conclusion (Grunnet and Brest Nielsen, 1969). These investigators found that many of the serotypes common in human sewage outfalls were different from those commonly found in animals or their feeds.

Recent observations in rural and metropolitan New York (Cherubin *et al.*, 1979; Timoney, 1978) suggest that the human and animal reservoirs of *S. typhimurium* (the most common serotype in humans and animals in this area) are essentially separate. The evidence supporting this conclusion is twofold: resistance to ampicillin appeared in strains from humans before it did in strains from animals and its prevalence declined between 1975 and 1977 when ampicillin-resistant strains in animals continued to increase (Cherubin *et al.*, in press). Many of the strains from animals found in New York were derived from veal calves, the retail market for which is New York City.

Epidemiological studies of salmonellosis in New York City have also provided definite evidence of the lateral spread of *S. typhimurium* (Cherubin *et al.*, 1969). This serotype was proportionately much more common in crowded and slum areas and in children than in other areas of the city or in older populations. Furthermore, *S. typhimurium* was isolated much less frequently from general, usually foodborne outbreaks of salmonellosis than from sporadic cases. The general outbreaks tended to be caused by other, less well known serotypes. There has been a similar finding on a national scale (Center for Disease Control, 1964-1967). Thus, there is good evidence, in the New York metropolitan area at least, that humans are an important immediate reservoir of *S. typhimurium* for infection of humans.

Comparisons of the frequency of antibiotic resistance of salmonellae from healthy poultry, swine, and bovines (Lakhotia and Stephens, 1973 b; McGarr *et al.*, 1977; Food and Drug Administration, 1973; Smith, 1970, Timoney, 1972) with that of isolates from humans (Bissett *et al.*, 1974; Neu *et al.*, 1975) show that resistance to antibiotics is much more common in strains from humans. This must be interpreted as suggesting either that the clones causing illness and disease in humans are different from the ones being carried in healthy livestock and/or that after transfer of strains from animals to humans, the therapeutic use of antibiotics in humans results in a selection pressure for antibiotic-resistant strains.

Thus, a considerable body of evidence indicates that, with the exception of large outbreaks of foodborne salmonellosis in adults, many *Salmonella* infections in humans are derived directly from humans.

It should be a relatively easy task to measure on a national scale the extent of transfer of salmonellae from the reservoir of animals to the reservoir of humans using data already on file at the Center for Disease Control (CDC) in Atlanta. Unfortunately, the format of CDC's *Salmonella* Surveillance Reports prevents any overall quantitative estimate of this transfer.

Occupation-Related Transfer

The occupation-related transfer of salmonellae is reviewed in a report of the National Academy of Sciences (1969). The *Salmonella* carrier rate is higher among food handlers than it is in the general population in the United States (Galton and Steele, 1961). There is also evidence that workers in abattoirs may carry salmonellae to their homes and subsequently infect members of their families (Public Health Laboratory Service, 1964).

Reports of *Salmonella* isolates from humans in urban and rural areas indicate that rural inhabitants appear to have a lower incidence of infection (Center for Disease Control, 1964-1976). This may partly reflect a difference in availability of laboratory services. However, close scrutiny of these reports reveals that there are annually from 4 to 5 times as many isolates from New York City as from upstate New York, a predominantly rural area served by excellent laboratory facilities at Albany. Also, the numbers of *Salmonella* isolates from humans in such states as Iowa, Indiana, Nebraska, and Oklahoma, where great numbers of livestock are raised, are among the lowest in the United States (Ryder *et al.*, 1976).

Transfer Via Food Contamination

Food contamination provides a major source of salmonellae that are transferred to humans (National Academy of Sciences, 1969). Processed foods, such as egg or milk products, are much more important in this regard than are fresh, unprocessed items (Center for Disease Control, 1976; Sanders *et al.*, 1963)--an indication that secondary contamination during and after processing is significant in the epidemiology of foodborne salmonellosis.

THE TRANSFER OF GENETIC DETERMINANTS FROM BACTERIA OF ANIMAL ORIGIN TO OTHER BACTERIA IN HUMANS

This subject will be dealt with by addressing the following questions: Is there a pool of resistance plasmids common to bacteria of human and animal origin? Are the genes for colonization and enterotoxin production the same in *E. coli* from animals and humans?

Resistance Plasmids and Resistance Genes in Bacteria from Humans and Animals

Similarity of resistance patterns is not an adequate criterion for establishing the identity of genes or plasmids from different sources because the same resistance pattern may be determined by different plasmids or combinations of different plasmids in the same host cell (Timoney, 1978). The evidence for similarity of plasmids from different sources must be based on DNA homology, incompatibility grouping studies, and endonuclease digestion studies.

Evidence from incompatibility testing and DNA homology studies indicates that resistance plasmids from bacteria isolated from humans and animals cannot be distinguished. Incompatibility (Inc) groups F, I, and N resistance plasmids are the same in animals and humans (Anderson *et al.*, 1975; Silver and Mercer, 1978). Inc H plasmids of *Salmonella typhimurium* from humans and animals are also similar (Anderson, 1977).

Furthermore, among resistance plasmids from the Enterobacteriaceae, the genes for TEM β-lactamase reside upon a 3.0 Mdal sequence of DNA that is transposable from one plasmid to another (Hedges and Jacob, 1974). This transposon has also been found in *Haemophilus influenzae* type b (De Graaff *et al.*, 1976) and in *Neisseria gonorrhoeae*

(Elwell et al., 1977). Thus, the same gene for resistance to ampicillin is widely distributed among the pathogenic bacteria.

Genes for tetracycline, kanamycin, chloramphenicol, trimethoprim, and streptomycin have also been found to be transposable (Silver and Mercer, 1978). This suggests that resistance genes can move freely among different bacteria and, presumably, between the reservoirs of these bacteria in humans and animals.

Although enteric resistance plasmids from bacteria isolated from humans and animals are identical, some evidence suggests that among the Enterobacteriaceae the host organism is an important determinant of the kinds of plasmids hosted. For instance, S. typhimurium and enteropathogenic E. coli strains from calves in the same geographic area can harbor substantially different populations of resistance plasmids (Sato and Terakado, 1977). (See Table 2.)

The data gathered in New York State from 1974 to 1978 indicate that Inc H plasmids carrying resistance to tetracycline, kanamycin, and some other antibiotics were present in 74% of resistant S. typhimurium strains from diseased calves whereas only 1% of similarly resistent enteropathogenic E. coli from calves harbored these plasmids. Interestingly, Smith et al. (1978) have also found only a low frequency of Inc H plasmids in multiresistant coliforms from sewage and river water in Britain.

Thus, although resistance plasmids may be similar in humans and animals, some unknown factors restrict the free flow of these plasmids from one group of enterobacteria to another.

Furthermore, it is unlikely that multiresistant E. coli from animals could be the source of the Inc H plasmids that are so common in strains of S. typhimurium and S. typhi from humans (Anderson, 1977; Taylor et al., 1978), not only because their occurrence in potential donor coliforms is so infrequent in comparison to plasmids of other incompatibility groups, but also because Inc H plasmids do not transfer at body temperature.

THE GENETIC DETERMINANTS FOR ENTEROTOXIN PRODUCTION IN *E. coli* FROM HUMANS AND ANIMALS

Toxigenic strains of E. coli synthesize two types of toxins. One is heat stable (ST); the other is heat labile (LT). The genetic determinants for these toxins can occur together on the same or on separate plasmids. Gyles et al. (1974) and Skerman

TABLE 2

The Occurrence of H Incompatibility Group Plasmids in Multiresistant *Salmonella typhimurium* and Enteropathogenic *Escherichia coli* from Calves in New York State, 1974-1978[a]

Strain (Number of Strains Tested)	Percentages of Strains Containing Group Plasmids			
	H only	H and Non H[b]	Non H only	No Transfer[c]
S. typhimurium (134)	37	37	16	10
E. coli (115)	1	0	69	30

[a] Unpublished data from Timoney, 1979.

[b] Plasmids of incompatibility groups other than H.

[c] Percentage of strains that did not transfer resistance(s) at either 28°C or 37°C.

et al. (1972) found that ST-LH plasmids from humans and swine were approximately the same size (55-60 Mdal) but that the molecular weight of ST plasmids was highly variable. Later, So *et al.* (1975) showed that ST plasmids in strains from swine had no homology with ST-LH plasmids from either swine or humans but that there was considerable homology between ST-LT plasmids from each of these sources. However, they found that these plasmids belonged to different incompatibility groups--the porcine ST-LH plasmid in F I and the human plasmid in F II. This difference in incompatibility group did not involve a substantial amount of DNA. So *et al.* (1976) demonstrated by DNA hybridization studies that ST-LH plasmids have a majority of nucleotides in common regardless of origin. Thus, there is good evidence that a substantial part of the ST-LH plasmid is common to strains of enterotoxigenic *E. coli* from both swine and humans. The DNA fragment in this plasmid, which encodes for LT toxin, is no greater than 3.0 kilobases (So *et al.*, 1978).

The ST determinant from a plasmid containing ST alone has been cloned in a DNA fragment of 3.4 kilobases and has been shown to be a transposon flanked by inverted repeats of IS 1 (So *et al.*, 1979). This transposability probably accounts for the differing molecular weight of ST plasmids.

These findings suggest that the ST genes in *E. coli* from a variety of hosts could be the same since they have the property of being able to transfer from one plasmid to another. Furthermore, there are indications that the genes for ST-LT are also located on a transposon. Inverted repeat sequences of bases are known to bound the area containing the genes on a plasmid with ST-LT function (Silva *et al.*, 1978).

SIMILARITY OF PLASMID-BASED GENES FOR COLONIZATION IN *E. coli* FROM ANIMALS AND HUMANS

A number of pilus- and capsule-associated antigens are known to be important in the colonization of the small intestine of pigs, calves, lambs, and humans by enteropathogenic *E. coli*. Included in this category are the K88 and K99 antigens, the pilus antigen of porcine *E. coli* 978 (Nagy *et al.*, 1978) and the colonization factor associated with the human *E. coli* strain H-10407 (Evans *et al.*, 1975). Only the genetic basis of the K88 antigen has been well studied. Shipley *et al.* (1978) have shown that the genes for the K88 antigen are located on 50- and 90-Mdal plasmids. The larger plasmid is self-transmissible, but the smaller one is not.

More recently, Mooi et al. (1979) have shown that the genes for $K88^{ab}$ synthesis lie on a DNA sequence of 4.3 Mdal or less. Studies to compare DNA sequences for K88 synthesis with DNA sequences from E. coli strains that colonize humans have not yet been reported. Since the K88 antigens have been found only on E. coli strains that are specific for swine (Moon et al., 1977), it is likely that the genes for factors with similar function in E. coli strains from humans will prove to be different.

Ørskov et al. (1975) found the K99 antigen on enteropathogenic E. coli from calves and lambs. Moon et al. (1977) reported finding the same antigen on porcine E. coli of O groups 101 and 64. These authors stated that the K99 antigen had not yet been found on human enteropathogenic strains. No studies on the characteristics of the K99 genes have yet been reported.

REFERENCES

Aaron, E., P. A. Gross, P. F. Wehrle, B. A. Kogan, and G. A. Heidbreder. 1971. Urban salmonellosis. Am. J. Public Health 61:337-343.

Anderson, E. S. 1968. The ecology of transferable drug resistance in the enterobacteria. Annu. Rev. Microbiol. 22:131-180.

Anderson, E. S. 1977. The geographical predominance of resistance transfer systems of various compatibility groups in salmonellae. Pp. 25-38 in J. Drews and G. Högenauer, eds. Topics in Infectious Diseases, Vol. 2. R-Factors: Their Properties and Possible Control. Symposium, Baden near Vienna, Austria, April 27-28, 1977. Springer-Verlag, Vienna and New York.

Anderson, E. S., G. O. Humphreys, and G. A. Willshaw. 1975. The molecular relatedness of R factors in enterobacteria of human and animal origin. J. Gen. Microbiol. 91:376-382.

Bettelheim, K. A., F. M. Bushrod, M. E. Chandler, E. M. Cooke, S. O'Farrell, and R. A. Shooter. 1974. *Escherichia coli* serotype distribution in man and animals. J. Hyg., Camb. 73:467-471.

Bettelheim, K. A., N. Ismail, R. Shinebaum, R. A. Shooter, E. Moorhouse, and W. Farrell. 1976. The distribution of serotypes of *Escherichia coli* in cow-pats and other animal material compared with serotypes of *E. coli* isolated from human sources. J. Hyg., Camb. 76:403-406.

Bissett, M. L., S. L. Abbott, and R. M. Wood. 1974. Antimicrobial resistance and R factors in *Salmonella* isolated in California (1971-1972). Antimicrob. Agents Chemother. 5:161-168.

Bruner, D. W., and J. H. Gillespie. 1973. Hagan's Infectious Diseases of Domestic Animals with Special Reference to Etiology, Diagnosis, and Biologic Therapy. Sixth Edition. Comstock Publishing Associates, a Division of Cornell University Press, Ithaca, N.Y. and London, England. 1,385 pp.

Center for Disease Control. 1964-1976. Salmonella Surveillance Annual Summaries, 1964-1976. Center for Disease Control, Atlanta, Ga.

Center for Disease Control. 1976. Milk-borne Salmonella infection--United Kingdom. From notes based on reports to the Public Health Laboratory Service from public health and hospital laboratories in the United Kingdom and the Republic of Ireland. Morbid. Mortal. Weekly Rep. 25:202-203.

Cherubin, C. E., T. Fodor, L. Denmark, C. Master, H. T. Fuerst, and J. Winter. 1969. The epidemiology of salmonellosis in New York City. Am. J. Epidemiol. 90:112-125.

Cherubin, C., M. F. Sierra, and J. Marr. 1979. Recent trends in Salmonella and Shigella in New York City and at Kings County Hospital. Bull. N.Y. Acad. Med. 55:303-312.

Cherubin, C. E., J. F. Timoney, M. F. Sierra, P. Ma, J. Marr, and S. Shin. 1980. A sudden decline in ampicillin resistance in Salmonella typhimurium. J. Am. Med. Assoc. 243:439-442.

Christopher, P. J., P. D. Claxton, D. C. Dorman, B. F. O'Connor, R. W. Proudford, and R. G. A. Sutton. 1974. Salmonellosis: An increasing public health hazard. Med. J. Aust. 1:337-341.

Cooke, E. M., I. G. T. Hettiaratchy, and A. C. Buck. 1972. Fate of ingested Escherichia coli in normal persons. J. Med. Microbiol. 5:361-369.

Cooke, M. D. 1976a. Antibiotic resistance among coliform and fecal coliform bacteria isolated from the freshwater mussel Hydridella menziesii. Antimicrob. Agents Chemother. 9:885-888.

Cooke, M. D. 1976b. Antibiotic resistance in coliform and faecal coliform bacteria from natural waters and effluents. N. Z. J. Mar. Freshwater Res. 10:391-397.

Davidson, I. 1972. A collaborative investigation of phages for typing bovine staphylococci. Bull. W. H. O. 46:81-98.

De Graaff, J., L. P. Elwell, and S. Falkow. 1976. Molecular nature of two beta-lactamase-specifying plasmids isolated from Haemophilus influenzae type b. J. Bacteriol. 126:439-446.

Dorn, C. R., R. K. Tsutakawa, D. Fein, G. C. Burton, and D. C. Blenden. 1975. Antibiotic resistance patterns of Escherichia coli isolated from families consuming home-raised meat. Am. J. Epidemiol. 102:319-326.

Dubos, R. J., and J. G. Hirsch, eds. 1965. Bacterial and Mycotic Infections of Man. Fourth Edition. J. B. Lippincott Company, Philadelphia, Pa. and Montreal, Quebec, Canada. 1,025 pp.

Elwell, L. P., M. Roberts, L. W. Mayer, and S. Falkow. 1977. Plasmid-mediated beta-lactamase production in Neisseria gonorrhoeae. Antimicrob. Agents Chemother. 11:528-533.

Evans, D. G., R. P. Silver, D. J. Evans, Jr., D. G. Chase, and S. L. Gorbach. 1975. Plasmid-controlled colonization factor associated with virulence in Escherichia coli enterotoxigenic for humans. Infect. Immun. 12:656-667.

Fein, D., G. Burton, R. Tsutakawa, and D. Blenden. 1974. Matching of antibiotic resistance patterns of Escherichia coli of farm families and their animals. J. Infect. Dis. 130:274-279.

Food and Drug Administration. 1973. Survey of Salmonella isolates for antibiotic resistance. Letter report to Special Assistant to the Director, Bureau of Veterinary Medicine, from Deputy Director, Division of Microbiology. Food and Drug Administration, Washington, D.C. 3 pp.

Galton, M. M., and J. H. Steele. 1961. Laboratory and epidemiological aspects of foodborne diseases. J. Milk Food Technol. 24:104-114.

Gangarosa, E. J., J. V. Bennett, C. Wyatt, P. E. Pierce, J. Olarte, P. Mendoza Hernandez, P. Vázquez, and D. Bessudo. M. 1972. From the Center for Disease Control. An epidemic-associated episome? J. Infect. Dis. 126:215-218.

Garrod, L. P. 1976. Defense against bacterial resistance. Br. Med. J. 2:933-936.

Gibbs, P. A., J. T. Patterson, and J. K. Thompson. 1978. Characterization of poultry isolates of Staphylococcus aureus by a new set of poultry phages. J. Appl. Bacteriol. 44:387-400.

Grunnet, K., and B. Brest Nielsen. 1969. Salmonella types isolated from the Gulf of Aarhus compared with types from infected human beings, animals, and feed products in Denmark. Appl. Microbiol. 18:985-990.

Guinée, P. A. M. 1963. Preliminary investigations concerning the presence of E. coli in man and in various species of animals. Zentralbl. Bakteriol. Parasitenkd. Infektionskr. Hyg. I. Abt. Orig. Reihe A 188:201-218.

Guinée, P., N. Ugueto, and N. van Leeuwen. 1970. Escherichia coli with resistance factors in vegetarians, babies, and nonvegetarians. Appl. Microbiol. 20:531-535.

Gyles, C., M. So, and S. Falkow. 1974. The enterotoxin plasmids of Escherichia coli. J. Infect. Dis. 130:40-49.

Hedges, R. W., and A. E. Jacob. 1974. Transposition of ampicillin resistance from RP4 to other replicons. Mol. Gen. Genet. 132: 31-40.

Hirsh, D. C., and N. Wiger. 1978. The effect of tetracycline upon the spread of bacterial resistance from calves to man. J. Anim. Sci. 46:1437-1446.

Hook, E. W. 1971. Disease caused by Salmonella. Pp. 576-581 in P. B. Beeson and W. McDermott, eds. Cecil-Loeb Textbook of Medicine. Thirteenth Edition. W. B. Saunders Company, Philadelphia, London, and Toronto.

Howe, K., and A. H. Linton. 1976. The distribution of O-antigen types of Escherichia coli in normal calves, compared with man, and their R plasmid carriage. J. Appl. Bacteriol. 40:317-330.

Kim, T. K., and J. F. Stephens. 1972. Drug resistance and transferable drug resistance of Escherichia coli isolated from "ready-to-cook" broilers. Poult. Sci. 51:1165-1170.

Lakhotia, R. L., and J. F. Stephens. 1973a. Drug resistance and R factors among enterobacteria isolated from eggs. Poult. Sci. 52:1955-1962.

Lakhotia, R. L., and J. F. Stephens. 1973b. Incidence of drug resistance and R-factor among salmonellae isolated from poultry. Poult. Sci. 52:2266-2270.

Linton, A. H., B. Handley, A. D. Osborne, B. G. Shaw, T. A. Roberts, and W. R. Hudson. 1977a. Contamination of pig carcasses at two abattoirs by Escherichia coli with special reference to O-serotypes and antibiotic resistance. J. Appl. Bacteriol. 42:89-110.

Linton, A. H., K. Howe, P. M. Bennett, M. H. Richmond, and E. J. Whiteside. 1977b. The colonization of the human gut by antibiotic resistant Escherichia coli from chickens. J. Appl. Bacteriol. 43:465-469.

Linton, A. H., K. Howe, C. L. Hartley, H. M. Clements, M. H. Richmond, and A. D. Osborne. 1977c. Antibiotic resistance among Escherichia coli O-serotypes from the gut and carcasses of commercially slaughtered broiler chickens: A potential public health hazard. J. Appl. Bacteriol. 42:365-378.

Live, I. 1972. Differentiation of Staphylococcus aureus of human and of canine origins: Coagulation of human and of canine plasma, fibrinolysin activity, and serologic reaction. Am. J. Vet. Res. 33:385-391.

Mallory, A., and E. J. Gangarosa. 1970. Salmonella surveillance--1968. J. Infect. Dis. 121:87-89.

McConnell, M. M., H. R. Smith, J. Leonardopoulos, and E. S. Anderson. 1979. The value of plasmid studies in the epidemiology of infections due to drug-resistant Salmonella wien. J. Infect. Dis. 139:178-190.

McGarr, C., W. R. Mitchell, H. C. Carlson, and N. A. Fish. 1977. Antimicrobial susceptibility of Salmonella isolates from the broiler chicken industry in Ontario. Can. J. Comp. Med. 41:107-111.

Mooi, F. R., F. K. de Graaf, and J. D. A. van Embden. 1979. Cloning, mapping and expression of the genetic determinant that encodes for the K88ab antigen. Nucleic Acids Res. 6:849-865.

Moon, H. W., B. Nagy, R. E. Isaacson, and I. Ørskov. 1977. Occurrence of K99 antigen on Escherichia coli isolated from pigs and colonization of pig ileum by K99$^+$ enterotoxigenic E. coli from calves and pigs. Infect. Immun. 15:614-620.

Moorhouse, E. C. 1971. Prevalence of R+ bacteria in infants in Ireland. Ann. N.Y. Acad. Sci. 182:65-71.

Nagy, B., H. W. Moon, R. E. Isaacson, C. C. To, and C. C. Brinton. 1978. Immunization of suckling pigs against enteric enterotoxigenic Escherichia coli infection by vaccinating dams with purified pili. Infect. Immun. 21:269-274.

National Academy of Sciences. 1969. An Evaluation of the Salmonella Problem. A Report of the U.S. Department of Agriculture and the Food and Drug Administration. Prepared by the Committee on Salmonella, Division of Biology and Agriculture, National Research Council. National Academy of Sciences, Washington, D.C. 207 pp.

Neu, H. C., C. E. Cherubin, E. D. Longo, B. Flouton, and J. Winter. 1975. Antimicrobial resistance and R-factor transfer among isolates of Salmonella in the northeastern United States: A comparison of human and animal isolates. J. Infect. Dis. 132:617-622.

Ørskov, I., F. Ørskov, H. W. Smith, and W. J. Sojka. 1975. The establishment of K99, a thermolabile transmissible Escherichia coli K antigen, previously called "KCo", possessed by calf and lamb enteropathogenic strains. Acta Pathol. Microbiol. Scand. Sect. B 83:31-36.

Public Health Laboratory Service. 1964. Salmonellae in abattoirs, butchers' shops and home-produced meat, and their relation to human infection. J. Hyg., Camb. 62:283-302.

Ryder, R. W., M. H. Merson, R. A. Pollard, Jr., and E. J. Gangarosa. 1976. From the Center for Disease Control. Salmonellosis in in the United States, 1968-1974. J. Infect. Dis. 133:483-486.

Sanders, E., F. J. Sweeney, Jr., E. A. Friedman, J. R. Boring, E. L. Randall, and L. D. Polk. 1963. An outbreak of hospital-associated infections due to Salmonella derby. J. Am. Med. Assoc. 186:984-986.

Sato, G., and N. Terakado. 1977. R factor types found in Salmonella typhimurium and Escherichia coli isolated from calves in a confined environment. Am. J. Vet. Res. 38:743-747.

Schroeder, S., B. Aserkoff, and P. S. Brachman. 1968. Epidemic salmonellosis in hospitals and institutions. A five-year review. N. Engl. J. Med. 279:674-678.

Shimizu, A. 1977. Establishment of a new bacteriophage set for typing avian staphylococci. Am. J. Vet. Res. 38:1601-1605.

Shipley, P. L., C. L. Gyles, and S. Falkow. 1978. Characterization of plasmids that encode for the K88 colonization antigen. Infect. Immun. 20:559-566.

Siegel, D. 1976. The Ecological Effects of Antimicrobial Agents on Enteric Florae of Animals and Man. Final Technical Report, FDA Contract Number 71-269. Food and Drug Administration, Rockville, Md. 404 pp.

Siegel, D., W. G. Huber, and F. Enloe. 1974. Continuous nontherapeutic use of antibacterial drugs in feed and drug resistance of the gram-negative enteric florae of food-producing animals. Antimicrob. Agents Chemother. 6:697-701.

Silva, M. L. M., W. K. Maas, and C. L. Gyles. 1978. Isolation and characterization of enterotoxin-deficient mutants of Escherichia coli. Proc. Nat. Acad. Sci. (USA) 75:1384-1388.

Silver, R. P., and H. D. Mercer. 1978. Use of drugs in animal feeds: An assessment of the animal and public health aspects. Pp. 649-664 in J. N. Hathcock and J. Coon, eds. Nutrition and Drug Interrelations. Academic Press, New York, San Francisco, London.

Sizemore, R. K., and R. R. Colwell. 1977. Plasmids carried by antibiotic-resistant marine bacteria. Antimicrob. Agents Chemother. 12:373-382.

Skerman, F. J., S. B. Formal, and S. Falkow. 1972. Plasmid-associated enterotoxin production in strains of Escherichia coli isolated from humans. Infect. Immun. 5:622-624.

Smith, H. W. 1969. Transfer of antibiotic resistance from animal and human strains of Escherichia coli to resident E. coli in the alimentary tract of man. Lancet 1:1174-1176.

Smith, H. W. 1970. The incidence of transmissible antibiotic resistance amongst salmonellae isolated from poultry in England and Wales. J. Med. Microbiol. 3:181-182.

Smith, H. W., Z. Parsell, and P. Green. 1978. Thermosensitive antibiotic resistance plasmids in enterobacteria. J. Gen. Microbiol. 109:37-47.

So, M., J. H. Crosa, and S. Falkow. 1975. Polynucleotide sequence relationships among Ent plasmids and the relationship between Ent and other plasmids. J. Bacteriol. 121:234-238.

So, M., H. W. Boyer, M. Betlach, and S. Falkow. 1976. Molecular cloning of an Escherichia coli plasmid determinant that encodes for the production of heat stable enterotoxin. J. Bacteriol. 128:463-472.

So, M., W. S. Dallas, and S. Falkow. 1978. Characterization of an Escherichia coli plasmid encoding for synthesis of heat-labile toxin: Molecular cloning of the toxin determinant. Infect. Immun. 21:405-411.

So, M., F. Heffron, and B. J. McCarthy. 1979. The E. coli gene encoding heat stable toxin is a bacterial transposon flanked by inverted repeats of IS1. Nature 277:453-456.

Taylor, D. E., M. Shermer, and R. B. Grant. 1978. Incidence of the H2 group of plasmids in chloramphenicol-sensitive Salmonella isolated in 1974 from clinical sources in Ontario. Can. J. Microbiol. 24:600-607.

Threlfall, E. J., L. R. Ward, and B. Rowe. 1978a. Epidemic spread of a chloramphenicol-resistant strain of Salmonella typhimurium phage type 204 in bovine animals in Britain. Vet. Rec. 103:438-440.

Threlfall, E. J., L. R. Ward, and B. Rowe. 1978b. Spread of multiresistant strains of Salmonella typhimurium phage types 204 and 193 in Britain. Br. Med. J. 2:997.

Timoney, J. 1972. The sensitivity of salmonellae of animal origin to chemotherapeutic agents in the Republic of Ireland. Irish Vet. J. 26:100-101.

Timoney, J. F. 1978. The epidemiology and genetics of antibiotic resistance of Salmonella typhimurium isolated from diseased animals in New York. J. Infect. Dis. 137:67-73.

Timoney, J. F., J. Port, J. Giles, and J. Spanier. 1978. Heavy-metal and antibiotic resistance in the bacterial flora of sediments of New York bight. Appl. Environ. Microbiol. 36: 465-472.

Walton, J. R., and L. E. Lewis. 1971. Contamination of fresh and cooked meats by antibiotic-resistant coliform bacteria. Lancet 2:255-257.

Wang, C. T. 1978. Bacteriophage typing of canine *Staphylococci*. I. Typing by use of the international phage sets for human and bovine *Staphylococci*. Jpn. J. Vet. Sci. 40:401-405.

Wells, D. M., and O. B. James. 1973. Transmission of infectious drug resistance from animals to man. J. Hyg., Camb. 71:209-215.

Wiedemann, B., and H. Knothe. 1971. Epidemiological investigations of R factor-bearing enterobacteria in man and animals in Germany. Ann. N.Y. Acad. Sci. 182:380-382.

APPENDIX G
TRANSMISSION OF FOOD-BORNE DISEASES
IMPLICATIONS OF THE SUBTHERAPEUTIC USE OF ANTIMICROBIALS

Jackson S. Kiser[1]

The major food-borne bacterial diseases in the United States are caused by salmonellae, staphylococci, and Clostridium botulinum (Center for Disease Control, 1977b) (Table 1). The number of outbreaks of food poisoning by salmonellae and staphylococci is without doubt greatly underestimated because many outbreaks are unreported and undiagnosed. Because of its acute onset and rapid course, staphylococcal food poisoning, in particular, is not often brought to the attention of any medical authority.

The statistics of C. botulinum food poisoning, because it is a much more serious disease in terms of its life-threatening potential, are much more accurate. However, since there is no known or suspected connection between C. botulinum food poisoning and the use of antibiotics at subtherapeutic levels in animal feeds, it will not be discussed further in this paper.

Salmonellosis is ubiquitous. It occurs usually as enterocolitis, usually of only a few days duration, and it is frequently caused by food-borne salmonellae. This form of salmonellosis is acutely uncomfortable and may cause humans to be absent from work for one or several days. The disease frequently involves a visit to a physician and, occasionally, hospitalization for a short period. It is generally agreed that antibiotic treatment is contraindicated since it does not shorten the course of the disease or lessen the severity of the symptoms (Hook and Johnson, 1972). Moreover, such treatment is likely to prolong the fecal excretion of the organisms (Aserkoff and Bennett, 1969).

SALMONELLOSIS IN FOOD ANIMALS AND HUMANS

Salmonellae infect both warm-blooded and cold-blooded animals. In 1977, 5,243 Salmonella isolates from nonhuman sources were reported to the U.S. Department of Agriculture (USDA) and the Center for Disease Control (CDC). Of the total nonhuman isolates, 28% (1,474) were obtained from chickens and turkeys, 25% (1,313) were of porcine origin, and 14% (713) were of bovine origin (CDC, 1979). Five of the 10 serotypes most frequently isolated

[1] Consultant, Agricultural Division of American Cyanamid Co., Princeton, N.J.

TABLE 1

Confirmed Outbreaks of Food-Borne Disease, by Etiology, 1976[a]

Organism	Outbreaks Number	Outbreaks %[b]	Cases Number	Cases %[b]
Salmonella	28	21.2	1,169	32.7
Staphylococcus	26	19.7	930	26.0
Clostridium botulinum	23	17.4	40	1.1
Clostridium perfringens	6	4.5	509	14.2
Shigella	6	4.5	273	7.6
Bacillus cereus	2	1.5	63	1.8
Yersinia enterocolitica	1	0.8	286	8.0
TOTAL	92	69.6	3,270	91.4

[a] From Center for Disease Control, 1977b.

[b] Percent of all (bacterial, chemical, parasitic, and viral) food-borne disease outbreaks in the United States.

from animals (Table 2) were also among the 10 serotypes most frequently isolated from humans (Table 3). S. typhimurium, including var. copenhagen, comprised 35.5% of the human isolates reported and 19.7% of the isolates from nonhuman sources. It is by far the most frequently isolated serotype.

Although the greatest number of isolates from nonhuman sources was obtained from swine, the incidence of Salmonella in healthy market-ready swine varies greatly from place to place. In 1975, a survey was conducted at a slaughterhouse in each of three hog-producing areas (Gustafson et al., 1976). The purpose of the survey was to determine the incidence of Salmonella in healthy swine at market and to see what percent of them might be harboring salmonellae with resistance to more than one antibiotic. Of 151 hogs sampled in Pennsylvania, 54 (35.7%) had salmonellae and none had multiply resistant salmonellae. Of 251 hogs sampled in Iowa, 26 (10.3%) had salmonellae and one had multiply resistant salmonellae. Of 256 hogs sampled in Georgia, 215 had salmonellae (83.9%) and 9 (3.5%) had multiply resistant salmonellae. These data suggest that only a few hogs harbor multiply antibiotic-resistant salmonellae.

THE EFFECT OF SUBTHERAPEUTIC TETRACYCLINES ON SALMONELLAE IN DOMESTIC ANIMALS

In April 1973, the Food and Drug Administration (FDA) issued a statement requiring the manufacturers of tetracyclines and certain other drugs to show, by April 20, 1974, that the use of these drugs in animal feeds did not increase the Salmonella reservoir in animals and poultry raised for meat (FDA, 1973).

The FDA Bureau of Veterinary Medicine (BVM) then issued a set of human health safety criteria for the drug manufacturers to meet in order to demonstrate that the Salmonella reservoir in meat animals was not increased by the subtherapeutic levels of the drugs in feed. BVM and the manufacturers designed protocols for experiments to determine the effect of the drug on the quantity, prevalence, and duration of shedding and the resistance characteristics of the Salmonella in animals consuming subtherapeutic levels of antibiotics in their feed. By April 20, 1974, these experiments had been conducted and the manufacturers had reported the results to the BVM.

The experiments that were published are described briefly below.

TABLE 2

10 *Salmonella* Serotypes Most Frequently Isolated from Nonhuman Sources, 1977[a]

Serotype	Number of isolates reported, by source					
	Feed	Chickens	Turkeys	Swine	Cattle	TOTAL[b]
typhimurium[c]	10	67	17	194	310	1,033
derby	25	5	14	264	1	378
cholerae-suis[d]	1	0	0	332	4	345
anatum	11	11	107	69	24	314
agona	3	25	35	28	85	271
heidelberg	1	75	113	3	1	236
saint-paul	3	2	182	7	1	219
panama	9	0	12	147	1	188
infantis	3	81	8	18	7	165
san-diego	0	1	104	1	0	112
TOTAL	66	267	592	1,063	434	3,261
PERCENT OF TOTAL OF ALL SEROTYPES ISOLATED	39	44	68	81	61	62
TOTAL OF ALL SEROTYPES ISOLATED	168	608	866	1,313	713	5,243

[a]From CDC, 1979.

[b]Also includes isolates from other animals and environmental samples.

[c]Includes var. copenhagen.

[d]Var. kunzendorf.

TABLE 3

10 *Salmonella* Serotypes Most Frequently Isolated from Human Sources, 1977[a]

Serotype	Number	Percent	Rank in 1976
typhimurium[b]	9,690	35.3	1
newport	2,187	8.0	4
heidelberg	1,741	6.3	2
enteritidis	1,472	5.4	5
infantis	1,304	4.7	6
agona	1,229	4.5	3
saint-paul	580	2.1	7
typhi	549	2.0	8
montevideo	470	1.7	12
oranienburg	440	1.6	9
TOTAL	19,662	71.6	
TOTAL OF ALL SEROTYPES	27,462	100	

[a] From CDC, 1979.

[b] Includes var. copenhagen.

EXPERIMENTS IN SWINE

Gutzmann *et al.* (1976) divided 30 5- to 6-week-old pigs, each weighing approximately 7 kg, into three groups of 10. One group was given chlortetracycline at 220 g/metric ton of feed. A second group was given AUREO S•P 250, at a level that supplied 110 g of chlortetracycline, 110 g of sulfamethazine, and 55 g of penicillin G per metric ton of feed.

The third group was given the nonmedicated basal ration. On the sixth day of medication, all three groups were given in their feed 100 billion cfu (colony-forming units) per pig of a nalidixic-acid-resistant, tetracycline-sensitive strain of *Salmonella typhimurium* of swine origin. A fourth group of 10 pigs from the same breeding was kept as an unmedicated, uninfected control. Fecal samples were taken at 1, 2, 6, 9, 15, 22, and 26 days after administration to detect and enumerate salmonellae.

As shown in Figure 1, chlortetracycline at 220 g/metric ton of feed substantially reduced the number of salmonellae shed. The effect of AUREO S•P 250 was somewhat less, but calculation of the total area under each curve, equivalent to the total number of salmonellae shed by each group, showed a 22.5% reduction in the number of salmonellae shed by the group on chlortetracycline and a 9.6% reduction in salmonellae shed by the group on AUREO S•P 250. The duration of shedding and number of animals shedding salmonellae was no different in the medicated than in the unmedicated groups. By plating the fecal samples on agar containing nalidixic acid and chlortetracycline, it was possible to learn whether the infecting salmonellae had acquired tetracycline resistance from the tetracycline-resistant *E. coli* which the pigs were known to have. Only a few tetracycline-resistant *Salmonella* were found in six of 172 fecal samples, and these occurred in unmedicated as well as medicated pigs. Thus, it could be concluded that the drug had not selected for resistance.

An experiment by another manufacturer (Evangelisti *et al.*, 1975; Girard *et al.*, 1976) was conducted in a manner very similar to that described above except that oxytetracycline at 150 g/ton of feed or oxytetracycline at 150 g plus neomycin at 150 g/ton of feed was given to medicated groups. Figure 2 shows the quantity of *Salmonella typhimurium* shed.

As in the previously described experiment the medicated groups shed substantially fewer salmonellae than did the unmedicated group.

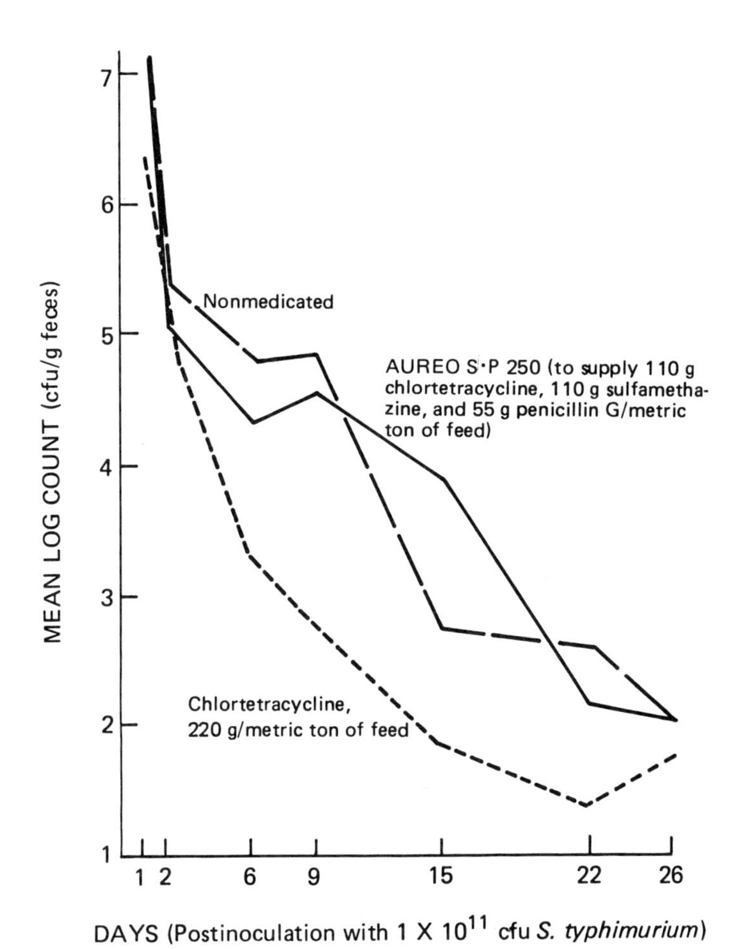

FIGURE 1. Summary of Salmonella typhimurium isolations from swine. From Gutzmann et al., 1976, with permission from the authors and the American Journal of Veterinary Research.

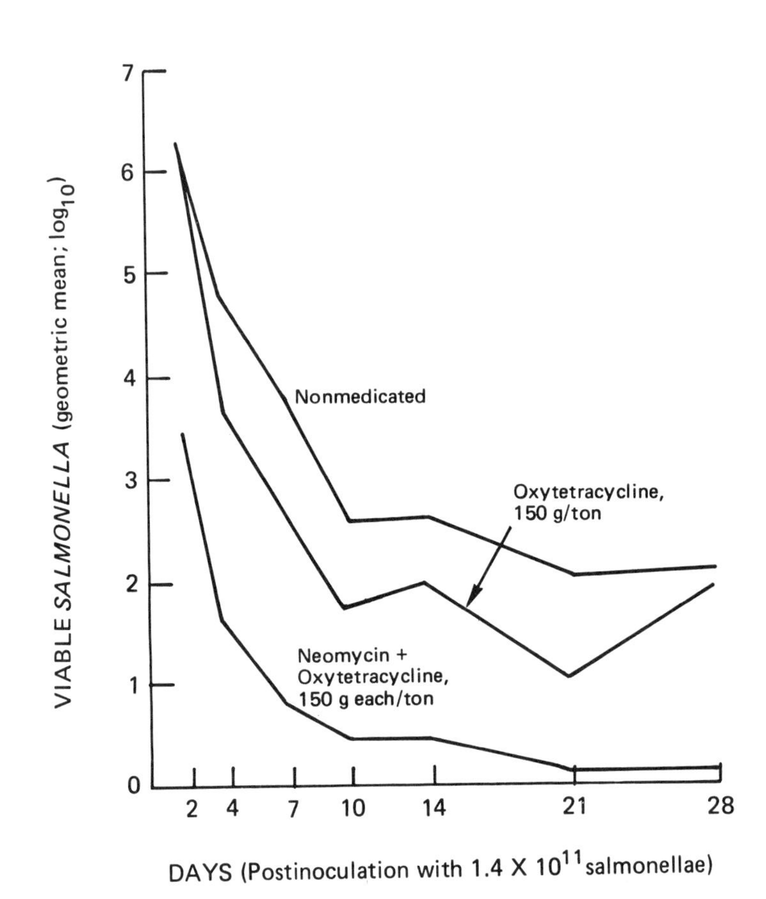

FIGURE 2. Number of salmonellae recovered from swine feces. From Evangelisti _et al._, 1975, and Girard _et al._, 1976.

There was no difference in duration of shedding between the medicated and unmedicated groups. Only two resistant isolates were detected in the medicated groups. None was seen in the unmedicated group.

EXPERIMENTS IN CALVES

Layton *et al.* (1975) divided 24 4-week-old calves into three groups of eight calves each. One group was given 350 mg of chlortetracycline per head per day in feed, and the other group was given 350 mg of chlortetracycline plus 350 mg of sulfamethazine per head per day in feed. These levels were supplied by a weighed amount of a concentrate containing the desired amount of the antimicrobial. The third group was not medicated. After 5 days of medication, each calf was infected orally via stomach tube with approximately 6.5 x 10^9 cfu of a nalidixic-acid-resistant, antibiotic-sensitive strain of *Salmonella typhimurium* of bovine origin. Fecal samples were obtained at 1, 2, 6, 9, 15, 22, and 26 days after infection and examined for the number of salmonellae. Figure 3 shows that the number of salmonellae from the medicated groups was lower than that from the unmedicated group at each sampling. The group on chlortetracycline shed 38.0% fewer salmonellae. The group on the combination shed 28.6% fewer salmonellae. The duration and prevalence of shedding was slightly greater in the unmedicated than in the medicated group. Salmonellae that were resistant to chlortetracycline were recovered from five calves in the unmedicated group, three calves in the chlortetracycline-medicated group, and one calf in the group on the combination. Only a very small fraction of the salmonellae in any of these samples was resistant, and in only two instances were resistant organisms isolated more than once from the same calf. In no instance did the resistant organisms become established in a calf.

In another experiment (Evangelisti *et al.*, 1975; Girard *et al.*, 1976), run in much the same way, three groups of 10 calves each, averaging approximately 85 kg per calf, were given feed containing oxytetracycline at 350 mg per head per day or oxytetracycline and neomycin in an amount calculated to give each calf 350 mg of each drug per head per day. One group was not medicated. The results of this experiment were very similar to the previously described experiment in calves. The number of salmonellae shed is shown in Figure 4. The duration and prevalence of shedding in the medicated groups were considerably less than in the unmedicated group. No tetracycline-resistant salmonellae were detected.

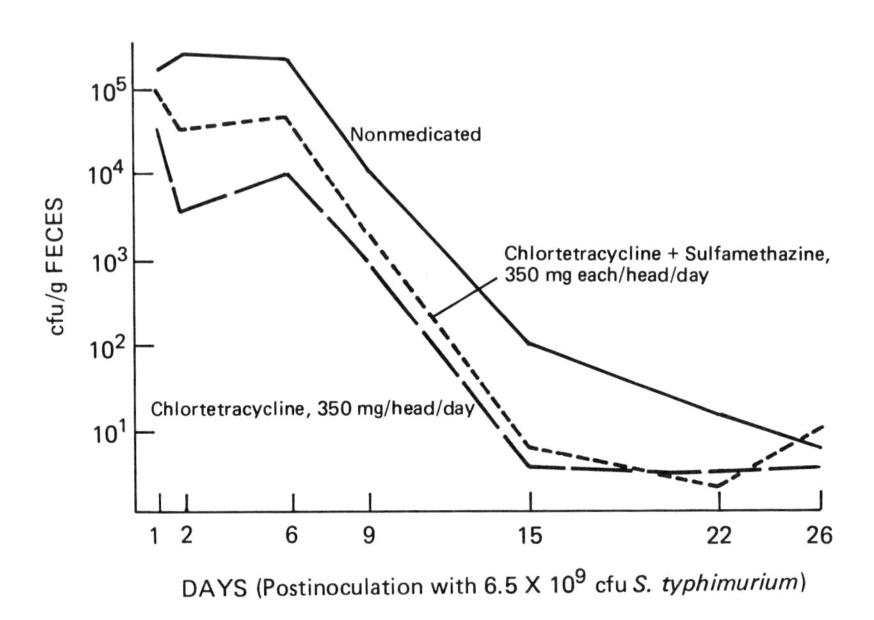

FIGURE 3. *Salmonella typhimurium* isolated from feces of infected calves (expressed as geometric means). From Layton *et al.*, 1975, with permission from the authors and *Zentralblatt fuer Veterinaermedizin Reihe B*.

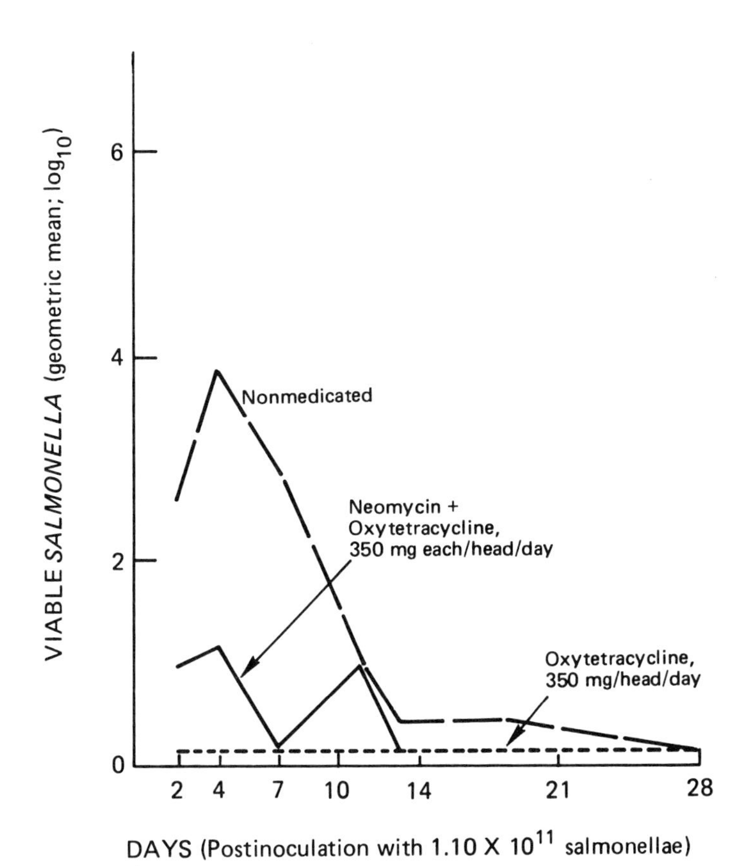

FIGURE 4. Number of salmonellae recovered from calves feces. From Evangelisti *et al.*, 1975, and Girard *et al.*, 1976.

EXPERIMENTS IN CHICKENS

In an experiment designed to meet the requirements of the BVM, Jarolmen *et al.* (1976) divided 112 1-day-old chicks into four groups of 28 each. Two groups were given feed containing 200 g chlortetracycline per ton of feed. The other two groups were given unmedicated feed. On the sixth day after medication had begun, each chick in one of the medicated and one of the unmedicated groups was infected orally with approximately 6.8×10^9 cfu of a nalidixic acid-resistant, antibiotic-sensitive strain of *Salmonella typhimurium* of chicken origin. Droppings from each bird in the infected groups were analyzed for *Salmonella* content at intervals for 57 days. Figure 5 shows the rate of disappearance and the number of *Salmonella* shed by medicated and unmedicated groups. Eight days after administration, the unmedicated group had shed 50 times as many salmonellae as did the medicated group. During the entire study the reduction in the number of salmonellae shed was highly signficant ($P = 0.01$).

Unlike the studies with swine and calves, many tetracycline-resistant salmonellae were isolated from both medicated and unmedicated groups. This was not unexpected since Walton (1966) had shown the *in-vivo* transfer of R factors in the guts of chickens that had been given 10 drops of an overnight broth culture of R-factor-containing *E. coli* by mouth immediately after hatching, while their intestinal tracts were still sterile, and the same amount of *S. typhimurium* by mouth 6 hours later.

Smith (1970) had also shown that resistance to tetracycline could be transferred from *E. coli* to *S. typhimurium* when newly hatched chicks were given large numbers of R-factor-containing *E. coli* in their drinking water for 3 days and then given 10^9 viable *S. typhimurium* by mouth. However, he had also shown that transfer occurred only when the *E. coli* used was a good colonizer of the chickens' intestine and was able to transfer resistance readily *in vitro*.

In the experiment by Jarolmen *et al.* (1976), the presence of chlortetracycline in the feed of the medicated chicks had insured that they would have large numbers of resistant *E. coli* in their intestines, and the unmedicated chicks had evidently become contaminated because they were in the same room. The numbers of both sensitive and resistant *S. typhimurium* decreased at about the same rate, even though the medicated birds continued to receive chlortetracycline throughout the experiment. The performance, in terms of final weight and kilogram of weight gain per kilogram of feed,

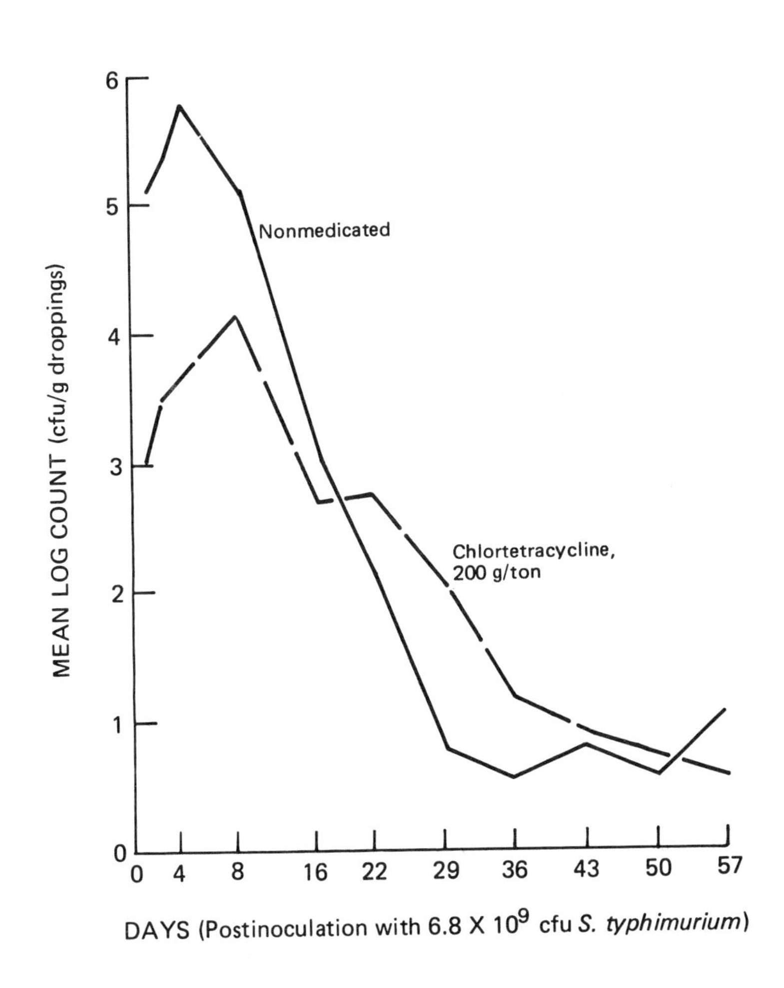

FIGURE 5. Salmonella typhimurium isolations from droppings of chickens inoculated with 6.8×10^9 cfu *S. typhimurium*. From Jarolmen *et al.*, 1976, with permission from the authors and the *Journal of Applied Bacteriology*.

was better in the medicated than in the unmedicated birds irrespective of whether they had been inoculated (Table 4).

In an independent experiment (Evangelisti *et al.*, 1975; Girard *et al.*, 1976) medication was started when the chickens were 8-days-old and thus had an established intestinal flora. One group of 10 birds that was given 200 g of oxytetracycline and another group of 10 birds given 200 g of oxytetracycline plus 200 g of neomycin per ton of feed shed far fewer *S. typhimurium* and stopped shedding earlier than did the group of 10 unmedicated controls (see Figure 6). Very few resistant *S. typhimurium* were detected.

A second type of experiment more nearly approximated natural conditions. Jarolmen *et al.* (1976) divided 100 1-day-old chicks into two groups of 50 each and housed the groups in separate buildings. Two chicks in each group were given oral doses of approximately 3.6×10^6 cfu of a nalidixic-acid-resistant, antibiotic-sensitive strain of *S. typhimurium*. One group was given feed containing 200 g of chlortetracycline per ton; the other group received unmedicated feed. Fecal samples were collected from each bird in each group once weekly for 8 weeks and analyzed for *Salmonella*.

The medicated, inoculated birds stopped shedding salmonellae within the first 2 weeks, whereas the unmedicated inoculated birds shed for 6 weeks. Figure 7 shows the percent of contact birds, i.e., uninoculated birds that have been exposed to birds infected with salmonellae, that were positive for *Salmonella* in each group at weekly intervals. The *Salmonella* spread quickly throughout the unmedicated group and maintained a level of infection of 90% or more for 6 weeks, when it dropped to 50%. In the medicated group, no more than 24% of the birds were infected and only 10% were positive at the end of the test. A tetracycline-resistant strain of *S. typhimurium* was isolated only once from a medicated bird, but it did not spread to other birds or recur in the same bird.

These experiments provide evidence that the use of subtherapeutic levels of tetracycline in the feed of swine, calves, and chickens do not increase the number of animals shedding *Salmonella* or the total number of salmonellae shed nor does it prolong the duration of shedding or select for resistant strains when the infecting organism is sensitive to antibiotics.

Williams *et al.* (1979) infected swine with *S. typhimurium* cells that were either sensitive or resistant to antibiotics. Some of the

TABLE 4

Final Weight and Ratio of Feed to Weight Gain of Chickens Inoculated with *Salmonella typhimurium* (6.8×10^9 colony forming units) Compared to Uninoculated Chickens When Receiving Medicated or Unmedicated Feed[a]

Type of Feed	Inoculated		Not Inoculated	
	Final Weight, kg	Feed:Gain	Final Weight, kg	Feed:Gain
Nonmedicated	1.95	2.2084	1.90	2.2712
Chlortetracycline	2.01	2.1758	2.04	2.2440

[a] From Jarolmen et al., 1976.

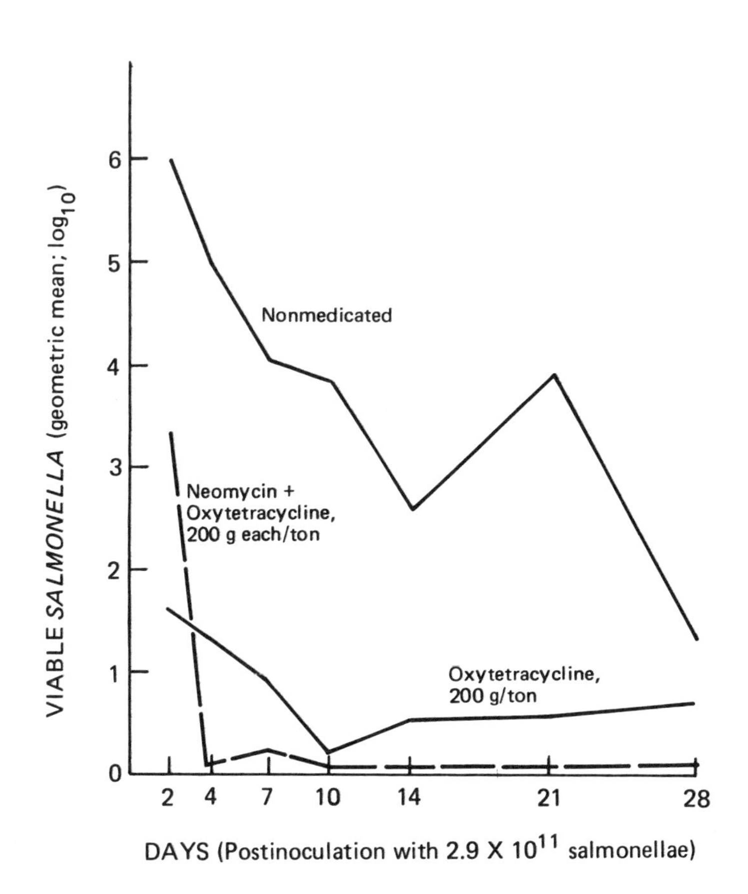

FIGURE 6. Number of salmonellae recovered from chickens feces. From Evangelisti _et al._, 1975, and Girard _et al._, 1976.

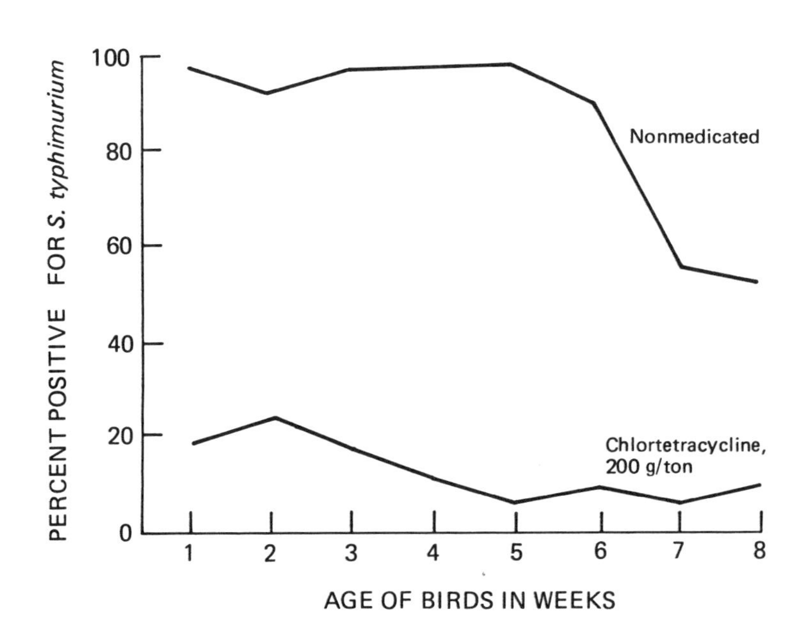

FIGURE 7. Percent of contact birds positive for *Salmonella typhimurium* by direct plating or after enrichment.

animals were given feed containing chlortetracycline at 110 mg/kg; others received unmedicated feed. The results obtained with the pigs infected with the sensitive strain were similar to those described previously. However, when the pigs were infected with an antibiotic-resistant strain and were then given feed containing chlortetracycline, they shed a greater quantity of salmonellae for a longer time than did the pigs on unmedicated feed. Salmonellae spread to uninfected pigs that were exposed to pigs with antibiotic-resistant salmonellae. The spread was greater when the recipients were receiving medicated feed. Five of 14 pigs infected with the antibiotic-sensitive strain died during the experiment. None of the pigs infected with the antibiotic-resistant strain died.

Garside *et al*. (1960) studied the emergence of resistant *S. typhimurium* in both unmedicated chicks and those that had been medicated with chlortetracycline. Resistant strains that emerged in the medicated groups were used to infect other groups of birds that were either medicated or unmedicated. Table 5 summarizes the mortality in five experiments conducted by Garside and his colleagues. The mortality in the birds infected with the resistant strains was not much less than it was in the groups infected with the sensitive strains, but the mortality in the groups infected with the resistant strains was reduced as much by medication with chlortetracycline as it was in the groups infected with sensitive strains.

INFECTION OF PIGS ON THE FARM

Williams *et al*. (1969) have shown that animal protein meal, when used as a constituent of pig feed, may be a source of salmonellae for hogs. Of 311 samples delivered to one feed mill over a 10-month period, 68% contained *Salmonella*. Of 206 lots of meat meal, 86% contained *Salmonella*.

Numerous other reports have incriminated the animal protein constituents of pig feed as sources of *Salmonella*. In 1977, 136 isolates of *Salmonella* from animal feeds were reported by various state health agencies to CDC (CDC, 1979). Of these, 22 were *S. derby*, the third most frequently isolated serotype from meat animals (Table 6). Only two isolates were obtained from vegetable protein. *S. derby* was not reported by the CDC as having been isolated from any food-borne outbreak of disease in humans in 1975, 1976, or 1977, although it was one of the three serotypes most frequently reported to the CDC as having been isolated from swine, cattle, turkeys, or chickens in each of those years (CDC, 1976b,

TABLE 5

Mortality of Chicks Infected with Strains of *Salmonella typhimurium* that were Sensitive or Resistant to Chlortetracycline When Receiving Feed Treated with Chlortetracycline or Unmedicated Feed[a]

Type of Feed	Mortality, by sensitivity of *Salmonella*	
	Sensitive	Resistant
nonmedicated	90/185[b] (48.6%)	92/217 (42.4%)
medicated	44/188 (23.4%)	26/164 (15.9%)

[a]From Garside et al., 1960.

[b]Number dead/total number.

TABLE 6

10 *Salmonella* Serotypes Most Frequently Isolated from Food Animals, 1975 through 1977[a]

1975		1976		1977	
Serotype	No. of Isolates	Serotype	No. of Isolates	Serotype	No. of Isolat
senftenberg	120	typhimurium	113	typhimurium	588
typhimurium[b]	86	derby	33	cholerae-suis	336
newport	17	panama	24	derby	284
derby	6	cubana	21	anatum	211
meleagridis	6	cholerae-suis	10	saint-paul	192
dublin	5	newington	10	heidelberg	192
cholerae-suis	3	dublin	8	agona	173
heidelberg	3	anatum	7	panama	160
muenchen	2	worthington	7	infantis	114
london	2	heidelberg	6	san-diego	106
TOTAL	250		239		2,356
PERCENTAGE OF ALL SEROTYPES ISOLATED	89		76		67
TOTAL OF ALL SEROTYPES ISOLATED	280		316		3,500

[a] From CDC, 1976b, 1977d, 1979.

[b] Includes var. copenhagen.

1977d, 1979). The state agencies also reported that *S. derby* was one of the serotypes most frequently isolated from human dietary items in 1976 and 1977 (Table 7). The figures reported by CDC have little significance since it probably receives reports on only a small number of the actual outbreaks of diseases. The fact that some few serotypes are reported year after year as the most frequently isolated serotypes suggests that they have some epidemiological significance. This is particularly true of the isolates from humans for which eight of the 10 most frequently reported serotypes were the same in 1975, 1976, and 1977 (Table 8). But because these serotypes are found so frequently in humans, it is highly speculative to assume that any particular serotype has come from animals. If phage typing were done and the phage type of the *Salmonella* from the animals were the same as the phage type of the *Salmonella* from the humans, the assumption would be more likely.

In an epidemiological study of *Salmonella* infection in swine in Ontario, only 3.2% of 380 carcasses were positive for *Salmonella* (Groves *et al.*, 1970). In a survey of five abattoirs, five carcasses out of 80 were positive in one abattoir and 10 out of 80 were positive at another. In the remaining three abattoirs, none of the carcasses were positive. However, 20.3% of the mesenteric lymph nodes from 462 hogs were positive. Of 190 environmental samples, 8.4% were positive, and of 101 feed samples, 7.8% were positive. *S. typhimurium*, *S. heidelberg*, *S. muenster*, and *S. anatum* were most frequently isolated from lymph nodes, but only *S. typhimurium* and *S. heidelberg* were isolated from carcasses. Antimicrobial resistance was detected in 11.7% of the 94 *Salmonella* isolates. Five of 14 isolates tested for R factors were positive. The other nine were resistant to only one antimicrobial agent. In one instance, *S. heidelberg* was isolated from feed samples and swine pens on a farm, from swine from the farm slaughtered in an abattoir, from the abattoir environment, and from the carcasses and washings of edible pork products in the abattoir. These data provide circumstantial evidence that swine serve as a reservoir for salmonellosis in humans, but the humans working in the abattoir were not sampled to determine whether they might be a source of *S. heidelberg*. Additionally, *S. heidelberg* is one of the most frequently isolated serotypes: phage typing of isolates from animals and from cases of salmonellosis in humans would be necessary to prove that the infections were caused by salmonellae of animal origin.

TABLE 7

10 *Salmonella* Serotypes Most Frequently Isolated from Dietary Items for Human Consumption, 1975 through 1977[a]

1975		1976		1977	
Serotype	No. of Isolates	Serotype	No. of Isolates	Serotype	No. of Isolate
kentucky	74	panama	22	newington	19
anatum	16	enteritidis	20	typhimurium	15
manhattan	16	derby	15	infantis	13
typhimurium	13	typhimurium	14	dublin	8
infantis	13	heidelberg	11	weltevreden	8
agona	12	mokola	10	agona	5
heidelberg	12	orion	10	derby	5
derby	9	muenster	7	senftenberg	5
saint-paul	7	anatum	6	tennessee	5
litchfield	7	lanka	6	bareilly	4
TOTAL	179		121		87
PERCENTAGE OF TOTAL ISOLATED FROM DIETARY ITEMS	77		70		66
TOTAL ISOLATED FROM DIETARY ITEMS	232		173		131

[a] From CDC, 1976b, 1977d, 1979.

TABLE 8

10 *Salmonella* Serotypes Most Frequently Isolated from Humans, 1975 through 1977[a]

75		1976		1977	
rotype	No. of Isolates	Serotype	No. of Isolates	Serotype	No. of Isolates
phimurium[b]	6,888	typhimurium	7,847	typhimurium	9,690
wport	1,550	heidelberg	1,962	newport	2,187
teritidis	1,519	agona	1,461	heidelberg	1,741
idelberg	1,474	newport	1,336	enteritidis	1,472
ona	1,333	enteritidis	1,219	infantis	1,304
fantis	1,194	infantis	1,014	agona	1,229
int-paul	833	saint-paul	545	saint-paul	580
phi	551	typhi	529	typhi	549
anienburg	446	oranienburg	465	montevideo	470
viana	426	muenchen	374	oranienburg	440
TAL	16,264		16,752		19,662
RCENTAGE OF TOTAL SERO- TYPES ISOLATED	69		72		72
TAL SEROTYPES ISOLATED	23,445		23,285		27,462

C, 1976b, 1977d, 1979.

cludes var. copenhagen.

CONTAMINATION OF CARCASSES AND MEAT BY *Salmonella*

Contamination of hog carcasses by *Salmonella* was recognized before antibiotics were used in animal feed. An extensive study by Galton *et al.* (1954) during 1951 and 1952 showed that 7% of 374 hogs on 28 Florida farms were positive for *Salmonella*. However, 18 of the 27 positive animals were from two farms. All pigs tested on 20 farms were negative. When hogs and carcasses were sampled for *Salmonella* at five abattoirs, the investigators found that extensive contamination and infection of the hogs had occurred during transport to the abattoir from the farm. A total of 1,883 rectal swabs were taken at the same point in the processing line of the five abattoirs. Results among the abattoirs ranged from 11% to 80% positive for *Salmonella*. There was a substantial difference in the efforts made by the abattoirs to prevent contamination and cross-contamination of the carcasses. This was evident from the fact that only 1% of environmental samples taken from the cutting and sausage rooms of one plant were positive, whereas 66% of the samples taken from the same types of locations in another plant were positive.

That pigs may be marketed virtually free of *Salmonella* infection was shown by Edel *et al.* (1974). They raised pigs in houses kept free of insects, birds, and rodents, and fed them pelletted feed. (Pelletting involves injecting steam into the feed to raise the temperature to 82 C. This temperature is maintained in the pellets long enough to kill most *Salmonella*.) Only 21 (1.6%) of 1,317 pigs slaughtered were *Salmonella*-positive, and of these, 14 (1.1%) were probably contaminated in the abattoir.

A study of salmonellae in cattle, their feed, and their relation to human infection was reported in England in 1965 (Ministry of Agriculture, Fisheries, and Food, 1965). This investigation showed that *S. dublin* was the serotype most frequently infecting cattle and calves but that there was also a high incidence of *S. typhimurium*. By the use of phage typing, the investigators showed that *S. typhimurium* spread from cattle, especially from calves, to humans. The infections in calves were exacerbated by shipping them long distances without proper food or rest, by subjecting them to chills, and by mixing them with calves from other sources. *S. typhimurium* was infrequently isolated from cattle feed. *S. dublin*, which was isolated from only two of 7,300 samples, was said to play only a small role in human infections.

Finlayson (1977) discussed the relationship between human infections and salmonellae in poultry products in Alberta, Canada. She reported that the great majority of human infections were "sporadic," involving only single cases or individual families, and that the vehicle of infection was seldom identified. There was circumstantial evidence that poultry products might be playing a role in human infections in that the serotypes most frequently isolated from humans were among those most frequently isolated from poultry. But again, this assumption would be strengthened if the isolates were of the same phage type. Cleaning procedures varied considerably from plant to plant. Hence, *Salmonella* contamination of the plants varied from 46% to 89% of the environmental samples taken. Eighty-seven percent of the strains examined were sensitive to antimicrobial agents commonly used in treatment of humans and livestock. In birds, resistance occurred mainly in strains specifically associated with turkeys (*S. saint-paul* and some types of *S. typhimurium*). Commoner *Salmonella* strains (*S. california* and *S. infantis*) were generally sensitive to antibiotics when isolated from turkeys.

FOOD-BORNE OUTBREAKS OF SALMONELLOSIS

In 1975 there were 25 reported outbreaks of salmonellosis involving an estimated 1,006 persons (CDC, 1976b), who comprised 4.3% of the 23,445 isolations reported that year. In 1976, there were 42 reported outbreaks affecting 1,915 persons. Of these, 571 had positive cultures, which was 2.4% of the 23,285 reported isolates (CDC, 1977d). In 1977, there were 40 reported outbreaks involving 1,632 persons. Of these, 364 had positive cultures, or 1.3% of the 27,462 isolates.

Of course, these figures are minimums since many outbreaks were not reported and, probably, many were not even diagnosed. From 1962 through 1977, 145 deaths were attributed to salmonellosis--a case fatality ratio of 0.36% (CDC, 1979). Table 9 lists the serotypes reported from 1975 to 1977 and the number of outbreaks from which they were isolated. *S. typhimurium* was isolated most frequently. *Heidelberg*, *thompson*, *newport*, and *saint-paul* were isolated in each of the 3 years. These serotypes, except for *thompson*, were among the seven most frequently isolated from humans in each of the 3 years.

From 1975 through 1977 outbreaks of salmonellosis were traced to commercially prepared precooked roast beef. Several of these outbreaks involved more than one state. In 1975, four outbreaks in New Jersey caused by *S. saint-paul* were attributed to roast beef that had been cooked at a temperature too low to destroy *Salmonella* after being injected with a fluid containing spices, flavorings,

TABLE 9

Isolates from Food-Borne Outbreaks of Salmonellosis, 1975 through 1977[a]

1975

Serotype	No. of Isolates
saint-paul	6
typhimurium	2
enteritidis	2
typhi	2
thompson	2
oranienburg	1
tennessee	1
reading	1
heidelberg	1
kottbus	1
litchfield	1
blockley	1
dublin	1
newport	1
singapore	1
TOTAL	25

1976

Serotype	No. of Isolates
typhimurium	15
typhi	5
heidelberg	5
enteritidis	3
saint-paul	2
bovis-morbificans	2
newport	2
typhimurium var. *copenhagan*	1
poona	1
muenchen	1
london	1
schwarzengrund	1
blockley	1
javiana	1
bredeney	1
san-diego	1
minnesota	1
thompson	1
infantis	1
give	1
Group E	1
TOTAL	48

1977

Serotype	No. of Isolat
typhimurium	8
infantis	4
agona	3
heidelberg	2
san-diego	2
typhi	2
bredeney	2
london	1
saint-paul	1
anatum	1
schwarzengrund	1
kottbus	1
bareilly	1
thompson	1
weltevreden	1
reading	1
newport	1
chester	1
oranienburg	1
muenchen	1
stanley	1
Group D	4
Group B	1
Other	2
TOTAL	44

[a] From CDC, 1976b, 1977d, 1979.

and, apparently, Salmonella. A second extensive outbreak, consisting of at least 200 identified cases in Pennsylvania, New Jersey, Connecticut, and Massachusetts, was due to S. bovis-morbificans (CDC, 1976a, 1977a). Epidemiological studies incriminated imported beef although Salmonella was not isolated from any of the beef at the site of purchase or processing. As a result of this outbreak, the USDA issued a regulation on September 2, 1977 requiring that all commercially prepared roasts of beef be cooked to an internal temperature of 63 C. In a third outbreak, which occurred in June, July, and August, 1977 (CDC, 1977c), S. newport was isolated from both the interior and exterior of roasts of beef before they had been carved. These cases were reported in Pennsylvania, New York, and New Jersey, and were all attributed to cooking the meat at too low a temperature.

In the first outbreak, the contamination was due to injecting the meat with a contaminated fluid. Since no salmonellae were found in the meat consumed in the second outbreak, the source of contamination has not been proven. In the third, no source of contamination was shown.

In 1977, the food-borne outbreaks of salmonellosis involved meat, milk, ice cream, or cheese (CDC, 1979). In July an outbreak in Michigan involving S. typhimurium was traced to home-made ice cream made with raw eggs (CDC, 1977e). Another outbreak involving S. typhimurium occurred in Kentucky where two children and their father were infected by raw milk used to make icing for a cake (CDC, 1977f). Salmonellae were isolated from the three patients, but not from the milk or icing. S. typhimurium with the same lysis pattern was isolated from a cow and a calf on the farm where the milk was produced. The organism was resistant to tetracycline, streptomycin, ampicillin, carbenicillin, and penicillin. There had been an oubreak of diarrheal illness of several months duration in the dairy herd, but the report of the outbreak (CDC, 1977f) did not document whether it had been treated with antibiotics.

Large amounts of ground beef, cold cuts, and frankfurters are consumed in the United States. Because the manufacture and sale of these products require more handling than do cuts of beef or pork, it is desirable to analyze CDC's food-borne disease surveillance data on these foods (CDC, 1975). From 1966 through 1973, 2,464 food-borne outbreaks were reported to CDC. In 1,827 (74%) of the outbreaks the food vehicle was identified. Ground beef, cold cuts, or frankfurters were responsible for 91 (5%) of the 1,827; 65 (3.6%) were caused by ground beef; 6 (0.3%) by cold cuts; and 20 (1.1%) by frankfurters. In 21 of the 91 outbreaks the proximate cause was determined: one was the result of a food-processing error before consumer purchase; the other 28 resulted from improper food handling after purchase.

The etiologic agent was identified in nine of the 65 outbreaks attributed to ground beef. Three of these were due to salmonellae other than *S. typhi*, one was due to *S. typhi*, two to *Clostridium perfringens*, one to *C. botulinum*, and two to chemicals.

Data concerning the place where ground beef was mishandled were available for 27 of the 65 outbreaks. The beef was mishandled in food-service establishments in 18 outbreaks and in private homes in eight of the outbreaks. The other instance of mishandling occurred in a food-processing establishment.

Of six outbreaks attributed to cold cuts, one was due to *S. anatum*.

From 1972 through 1975, the USDA intermittently surveyed ground beef, luncheon meat, and frankfurters for salmonellae. Three contaminated beef patties were found. No salmonellae were found in luncheon meat or in frankfurters (CDC, 1975) (Table 10).

Data on food-borne outbreaks of salmonellosis in England and Wales for 1973 through 1975 are of interest for comparative purposes (Vernon, 1977). Table 11 lists the 10 most frequently isolated serotypes from humans in England and Wales and in the United States. Six of the 10 most frequently isolated serotypes are the same in both lists as are three of the first four ranked. These four serotypes (*S. typhimurium*, *S. newport*, *S. heidelberg*, and *S. enteritidis*) accounted for 60% and 55% of the total reported isolates in England and Wales and the United States, respectively. If one used the same logic that was used to link the isolates of *Salmonella* from animals with those from humans, i.e., the fact that several serotypes are among those most often isolated from each other, then one might argue that salmonellosis in England and Wales is transferred from humans in the United States. It is doubtful that many epidemiologists would subscribe to that proposition. There were 1,685 reported outbreaks of salmonellosis in England and Wales from 1973 to 1975 of which 407 were general outbreaks (i.e., involving more than one family) and 1,278 were outbreaks within a single family.

Hospitals accounted for 157 (39%) of the general outbreaks. There were 15,084 sporadic cases reported. The presumed causal agents were identified in 107 of the general and family outbreaks.

TABLE 10

Surveys of Salmonellae in Raw Beef Patties, Luncheon Meat, and Frankfurters, 1972 through 1975[a]

Product	Samples Examined	Samples Positive
Raw beef patties		
Raw trimmings	690	1
Raw finished patties	735	3
Frankfurters		
Raw trimmings	842	56
Cooked finished frankfurters	690	0
Sliced luncheon meat		
Raw trimmings	936	69
Cooked, sliced luncheon meat	456	0

[a]From CDC, 1975.

TABLE 11

10 Most Frequently Isolated *Salmonella* Serotypes from Humans in England and Wales and in the United States[a]

England and Wales, 1973-1975		United States, 1977	
Serotype	No. of Isolates	Serotype	No. of Isolates
typhimurium	8,396	typhimurium	9,690
agona	3,685	newport	2,187
enteritidis	2,602	heidelberg	1,741
heidelberg	1,178	enteritidis	1,472
anatum	1,009	infantis	1,304
indiana	931	agona	1,229
newport	908	saint-paul	580
infantis	698	typhi	549
hadar	512	montevideo	470
bredeney	494	oranienburg	440
TOTAL	20,413		19,662
PERCENTAGE OF ALL SEROTYPES ISOLATED	77		72
TOTAL SEROTYPES ISOLATED	26,574		27,462

[a] From Vernon, 1977, and CDC, 1979.

Meat was incriminated in 27 outbreaks of which 11 were attributed to ham and bacon. Poultry was responsibile for 49, milk and cream for 30, and sweet desserts for one.

Several things seem clear from the above discussion on salmonellosis. First, domestic animals are a significant reservoir of *Salmonella*. Second, this reservoir is expanded in the holding pens at slaughterhouses. Third, carcasses and meat are contaminated with *Salmonella* during the killing and dressing process. It is less clear how much of this *Salmonella* actually reaches the consumer. However, when it does reach the consumer, mishandling of meat and meat products can result in multiplication of the organisms to the point that the consumer becomes infected and an outbreak occurs. But examination of the information on which these conclusions are based produces no evidence that the use of subtherapeutic levels of tetracyclines or penicillin in animal feed played any role in the size of the reservoir, the spread of the salmonellae, or in any of the steps in transmission to the consumer.

The factors that contribute to outbreaks of food-borne disease were reviewed by Bryan (1978). Inadequate cooling was the single most frequent factor: either failure to refrigerate or storing such large amounts that they cooled too slowly. Handling of cooked foods by infected persons and cross-contamination were other important factors. Antibiotic sensitivity is seldom mentioned in the articles reviewed by Bryan, and in no instance was the subtherapeutic use of antibiotics in animal feed shown to be a factor. Occasionally, however, there were speculations that subtherapeutic use might increase the number of resistant *Salmonella* reaching the human population. In the Kentucky outbreak discussed above (CDC, 1977f), resistance of the organism was probably due to treatment of the dairy herd for a prolonged episode of diarrheal illness, although this was not documented.

ANTIBIOTIC RESISTANCE IN SALMONELLAE

There have been a number of surveys of antibiotic-resistant *Salmonella* in humans and animals in the United States. One such survey (Neu *et al.*, 1975) compared the antibiotic resistance and R-factor transmissibility of 718 isolates from humans in the northeastern United States with that of 688 isolates from animals in the eastern and midwestern states. The isolates from animals, like those from humans, were obtained from sick individuals. The animals, and perhaps the humans, had probably been treated with antibiotics. The percentage of *S. typhimurium*, *S. heidelberg*, and *S. saint-paul* from animals with resistance to streptomycin, sulfisoxazole, and tetracycline was greater than that for the strains from humans (Table 12). Resistance to kanamycin was high in the strains from the animals, but this may have been due to the fact that resistance to kanamycin and neomycin are often linked and neomycin is frequently used both therapeutically and prophylactically in animals. The percentage of *S. saint-paul* and *S. enteritidis* strains from animals with resistance to ampicillin was greater than that for the corresponding strains from humans. Ampicillin is not approved by FDA for use in animal feed but has been approved for therapeutic use in calves and swine since 1973.

The therapeutic use of antibiotics has been shown to elicit antibiotic resistance somewhat more rapidly than do prophylactic levels. Luther *et al.* (1974) gave 6-day-old chicks oxytetracycline in drinking water and measured the development of resistance in the *Escherichia coli* of their intestinal flora. One group of birds received 50 ppm of oxytetracycline in drinking water. This amount is equivalent to 100 ppm in the feed, which is a subtherapeutic level (Table 13). Resistance of 100% of the isolates to tetracycline, dihydrostreptomycin, and sulfamethazine developed in 3 days. Another group of birds was given 500 ppm in drinking water. This is equivalent to 1,000 ppm in feed, a therapeutic level. In this group of chicks, resistance of all isolates to tetracycline and dihydrostreptomycin developed in 2 days. Some resistance to ampicillin emerged in the chicks on 50 ppm, presumably because of linkage of resistance genes, but not in those on 500 ppm.

On the basis of resistance patterns of salmonellae from humans and animals, Neu *et al.* (1975) suggested that animals might be contributing to the pool of resistant organisms in humans. Cherubin *et al.* (1972) thought that unlikely. They said, "An urban reservoir of resistance transfer factor could exist equally as well as the postulated animal reservoir. It is difficult to reconcile the knowledge that the highest incidence of salmonellosis occurs in young children and infants in slum areas in New York City and the finding that the highest frequency of resistant *Salmonella* strains occurs in municipal hospitals serving these areas, with the hypothesis that *Salmonella* in general and resistant strains (or the resistance transfer factor) in particular, originate in farm animals. Unless one accepts the doubtful proposition that meat, poultry, eggs, milk and processed foods derived from them are preferentially consumed by the

TABLE 12

Resistance of Four *Salmonella* Serotypes from Humans and Animals to Individual Antimicrobial Agents[a]

Antibiotic	Percentage of Strains Resistant, by Serotype (No. of Strains Tested)							
	typhimurium		*heidelberg*		*saint-paul*		*enteritidis*	
	(241) human	(484) animal	(30) human	(72) animal	(44) human	(77) animal	(102) human	(27) animal
Ampicillin	36.9	31.0	30.0	11.0	13.6	19.5	0.9	7.4
Cephalothin	2.1	1.6	3.3	0	0	1.3	0.9	0
Chloramphenical	2.9	0.8	0	0	0	0	0	0
Gentamicin	0	0	0	0	0	0	0	0
Kanamycin	29.4	46.0	30.0	19.0	2.2	36.0	0.9	7.4
Streptomycin	45.6	64.0	16.6	32.0	11.3	45.0	2.9	0
Sulfisoxazole	30.9	73.0	6.6	22.0	2.2	27.0	2.9	0
Tetracycline	44.8	61.0	20.0	18.0	9.0	35.0	1.9	0
Trimethoprim	0	0	0	0	0	0	0.9	0
PERCENTAGE OF ALL STRAINS ISOLATED WITH RESISTANCE TO AN ANTIBIOTIC	57.6	80.0	30.0	41	15.9	61	5.8	7

[a] From Neu et al., 1975, with permission from the authors and the Journal of Infectious Diseases.

TABLE 13

Effect of Oxytetracycline (OTC) Water Medication on the Rate of Development of *Escherichia coli* Resistance *In Vivo* to Tetracyclines, Dihydrostreptomycin, Sulfamethazine, and Ampicillin[a]

	No OTC				OTC, 50 ppm				OTC, 500 ppm			
	Percentage Resistant				Percentage Resistant				Percentage Resistant			
Day	Tc[b]	Dhs[c]	Smz[d]	Amp[e]	Tc	Dhs	Smz	Amp	Tc	Dhs	Smz	Amp
-6	0	0	0	0	0	0	0	0	0	0	0	0
-2	3	6	6	6	0	0	0	0	0	0	0	0
0	-[f]	-	-	-	0	0	0	0	0	0	0	0
+1	0	0	3	0	55	50	55	23	66	66	0	13
+2	0	0	0	0	94	94	94	16	100	100	0	0
+3	19	19	16	9	100	100	100	3	100	100	0	0
+4	3	0	0	0	97	97	97	19	100	100	3	0
+5	0	0	0	0	100	100	100	13	100	100	0	0
+6	0	0	0	0	94	94	94	3	100	100	0	0

[a]From Luther et al., 1974, with permission from the authors and Miles Laboratories, Ltd.

[b]Tc = tetracyclines

[c]Dhs = dihydrostreptomycin

[d]Smz = sulfamethazine

[e]Amp = ampicillin

[f]Dashes indicate that no measurements were taken.

young and the poor, we would expect that the hypothesis of an animal origin would require that salmonellosis and resistant _Salmonella_ isolates occur most frequently in adults and in the affluent."

Another frequently mentioned survey of antibiotic resistance in animals is that of Pocurull _et al_. (1971). They tested 1,251 strains of _Salmonella_ isolated from sick animals at the National Animal Disease Laboratory in Ames, Iowa. Of these, 935 (75%) were resistant to one or more of the 11 antimicrobials used in the survey. Here again it is likely that this resistance resulted from therapeutic use rather than subtherapeutic use in feed since these isolates were obtained from sick animals. It is unusual for a veterinarian to take samples for antibiotic sensitivity testing before beginning treatment.

Timoney (1978) provided further evidence that the pool of resistant _Salmonella_ in humans may be different from that in calves. From 1973 to 1976 he tested 249 strains of _S. typhimurium_ isolated from diseased animals in New York State for sensitivity to six commonly used antibiotics. Only 12% were sensitive to all six. Virtually all of the 135 strains isolated from calves during this time were resistant to kanamycin, neomycin, streptomycin, and tetracycline (Table 14). An interesting observation was that resistance to ampicillin, which was first approved for therapeutic use in calves in 1973, increased steadily during the 4 years. Moreover, the resistance to chloramphenicol also increased during that 4-year-period although to a much smaller degree. Chloramphenicol is not approved for any use in livestock. The emergence of resistance to ampicillin in calves is reminiscent of a similar increase in resistance to this antibiotic in strains from humans in the northeastern United States during the late 1960's following widespread use of the drug after its introduction in 1964 (Neu _et al_., 1971). The development of resistance to ampicillin in _S. typhimurium_ in calves and in humans would seem to be separate phenomena, and neither the use of antibiotics in feed nor therapeutic use in calves has influenced resistance in strains of _S. typhimurium_ from humans in the northeastern United States. Further evidence of the separation of human and calf pools of _S. typhimurium_ is reported by Cherubin _et al_. (1980), who showed that resistance to ampicillin in _S. typhimurium_ from two New York City hospitals has returned to 1965 levels (Table 15). Resistance to tetracycline in these strains of _S. typhimurium_ has also decreased, although not as markedly.

TABLE 14
Antibiotic-Resistant Strains of *Salmonella typhimurium* Isolated from Calves[a]

Year	No. of Isolates	Percentage resistant						Percentage with transferable R-factors
		Amp[b]	Coli[c]	Km[d]	Nm[e]	Sm[f]	Tc[g]	
1973	37	16	3	95	95	100	100	38
1974	40	33	3	87	83	97	95	49
1975	35	43	5	80	69	78	86	60
1976	23	74	9	96	87	100	100	87

[a] From Timoney, 1978, with permission from the author and the University of Chicago Press.

[b] Amp = ampicillin

[c] Coli = chloramphenicol

[d] Km = kanamycin

[e] Nm = neomycin

[f] Sm = streptomycin

[g] Tc = tetracycline

TABLE 15

Antibiotic-Resistant *Salmonella typhimurium*

Antibiotic	Percentage of Resistant Isolates, by Study (Total of Isolates Tested)			
	1968-1969[a] (128)	1970[b] (85)	1973[c] (241)	1975-1978[d] (161)
Ampicillin	23.4	12.9	36.9	4.3
Tetracycline	12.5	23.5	44.8	21.1
Streptomycin	27.3	29.4	45.6	59.6
Chloramphenicol	0.0	0.0	2.9	0.0

[a] From Neu et al., 1971.

[b] From Cherubin et al., 1972.

[c] From Neu et al., 1975.

[d] From Cherubin et al., 1980.

NOTE: Table reproduced with permission from the authors and the Journal of the American Medical Association 243:439-442, February 1, 1980, ©1980, American Medical Association.

There were no reports of Salmonella agona in humans before 1970, but by 1976, it had become the third most frequently isolated serotype (Table 16) (CDC, 1976b, 1977d, 1979). Few isolates were reported from nonhuman sources until 1977 when 271 were reported. Of these, 173 were from pigs, cattle, chickens, and turkeys, 45 were from horses, and 10 were from miscellaneous animal sources. This suggests independent pools in humans and animals. S. agona was the second most frequently isolated serotype from humans in England and Wales from 1973 to 1975. It was also isolated frequently from poultry, sausage, and feedstuffs.

Salmonella typhimurium IN ENGLAND

An epidemic of antibiotic-resistant Salmonella typhimurium phage type 29 occurred in calves in England starting in 1964, peaking in 1965, and subsiding in 1966. This infection spread to humans. Of 2,544 cultures of S. typhimurium from humans submitted in 1965 to the Enteric Reference Laboratory in the United Kingdom, 576 (23%) were phage type 29 and 555 (22%) were resitant to antibiotics (Anderson, 1968b). In the testing of 1,772 cultures of S. typhimurium from bovines, 1,297 (73%) were phage type 29 and 1,294 were resistant to antibiotics. Thus, the phage type 29 strain played a much larger role in calves than in humans, but many human cases were involved. Since many of the infected humans had been in close contact with infected calves, it is likely that the infection was transferred from the calves. This epidemic was most severe in calves intended for "intensive" or confined rearing (Anderson, 1968a). This was a highly profitable business and calves were bringing high prices. In this method of rearing the calves were gathered from various farms, often only hours after birth, shipped to a collecting point, and then transported to a farm where they were to be fed for several months before slaughter. Some of the dealers were very careless in their management and hygiene. Calves were crowded into dirty vehicles and the conditions were ideal for the spread of disease.

When the epidemic was at its height, large amounts of antibiotics were used in an attempt to prevent or treat the disease. These attempts were largely futile because the organisms had become resistant to most of the commonly used drugs. This outbreak of disease can hardly be viewed as an indictment of the use of antibiotics in animal feed since it was really due to bad management. Specifically, calves were deprived of colostrum, without which no antibiotic will be effective in calves. Moreover, calves from various sources were mixed, which enabled the disease to spread

TABLE 16

Salmonella agona Isolated from Human and Nonhuman Sources, 1969-1977[a]

Year of Study	Number of Isolates	
	Human	Nonhuman
1969	0	3
1970	4	5
1971	44	34
1972	524	NA[b]
1973	864	NA
1974	1,037	NA
1975	1,333	45
1976	1,461	40
1977	1,229	271

[a]From CDC, 1976b, 1977d, 1979.

[b]NA = Data not available.

when the calves were moved to new farms. These animals were not kept adequately clean or warm nor were they fed or watered properly.

At the time of these outbreaks, antibiotics were not legally permitted in the feed of calves in England but were allowed in feed for pigs and chickens. Because of this epidemic the Swann Committee was appointed by the government of the United Kingdom. As a result of its recommendations (Swann *et al.*, 1969), tetracyclines, penicillin, and other antimicrobials were banned from the feed of pigs and chickens except on veterinary prescription. The ban on subtherapeutic use was not justified on the basis of evidence of incidents involving pigs or chickens since there had been no outbreaks of disease attributable to such use.

The restrictions based on the Swann recommendations were implemented in March 1971. In 1978, there was an outbreak of antibiotic-resistant *S. typhimurium* in calves in England that was similar to the 1965 outbreak (Threlfall *et al.*, 1978). Again, the disease was spread by crowding very young calves into dirty vehicles, transporting them long distances without adequate food, water, or warmth, and trying to cover these bad management practices with heavy doses of antibiotics. Again, the motivating force was high prices for calves. It would seem that the Swann recommendations missed their mark.

In summary, there is a large pool of *Salmonella* in domestic animals and a similarly large pool in humans. It is not clear that the second pool receives much contribution from the first. Food-borne outbreaks of salmonellosis are not uncommon, but what, if any, role antibiotic resistance plays in them seems impossible to determine from the evidence at hand. Finally, there seems to be no evidence that the use of tetracyclines and penicillin in animal feed play any adverse role in the development of salmonellosis in animals or humans or in food-borne outbreaks of salmonellosis in humans.

ANTIBIOTIC-RESISTANT *Escherichia coli* IN HUMANS AND DOMESTIC ANIMALS

In the Statement of Policy and Interpretation Regarding Animal Drugs and Medicated Feeds (FDA, 1973), the Commissioner of the FDA said that a theoretical hazard was posed by the possible colonization of the intestines of humans by R-factor-bearing *E. coli* from animals and by the possible linkage of an R-factor plasmid with a plasmid for the production of enterotoxin in *E. coli* of animal origin, thus enhancing its pathogenicity.

The first of these questions was addressed by Levy *et al.* (1976), who inoculated chickens in the cloaca with a strain of *E. coli* carrying a marked plasmid with resistance to tetracycline, streptomycin, and sulfonamides. These chickens were then placed in two cages with other, uninoculated chickens. The chickens in one of the cages were given feed containing oxytetracycline; those in the other were not. The resistant *E. coli* spread to other chickens in the cage with the feed containing the antibiotic. It was not isolated from the chickens in the cage with unmedicated feed. Two other cages of uninoculated birds were in the same room. The birds in one of these cages were given feed containing oxytetracycline; the other plain feed. The *E. coli* with the marked plasmid was isolated from birds in the cage on antibiotic feed but not from those on plain feed.

On two occasions the labelled *E. coli* was recovered from fecal samples of people who worked in proximity to the chickens. An antibiotic-resistant *E. coli* that was isolated from one fecal sample taken from a young boy who cleaned the cages was resistant to streptomycin and sulfonamides but not to tetracycline. The second antibiotic-resistant *E. coli* was isolated from a young lady who took fecal samples from the chickens. This *E. coli* had the same resistance characteristics as that of the chickens. However, she also worked with the culture in the laboratory. Since the organism was isolated from her feces 7 days after she had handled the chickens, it is quite possible that she had acquired the organism in the laboratory rather than from the chickens. Because the organism was isolated only once from each person, it could not be said to have colonized their intestines.

In a study of calves, Hirsh and Wiger (1977) used a labelled *E. coli* of bovine origin containing a labelled plasmid. This plasmid carried resistance to gentamicin, tetracycline, streptomycin, and sulfonamides. The calves were fed the organism and/or were given tetracycline twice a day orally. The tetracycline did not affect the prevalence of antibiotic resistance in *E. coli* from isolates from the feces of the calves: the prevalance was as great when the calves were not receiving tetracyclines as when they were. The marked organism with the marked plasmid was isolated once from each of three of the animal attendants. The plasmid did not transfer to the indigenous flora, did not persist, nor did it recur.

Two groups of investigators in England have studied the colonization of the human intestine by E. coli of animal origin. Shooter et al. (1970) at St. Bartholomew's Hospital in London isolated antibiotic-resistant E. coli of the same O-serotype from animals and poultry at slaughter, from the meat as it came into the hospital kitchen, from the kitchen itself, especially from the water used to wash dishes, from the dishes, from the food as it was prepared for delivery to patients, and from the feces of the patients (Cooke et al., 1971; Shooter et al., 1970). This study suffers from two serious flaws. First, Guinée (1963) has said, based on a study of more than 1,000 strains of E. coli from humans and animals, "The results of our investigation show that with an extensive serological and biochemical study a relatively large number of serofermentation types can be found within one O-group, so that epidemiological conclusions based exclusively on the determination of the O-antigen can be quite deceptive." Shooter's study was based exclusively on the determination of the O-antigen. Guinée also said, "...the results of the investigation reported above do not justify any conclusions on the problem of whether or not the strains of E. coli originating from animals are of any importance as pathogenic agents for man, or vice versa." Moreover, Shooter and his colleagues sampled the environment of the hospital kitchen, the articles used in the preparation of the food, and the food itself, but they failed to sample any of the people working in the kitchen to see what strains of E. coli they might possibly be contributing to the food.

At the University of Bristol in England, a second group investigated the possible colonization of human intestines by E. coli of animal origin. Initially, these investigators determined only the O-groups, but they later determined O-serotypes and resistance patterns of E. coli from animals and humans. If the two were the same, they also determined H and K antigens to establish conclusively the identity of the strains. In one study (Linton et al., 1977), 15 chickens were purchased from a local retailer over a 3-month period and were distributed to five volunteers who prepared and ate them. After the chickens were thawed prior to cooking, swabs from them were cultured for E. coli. Prior to and after the chickens had been consumed, fecal samples from the volunteers were also cultured for E. coli. When strains from the chickens and the humans had the same O-serotype and antibiotic resistance pattern, the H and K antigens were also determined. No evidence of transfer occurred in 14 of the 15 chickens or in four of the five volunteers. Five strains of E. coli with similar serological and antibiotic resistance characteristics were isolated from one of the chickens and from one volunteer. Two of these strains were isolated only on 1 day, the third after preparation of the chicken for eating. This could hardly be termed colonization. One strain was isolated the 10th and 11th days after preparation. There were 13 isolates of this strain from the human and only one from the chicken, suggesting that a strain from the human had contaminated the chicken. Two strains were isolated on the second, third, and fourth days after preparation in roughly equal numbers from each source. Therefore, if one defines colonization as the isolation of a particular strain on three consecutive days from a particular individual, these strains could be said to have colonized this individual.

These experiments suggest that the colonization of the human intestine by *E. coli* of animal origin is a rare event.

R-FACTOR TRANSFER *In Vivo*

The transfer of R factors *in vivo* is not easily accomplished in normal animals and humans. One experiment demonstrating this fact was conducted by Anderson *et al.* (1973). They used *E. coli* isolated from the humans who were subjects of these experiments. The *E. coli* was isolated from the fecal flora of each subject, chromosomally labelled so it could be identified, and fed back to the same subject. Some strains also had an R factor introduced so that they might serve as donors in experiments on the *in-vivo* transfer of R factors.

Anderson *et al*. concluded that "No R-factor transfer could be detected in the absence of antibiotic therapy, even though the R-factors concerned could be transferred in laboratory studies from the potential donors to many different enteric organisms as recipients, including the genetically marked potential recipients used in these experiments." When the subjects were treated with ampicillin or tetracycline, the organism containing the R factor would persist for a short time in the subjects' intestine allowing R-factor transfer to be demonstrated. This work was conducted with strains indigenous to the human gut flora as both donor and acceptor.

An early attempt to demonstrate *in-vivo* transfer of antibiotic resistance from an *E. coli* of animal origin to an indigenous human strain was reported by Smith (1969). The investigator characterized the principal resident *E. coli* in the alimentary tract of a volunteer and showed that it remained stable throughout the 2-year study. The organism did not contain an R factor but was capable of receiving an

R factor *in vitro*. This volunteer ingested a series of 18 different R-factor-containing *E. coli* isolates--14 of animal origin and four of human origin--at different times during the 2-year period. The animal strains were from pigs, oxen, and fowl. They were shown to be capable of transferring their R factors to the resident strain *in vitro*.

In this study, Smith showed that none of the donor strains was capable of colonizing the alimentary tract permanently (Table 17). When administered in a dose of 10^9 organisms, some of the strains of animal origin could be recovered from the feces for periods of 1 to 11 days, but when the dose was 10^6 organisms they could not be recovered even 1 to 2 days after administration. When the strains were of human origin, colonization for as long as a month was achieved when the dose was 10^9 organisms.

Smith also reported that when temporary colonization occurred, transfer of R factors to the resident *E. coli* took place at an extremely low rate. Only about one to 10 colonies of the resident strain with an R factor were recovered after doses of 10^9 donor organisms had been administered. These resident bacteria to which R factors had been transferred did not persist as a permanent part of the *E. coli* microflora. This suggests that the presence of the R factor reduced the survival potential of the strains in competition with their drug-sensitive forms. No R-factor transfer occurred with any donor strain when the dose of organisms was 10^6 cells.

There is no doubt that carcasses are contaminated with coliform organisms at the abattoir. There are many references attesting to this. Those showing contamination with salmonellae at the abattoir are relevant for *E. coli* as well. A typical reference for the contamination of carcasses with antibiotic-resistant *E. coli* is that of Walton (1970).

The most important question is how much of the contamination persists in the retail store and in cooked food. Walton addressed this question in another study (Walton and Lewis, 1971) in which 25 samples from fresh minced beef and sausage and 25 from cooked boiled ham and roast pork obtained from 25 butcher shops were examined for contamination with antibiotic-resistant fecal coliform organisms.

Eleven sausages, three samples of minced beef, two of roast pork, and none of the boiled ham yielded antibiotic-resistant coliform bacteria. All samples, fresh and cooked, were heavily contaminated with other types of bacteria. There were up to 10^6

TABLE 17

Transfer of Antibiotic Resistance from Animal and Human Strains of ***E.*** *coli* Taken by Mouth, to the Resident *E. coli* in the Alimentary Tract of a Human[a]

Origin of Donor Strain	Dose	No. of Days Colonization $>20\%$	$<20\%$	Transfer of Resistance to Resident Strain[b] No. of Days on Which it was Detected	No. of Resident Colonies Per Plate
Pig	10^4, 10^5, 10^6 once, 10^5, 10^6 daily for 7 days	0-8	0-4	None	None
Ox	10^5, 10^6 once, 10^6 daily for 7 days	0	0-2		
Fowl	10^6 once, 10^6 daily for 7 days	0	0		
Human	10^6 once, 10^6 daily for 7 days	0	0-7		
Pig	10^9 once	2-3	2-5	0-2	0-1
Ox	10^9 once, 10^9 daily for 7 days	0-2	1-11	0-18	0-10,000
Fowl	10^9 once	0-8	0-4	0-3	0-5
Human	10^9 once	0-25	10-35	0-4	0-35

[a] From Smith, 1969.

[b] Ranges reflect results obtained from replicated rests.

organisms per gram in the boiled ham and 10^5 organisms per gram in the roast pork. Approximately 40% of the fresh meat and from 4% to 12% of cooked meat samples carried drug-resistant coliform organisms. Of 100 samples, only two yielded *E. coli* with transferable drug resistance. There was very little evidence of contamination of meats with drug-resistant fecal *E. coli*, but the meat was heavily contaminated with other organisms, suggesting that the contamination was not from the animals but from humans and the environment.

In summary, it seems likely that the *E. coli* from animals does not play a significant role in colonizing the human intestine. If these organisms should do so, and if they contained R factors, it is unlikely that the R factor would be transferred to the indigenous microflora. Carcasses are contaminated at the abattoir with fecal *E. coli*, some with transferable R factors, but it is likely that not much of the contamination reaches the retailer or the consumer. The organisms on the meat at the time of purchase by the consumer are more likely to be from humans or the environment.

LINKAGE OF PLASMIDS FOR ENTEROTOXIN PRODUCTION AND ANTIBIOTIC RESISTANCE

Falkow and Gyles (1973) have shown that a plasmid coding for enterotoxin production (Ent) could be transferred into an *E. coli* containing a plasmid for tetracycline resistance. They used 3-week-old weanling pigs in these experiments and doses of donor and recipient organisms that were greater than 10^{12} organisms. The recipient was given 1 or 4 hours after the donor. Neither organism persisted much longer than 48 hours in the intestines of the pigs in the experiments where transfer took place. The presence of a K88ac plasmid, which enhances colonization, seemed to prevent transfer of the Ent plasmid. The presence of 50 g of oxytetracycline per ton of feed seemed to have no effect on numbers of either donor or recipient recovered from the pigs. No attempt was made to show whether the Ent and resistance plasmids would transfer together. Walton (1977) used established donors of enterotoxin-plasmids to attempt the simultaneous transfer of Ent plasmids and R factors. The transfer of Ent plasmids from *E. coli* that contained R plasmids was not detected when antibiotic-resistant transconjugants were selected.

Gyles *et al.* (1977) isolated a naturally occurring strain of *E. coli* from a piglet with diarrhea. This strain, which was resistant to tetracycline, streptomycin, and sulfonamides and which was capable of producing both heat-stable and heat-labile enterotoxin, could transfer all of these characteristics en bloc to other *E. coli*. However, such a strain would have no selective advantage in pigs receiving antibiotics in their feed since a high proportion of the *E. coli* in those pigs would already be resistant to antibiotics.

Falkow *et al*. (1976) have shown that organisms of a strain of *E. coli* carrying an Ent plasmid will survive longer and in greater numbers than would those of a homogenic strain without the Ent plasmid. The presence of a K99 plasmid, which confers the ability to colonize the intestinal tract of young calves, did not greatly increase the ability of the *E. coli* with the Ent plasmid to survive in the calves.

Food-borne outbreaks of disease due to *E. coli* are not reported by the CDC in its annual summaries (CDC, 1977b). Such outbreaks are reported in England, but since they are difficult to identify most of them are probably not detected. Enterotoxigenic *E. coli* is generally recognized as the cause of traveler's diarrhea (Sack, 1978). This disease is usually attributed to the eating of raw foods or the drinking of polluted water. It is usually not a very serious disease in otherwise healthy adults. Enterotoxigenic *E. coli* causes two more serious diseases, a choleralike syndrome and infantile diarrhea.

Infantile diarrhea is a leading cause of death in children under 5 years of age. Sack *et al*. (1975) established that diarrheal disease in 59 Apache children, all under 4 years of age, was associated with enterotoxigenic *E. coli* rather than the so-called enteropathogenic serotypes that are often associated with infantile diarrhea. The investigators did not investigate the mode of spread of the disease since these children already had the disease when they were admitted to the hospital.

Ryder *et al*. (1976) investigated an outbreak of diarrheal illness in a hospital special care nursery. Of 205 infants admitted to this nursery between December 1974 and September 1, 1975, 55 (27%) of them had diarrheal illness. The diarrhea had a short incubation period, sometimes less than 48 hours, and a short duration (mean of 4 days), but it was associated with definite morbidity. Symptomatic, culture-positive infants had a mean hospital stay of 32 days compared to 15 days for asymptomatic culture-negative infants. This illness was associated with the presence of a strain of *E. coli* of serotype 078:K80:H12, which is resistant to chloramphenicol, ampicillin, carbenicillin, kanamycin, sulfonamides, cephalothin, and tetracycline but is sensitive to gentamicin and colistin. A factor specifying a pilus facilitating colonization was also shown to be present. This strain produced a heat-stable enterotoxin. Of the possible risk factors examined in this outbreak, only oral consumption of formula was associated with illness, and it was only from this source that the epidemic strain was isolated. Unopened formula was sterile, but cultures taken from several locations in the nurseries and from the hands of one of the nurses were positive for the organism.

A 5-day course of prophylactic colistin was ineffective in preventing spread of the organism. There were no deaths in this outbreak, but several infants required rehydration.

Apparently, antibiotic resistance in enterotoxigenic *E. coli*, especially from adults, is not common (DuPont *et al.*, 1978). Table 18 shows the antibiotic susceptibility of 126 strains of enterotoxigenic *E. coli* isolated from children in Houston, Texas, students attending a Mexican University, and adults in Bangladesh. All of the strains were sensitive to nalidixic acid, oxolinic acid, and cinoxacin, which are related compounds that are not very important in the therapy of bacterial infections. Of the 126 strains that were isolated, 119 (92%) were sensitive to sulfamethoxazole-trimethoprim. All of the strains from the Mexican students that produced stable toxin only were sensitive to the 10 antimicrobials tested. The greatest incidence of resistance occurred in strains that produced labile toxin in the Texas children. The authors suggested that naladixic acid or related compounds might be useful in preventing diarrhea due to enterotoxigenic *E. coli*.

In summary, plasmids for antibiotic resistance and for the production of enterotoxin can coexist in an *E. coli* cell and can be transferred together experimentally. Cells containing both plasmids would have no survival advantage over cells containing the R factor alone in animals receiving antibiotics in their feed since a high percentage of the cells would already be resistant.

Enteropathogenic *E. coli* causes three kinds of disease--a cholera-like disease, traveler's diarrhea, and infantile diarrhea. None of these is particularly common in the United States. There seems to be no connection between these diseases and the use of antibiotics in animal feed.

STAPHYLOCOCCAL FOOD POISONING

Staphylococcal enterotoxin is one of the two most frequently reported causes of outbreaks of food-borne disease. In 1974 and

TABLE 18

Antimicrobial Susceptibility of *Escherichia coli* Strains that Produce Heat-Labile (LT) or Heat-Stable ('ST-only') Enterotoxins[a]

Study Group	Number of Patients Studied	Number (and Percentage) of Patients with Antimicrobial Susceptibility							
		Sm[b]	Tc[c]	Amp[d]	Km[e]	TSx[f]	Coli[g]	Cf[h]	NA,[i] OA,[j] Ci[k]
Pediatric patients									
Houston									
LT-E. coli	9	8(89)	8(89)	9(100)	9(100)	9(100)	9(100)	9(100)	9(100)
ST-only	1	0	0	0	0	1	0	0	1
Mexico									
LT-E. coli	6	4(67)	3(50)	5(83)	4(67)	6(100)	5(83)	6(100)	6(100)
ST-only	22	13(59)	5(23)	14(64)	14(64)	18(82)	11(50)	20(91)	22(91)
Adult patients									
Mexico									
LT-E. coli	44	25(57)	28(64)	44(100)	44(100)	42(95)	39(89)	43(98)	44(100)
ST-only	10	10(100)	10(100)	10(100)	10(100)	10(100)	10(100)	10(100	10(100)
Bangladesh									
LT-E. coli	34	29(85)	32(94)	34(100)	34(100)	31(91)	34(100)	33(97)	34(100)

[a]From DuPont et al., 1978, with permission from the authors and the Journal of Antimicrobial Chemotherapy.
[b]Sm = streptomycin
[c]Tc = tetracycline
[d]Amp = ampicillin
[e]Km = kanamycin
[f]TSx = trimethoprim plus sulfamethoxazole
[g]Coli = chloramphenicol
[h]Cf = cephalosporin
[i]NA = nalidix acid
[j]OA = oxolinic acid
[k]Ci = cinoxacin

1975 outbreaks of disease from *Staphylococcus* exceeded those from *Salmonella*, although *Salmonella* ranked first in 1976. Because staphylococcal enterotoxin is heat-stable, it is not destroyed by cooking. While meat products are frequently implicated in outbreaks of staphylococcal food-poisoning, investigation frequently reveals that the food has been contaminated by a food handler who is a carrier of an enterotoxin-producing strain of staphylococcus or who has a staphylococcus-infected wound (Bryan, 1978; CDC, 1977b).

This contamination of meat by staphylococci of human origin was confirmed in a study by Sinell *et al.* (1975) in the Federal Republic of Germany. These investigators examined 3,065 cultures of staphylococci from slaughtered pigs, meat plant equipment, and other sources including human beings. Strains originating from swine produced significantly less (21%) enterotoxin than did strains from clinical specimens obtained in hospitals (approximately 40%). Enterotoxin was not produced by any of 39 phage group II strains, a group that is considered to be specific to animals. The strains from animals were more frequently resistant to antibiotics than were the strains from the hospital. In 1973, before the German government banned the use of tetracycline in animal feed, there was a high incidence of resistance to tetracycline. In 1974, after the ban, a survey showed that the incidence of resistance to tetracycline in cultures from pigs had dropped but that the incidence of resistance to bacitracin had become very high. Strains of staphylococci isolated in a meat plant in 1974 continued to have a high incidence of resistance to both tetracycline and bacitracin.

Domestic animals and pets can become carriers of strains of staphylococci of phage types that are frequently associated with human disease (Pagano *et al.*, 1960). During the school year 1956-1957 an unusual number of senior students at the University of Pennsylvania School of Veterinary Medicine were afflicted with furuncles, deep cutaneous abscesses, cellulitis, and paronychia. The epidemic continued through the following 2 years. *Staphylococcus aureus* phage type 80/81 was repeatedly isolated from these lesions. This strain was resistant to penicillin, streptomycin, the tetracyclines, and, occasionally, to erythromycin but was sensitive to chloramphenicol and novobiocin.

A survey of students, faculty, and other employees of the school revealed that only the senior students who spent much of their time in the clinic and the faculty of the clinic had a high incidence of this strain in their external nares. They frequently became carriers after contact with a student with an active lesion.

Sporadic culturing of swabs from lesions of animals in the clinic revealed the existence of type 80/81 strain on only three occasions, whereas random swabbing of the nostrils of the animals failed to show it. In 1959 a systematic swabbing of the nostrils of the animals showed the strain to be present in cows, horses, goats, and, most frequently, in dogs. There was no proof that the organism was transmitted from an animal to a human.

The animal-to-person transfer of antibiotic-resistant *S. aureus* of human type 80/81 was suggested by Wallace *et al.* (1962). Eight of 287 cows tested yielded staphylococci type 80/81 with resistance to streptomycin, tetracycline, and penicillin, and sensitivity to chloramphenicol, neomycin, novobiocin, oleandomycin, and carbomycin. The cows all had mastitis. Some cases were so severe that the animals had to be destroyed.

Three people in the family that operated the dairy studied by Wallace *et al.* also yielded type 80/81 with the same resistance pattern when swabs were taken from their nares and from two boils on the father at different times and from one boil and the sore throat of an 18-month-old child. Here again the spread from animal to person is putative. The organism could have spread from the humans to the animals. Antibiotic resistance in staphylococci from mastitic cows is common because large amounts of antibiotics are used in intramammary infusions to treat the mastitis, which may clear up but frequently recurs.

Another study on antibiotic-resistant *S. aureus* from dairy herds was reported by Devriese and Hommez (1975). In 1971 and from July 1972 to June 1973 they isolated 68 methicillin-resistant strains of *S. aureus* from milk samples from mastitic cows in 20 Belgian dairy herds. In the 1972-1973 survey 52 methicillin-resistant strains were isolated on nine farms, representing 50% of all *S. aureus* isolated on those farms. A determination of the biological and phagetypes of the methicillin-resistant strains suggested that they were actually strains from humans and might have had a common human source, but that seems highly speculative.

In summary, food poisoning due to *Staphylococcus aureus* enterotoxin is frequently reported in the United States, England, and Wales. It often involves meat products, but upon investigation it is frequently found that the food was contaminated by a human carrier or one with a staphylococcal lesion. There is no evidence that the use of antibiotics in animal feed is in any way involved.

Frequently, staphylococci of phage types usually considered to be of human origin have been found in pets and dairy cows. It is likely that these organisms were transferred from humans and were resistant when they were acquired by the cows, but they may have become resistant during treatment for mastitis by antibiotic intramammary infusion. It is highly unlikely that the resistance arose due to the use of antibiotics in the feed of the cows since that is a rather uncommon practice in the dairy industry in the United States.

CONCLUSIONS

Salmonellosis is the most important of the food-borne diseases that may be transmitted from animals to humans. There is a large pool of *Salmonella* in domestic animals, carcasses are contaminated with *Salmonella* at the slaughterhouse, and outbreaks of food-borne salmonellosis due to contaminated food of animal origin are a serious threat to human health and an economic problem. It is not clear that the *Salmonella* on the food originated in the animals. Moreover, when antibiotic resistance has occurred, it does not seem to have been due to the use of antibiotics in animal feed.

It seems likely that antibiotic-resistant *E. coli* in animals does not play a significant role in colonizing the human intestine. If these organisms do colonize temporarily, it is unlikely that they transfer their R factor to the human flora. Carcasses are contaminated at the slaughterhouse with *E. coli*--some of which is resistant to antibiotics, but it is doubtful that more than a few of these organisms reach the consumer. The organisms on the meat are probably of human or environmental origin.

Plasmids for antibiotic resistance and enterotoxin production can coexist in an *E. coli* cell and can be transferred together experimentally. Cells containing both genes would have no survival advantage over cells containing the R factor alone in animals receiving antibiotics in feed since a high percentage of the cells would already be resistant.

Food poisoning in the United States due to *Staphylococcus* enterotoxin is second only to salmonellosis as a food-borne disease. It often involves meat products, but upon investigation, it is frequently found that the food was contaminated by a human carrier or one with a *Staphylococcus*-infected lesion. Staphylococci of phage types usually considered to be of human origin have been found in pets and dairy cows. There is no evidence that the use of antibiotics in animal feed is in any way involved.

REFERENCES

Anderson, E. S. 1968a. Drug resistance in Salmonella typhimurium and its implications. Br. Med. J. 3:333-339.

Anderson, E. S. 1968b. Transferable drug resistance. Sci. J. 4: 71-76.

Anderson, J. D., W. A. Gillespie, and M. H. Richmond. 1973. Chemotherapy and antibiotic-resistance transfer between enterobacteria in the human gastro-intestinal tract. J. Med. Microbiol. 6:461-473.

Aserkoff, B., and J. V. Bennett. 1969. Effect of antibiotic therapy in acute salmonellosis on the fecal excretion of salmonellae. N. Engl. J. Med. 281:636-640.

Bryan, F. L. 1978. Factors that contribute to outbreaks of foodborne disease. J. Food Protection 41:816-827.

Center for Disease Control. 1975. Current trends. Microbiologic standards for raw ground beef, cold cuts and frankfurters. Reported by the U. S. Department of Agriculture and the Center for Disease Control. Morbid. Mortal. Weekly Rep. 24:229-230.

Center for Disease Control. 1976a. Salmonella bovis-morbificans in precooked roasts of beef. Reported by P. J. Checko, J. N. Lewis, R. Altman, K. Black, H. Rosenfeld, W. Parkin, the U.S. Department of Agriculture, and the Center for Disease Control. Morbid. Mortal. Weekly Rep. 25:333-334.

Center for Disease Control. 1976b. Salmonella Surveillance Annual Summary 1975. Center for Disease Control, Atlanta, Ga. 51 pp.

Center for Disease Control. 1977a. Follow-up on salmonellae in precooked roasts of beef. Reported by J. N. Lewis, R. Altman, D. O. Lyman, W. E. Parkin, the U. S. Department of Agriculture, the Food and Drug Administration, and the Center for Disease Control. Morbid. Mortal. Weekly Rep. 26:394-399.

Center for Disease Control. 1977b. Food Borne and Water Borne Disease Outbreaks. Annual Summary 1976. Center for Disease Control, Atlanta, Ga. 82 pp.

Center for Disease Control. 1977c. Multi-state outbreak of Salmonella newport transmitted by precooked roasts of beef. Reported by P. J. Checko, J. N. Lewis, R. Altman, G. Halpin, R. Inglis, M. Pierce, K. Pilot, J. Prince, W. Rednor, M. Fleissner, D. O. Lyman, W. E. Parkin, the U. S. Department of Agriculture, and the Center for Disease Control. Morbid. Mortal. Weekly Rep. 26:277-278.

Center for Disease Control. 1977d. Salmonella Surveillance Annual Summary 1976. Center for Disease Control, Atlanta, Ga. [23] pp.

Center for Disease Control. 1977e. Salmonellosis associated with home-made ice cream--Michigan. Reported by R. Locey, P. Owens, G. Markakis, R. P. Daniels, D. F. Fuller, Jr., D. Muentener, N. S. Hayner, K. S. Read, and the Center for Disease Control. Morbid. Mortal. Weekly Rep. 26:94-99.

Center for Disease Control. 1977f. Salmonellosis--Kentucky. Reported by R. N. McLeod, W. L. Adams, L. M. Mullins, M. A. Shepherd, R. K. Bonner, B. F. Brown, N. J. Cambron, C. Hernandez, G. E. Killgore, J. W. Skaggs, [Kentucky] Epidemiological Notes and Reports 12(4): 1, and the Center for Disease Control. Morbid. Mortal. Weekly Rep. 26:239.

Center for Disease Control. 1979. Salmonella Surveillance Annual Summary 1977. Center for Disease Control, Atlanta, Ga. [21] pp.

Cherubin, C. E., M. Szmuness, and J. Winter. 1972. Antibiotic resistance of Salmonella. Northeastern United States--1970. N. Y. State J. Med. 72:369-372.

Cherubin, C. E., J. F. Timoney, M. F. Sierra, P. Ma, J. Marr, and S. Shin. 1980. A sudden decline in ampicillin resistance in Salmonella typhimurium. J. Am. Med. Assoc. 243:439-442.

Cooke, E. M., A. L. Breaden, R. A. Shooter, and S. M. O'Farrell. 1971. Antibiotic sensitivity of Escherichia coli isolated from animals, food, hospital patients, and normal people. Lancet 2:8-10.

Devriese, L. A., and J. Hommez. 1975. Epidemiology of methicillin-resistant Staphylococcus aureus in dairy herds. Res. Vet. Sci. 19:23-27.

DuPont, H. L., H. West, D. G. Evans, J. Olarte, and D. J. Evans, Jr. 1978. Antimicrobial susceptibility of enterotoxigenic Escherichia coli. J. Antimicrob. Chemother. 4:100-102.

Edel, W., M. van Schothorst, P. A. M. Guinée, and E. H. Kampelmacher. 1974. Preventive measures to obtain Salmonella-free slaughter pigs. Zentralbl. Bakteriol. Parasitenkd. Infektionskr. Hyg., I Abt. Orig. Reihe B 158:568-577.

Evangelisti, D. G., A. R. English, A. E. Girard, J. E. Lynch, and I. A. Solomons. 1975. Influence of subtherapeutic levels of oxytetracycline on Salmonella typhimurium in swine, calves, and chickens. Antimicrob. Agents Chemother. 8:664-672.

Falkow, S., and C. Gyles. 1973. Studies on in vivo transfer of the Ent plasmid. Progress Report. FDA contract number 73-210 M #1. Food and Drug Administration, Rockville, Md.

Falkow, S., L. P. Williams, Jr., S. L. Seaman, and L. D. Rollins. 1976. Increased survival in calves of Escherichia coli K-12 carrying an Ent plasmid. Infect. Immun. 13:1005-1007.

Finlayson, M. 1977. Salmonella in Alberta poultry products and their significance in human infections. Pp. 156-180 in Proceedings of the International Symposium on Salmonella and Prospects for Control, June 8-11, 1977, University of Guelph, Guelph, Ontario, Canada.

Food and Drug Administration. 1973. Antibiotic and sulfonamide drugs in the feed of animals. Fed. Reg. 38:9811-9814.

Galton, M. M., M. V. Smith, H. B. McElrath, and A. B. Hardy. 1954. Salmonella in swine, cattle and the environment of abattoirs. J. Infect. Dis. 95:236-245.

Garside, J. S., R. F. Gordon, and J. F. Tucker. 1960. The emergence of resistant strains of Salmonella typhimurium in the tissues and alimentary tracts of chickens following the feeding of an antibiotic. Res. Vet. Sci. 1:184-199.

Girard, A. E., A. R. English, D. G. Evangelisti, J. E. Lynch, and I. A. Solomons. 1976. Influence of subtherapeutic levels of a combination of neomycin and oxytetracycline on Salmonella typhimurium in swine, calves, and chickens. Antimicrob. Agents Chemother. 10:89-95.

Groves, B. I., N. A. Fish, and D. A. Barnum. 1970. An epidemiological study of Salmonella infection in swine in Ontario. Can. J. Public Health 61:396-401.

Guinée, P. A. M. 1963. Preliminary investigations concerning the presence of E. coli in man and in various species of animals. Zentralbl. Bakteriol. Parasitenkd. Infektionskr. Hyg., I. Abt. Orig. Reihe A 188:201-218.

Gustafson, R. H., J. D. Kobland, and P. H. Langner. 1976. Incidence and antibiotic resistance of Salmonella in market swine. P. M2 in Proceedings of the International Pig Veterinary Society, 4th International Congress, June 22-24, 1976, Ames, Ia. International Pig Veterinary Society, Ames, Ia.

Gutzmann, F., H. Layton, K. Simkins, and H. Jarolmen. 1976. Influence of antibiotic-supplemented feed on occurrence and persistence of Salmonella typhimurium in experimentally infected swine. Am. J. Vet. Res. 37:649-655.

Gyles, C. L., S. Palchaudhuri, and W. K. Maas. 1977. Naturally occurring plasmid carrying genes for enterotoxin production and drug resistance. Science 198:198-199.

Hirsh, D. C., and N. Wiger. 1977. Effect of tetracycline upon transfer of an R plasmid from calves to human beings. Am. J. Vet. Res. 38:1137-1139.

Hook, E. W., and W. D. Johnson. 1972. Nontyphoidal salmonellosis. Pp. 583-591 in P. D. Hoeprich, ed. Infectious Diseases. A Guide to the Understanding and Management of Infectious Processes. Harper and Rowe, Hagerstown, Md.

Jarolmen, H., R. J. Sairk, and B. F. Langworth. 1976. Effect of chlortetracycline feeding on the Salmonella reservoir in chickens. J. Appl. Bacteriol. 40:153-161.

Layton, H. W., B. F. Langworth, H. Jarolmen, and K. L. Simkins. 1975. Influence of chlortetracycline and chlortetracycline + sulfamethazine supplemented feed on the incidence, persistence and antibacterial susceptibility of Salmonella typhimurium in experimentally inoculated calves. Zentralbl. Veterinaermed. Reihe B 22:461-472.

Levy, S. B., G. B. FitzGerald, and A. B. Macone. 1976. Spread of antibiotic-resistant plasmids from chicken to chicken and from chicken to man. Nature 260:40-42.

Linton, A. H., K. Howe, P. M. Bennett, M. H. Richmond, and E. J. Whiteside. 1977. The colonization of the human gut by antibiotic-resistant Escherichia coli from chickens. J. Appl. Bacteriol. 43:465-469.

Luther, H. G., W. G. Huber, D. Siegel, and H. G. Luther, Jr. 1974. Antibacterial feed additives: Residues and infectious drug resistance. Pp. 89-134 in W. W. Hawkins, ed. Drug-Nutrient Interrelationships. Nutrition and Pharmacology--An Interphase of Disciplines. Proceedings of the Miles Symposium '74, presented by The Nutrition Society of Canada, June 24, 1974, McMaster University, Hamilton, Ontario, Canada

Ministry of Agriculture, Fisheries, and Food. 1965. Salmonellae in cattle and their feedingstuffs, and the relation to human infection. A report of the Joint Working Party of the Veterinary Laboratory Services of the Ministry of Agriculture, Fisheries, and Food, and the Public Health Laboratory Service. J. Hyg., Camb. 63:223-241.

Neu, H. C., E. B. Winshell, J. Winter, and C. E. Cherubin. 1971. Antibiotic resistance of Salmonella in the northeastern United States, 1968-1969. N. Y. State J. Med. 71:1196-1200.

Neu, H. C., C. E. Cherubin, E. D. Longo, B. Flouton, and J. Winter. 1975. Antimicrobial resistance and R-factor transfer among isolates of Salmonella in the northeastern United States: A comparison of human and animal isolates. J. Infect. Dis. 132: 617-622.

Pagano, J. S., S. M. Farrer, S. A. Plotkin, P. S. Brachman, F. R. Fekety, and V. Pidcoe. 1960. Isolation from animals of human strains of staphylococci during an epidemic in a veterinary school. Science 131:927-928.

Pocurull, D. W., S. A. Gaines, and H. D. Mercer. 1971. Survey of infectious multiple drug resistance among Salmonella isolated from animals in the United States. Appl. Microbiol. 21:358-362.

Ryder, R. W., I. K. Wachsmuth, A. E. Buxton, D. G. Evans, H. L. DuPont, E. Mason, and F. F. Barrett. 1976. Infantile diarrhea produced by heat-stable enterotoxigenic Escherichia coli. N. Engl. J. Med. 295:849:853.

Sack, R. B. 1978. The epidemiology of diarrhea due to enterotoxigenic *Escherichia coli*. J. Infect. Dis. 137:639-640.

Sack, R. B., N. Hirschhorn, I. Brownlee, R. A. Cash, W. E. Woodward, and D. A. Sack. 1975. Enterotoxigenic *Escherichia-coli*-associated diarrheal disease in Apache children. N. Engl. J. Med. 292:1041-1045.

Shooter, R. A., S. A. Rousseau, E. M. Cooke, and A. L. Breaden. 1970. Animal sources of common serotypes of *Escherichia coli* in the food of hospital patients. Possible significance in urinary-tract infections. Lancet 2:226-228.

Sinell, H. J., D. Kusch, and F. Untermann. 1975. Enterotoxin-producing *Staphylococci* in meat processing plants: Origin, biochemical properties, resistance to antibiotics. Eur. J. Appl. Microbiol. 1:239-245.

Smith, H. W. 1969. Transfer of antibiotic resistance from animals and human strains of *Escherichia coli* to resident *E. coli* in the alimentary tract of man. Lancet 1:1174-1176.

Smith, H. W. 1970. The transfer of antibiotic resistance between strains of enterobacteria in chickens, calves and pigs. J. Med. Microbiol. 3:165-180.

Swann, M. M., K. L. Blaxter, H. I. Field, J. W. Howie, I. A. M. Lucas, E. L. M. Millar, J. C. Murdoch, J. H. Parsons, and E. G. White. 1969. Report of the Joint Committee on the Use of Antibiotics in Animal Husbandry and Veterinary Medicine. Cmnd. 4190. Her Majesty's Stationery Office, London. 83 pp.

Threlfall, E. J., L. R. Ward, and B. Rowe. 1978. Epidemic spread of a chloramphenicol-resistant strain of *Salmonella typhimurium* phage type 204 in bovine animals in Britain. *Vet. Rec.* 103: 438-440.

Timoney, J. F. 1978. The epidemiology and genetics of antibiotic resistance of *Salmonella typhimurium* isolated from diseased animals in New York. J. Infect. Dis. 137:67-73.

Vernon, E. 1977. Food poisoning and Salmonella infections in England and Wales, 1973-75. Public Health, London 91:225-235.

Wallace, G. D., W. B. Quisenberry, R. H. Tanimoto, and F. T. Lynd. 1962. Bacteriophage type 80/81 staphylococcal infection in human beings associated with mastitis in dairy cattle. Am. J. Public Health 52:1309-1317.

Walton, J. R. 1966. In vivo transfer of infectious drug resistance. Nature 211:312-313.

Walton, J. R. 1970. Contamination of meat carcasses by antibiotic-resistant coliform bacteria. Lancet 2:561-563.

Walton, J. R. 1977. The relationship between the transferability of enterotoxin plasmids and the simultaneous transfer of antibiotic resistance plasmids. Zentralbl. Veterinaermed. Reihe B 24:317-324.

Walton, J. R., and L. E. Lewis. 1971. Contamination of fresh and cooked meats by antibiotic-resistant coliform bacteria. Lancet 2:255-257.

Williams, L. P., Jr., J. B. Vaughn, A. Scott, and V. Blanton. 1969. A ten-month study of Salmonella contamination in animal protein meals. J. Am. Vet. Med. Assoc. 155:167-174.

Williams, R. D., L. D. Rollins, D. W. Pocurull, M. Selwyn, and H. D. Mercer. 1978. Effect of feeding chlortetracycline on the reservoir of Salmonella typhimurium in experimentally infected swine. Antimicrob. Agents Chemother. 14:710-719.

APPENDIX H

FOOD CONTAMINATION

William E. Pace[1]

When considering the effects on human health of subtherapeutic use of antibiotics in animal feeds, the food scientist must first consider the order of events that could lead to possible adverse effects. To develop a systematic approach, one must face a number of questions that are ultimately related but do not lend themselves to a simple sequential consideration. Among these are:

- With what potential human health effects should we be concerned?

- Do epidemiological data indicate that real problems exist today or could exist in the future?

- What diseases may be involved?

- Might the use of antibiotics in animal feeds play a direct or indirect role in increasing the incidence or in complicating the treatment of diseases?

- What lines of communication connect animals and humans in the chain of events that might result in manifestation of adverse effects?

- Do processing and storage significantly decrease antibiotic residues?

- Are there beneficial effects from the presence of antibiotics in foods?

- Is the attention given to foods of foreign origin similar to that given to foods originating in the United States?

- What recommendations should be made regarding antibiotic use?

---

[1]Office of the Surgeon General, Headquarters, U.S. Air Force, Bolling Air Force Base, Washington, D.C.

CONCERNS

There are two general areas of concern: the toxic effect of antibiotic residues and the potentiation of disease by antibiotic-microorganisms. The former is far simpler to approach than is the latter.

TOXIC EFFECTS

Manifestation of a toxic effect requires only that a susceptible individual be exposed to the antibiotic residues. Mercer (1975) reported that approximately 7.2% of a test population was hypersensitive to penicillin and that ingestion of as little as 10 units has produced mild reactions. Furthermore, he stated that neomycin has cross-sensitization properties with streptomycin and that 5.7% of a test population was sensitive to neomycin. These data alone are adequate to indicate that there is a strong and definite potential for toxic effects from antibiotic residues. However, measures to control or eliminate such effects are relatively simple to define. Although the susceptibility of a population cannot be changed easily, steps can be taken to avoid or to minimize exposure. Most if not all of those steps are already in routine use.

APPROVAL OF USE

The use of antibiotics in animal feeds must be limited to those that are safe, have proven efficacy, and can readily be detected in the tissues or products of the animals receiving them. All of these criteria must be met before the Food and Drug Administration (FDA) will approve a New Animal Drug Application (NADA). After approval has been granted, our concerns must then turn to detecting illicit use (concentrations in feed exceeding those authorized, inadequate or improper mixing procedures, combining with unapproved additives, etc.), ensuring adherence to prescribed withdrawal periods, and sampling of market-ready products for residue analyses. Responsibility for residue analysis of meats, poultry, and their products is vested in the U.S. Department of Agriculture (USDA). The FDA is responsible for analysis of dairy products.

SAMPLING FOR RESIDUE ANALYSES

Mussman (1973) stated that two types of sampling programs are used by the USDA. Each is designed to provide a different kind of information. One, an "objective" program, is aimed at determining the nationwide extent of a specific residue and identifying herds or flocks that require detailed examination. The other, a "selective" program, is designed to define problems identified by the objective program. Analysis for specific antibiotics involves the combined use of bioassay and thin-layer or gas chromatographic techniques.

EFFECTS OF PROCESSING AND STORAGE ON RESIDUES

Morrison and Munro (1969) have commented on the destruction of drug residues in foods by food processing and storage. Literature cited by them indicates that cooking causes significant reductions of tetracyclines in chicken, fish, and beef. Data presented by Mercer (1975) indicate a marked reduction in levels of penicillin in the kidney, liver, and muscle of chickens, swine, and lambs following frozen storage for as short a time as 8 days. In the United States, fresh poultry reaches the market within 1 to 2 days whereas fresh beef and pork require from 1 to 3 weeks. By intention, frozen products reach the market weeks or even months after processing. The changes in levels of antibiotic residues during storage and preparation add an additional margin of safety for the antibiotic-susceptible consumer. Assays must continue to be performed as quickly as possible after slaughter when residue levels are highest and most readily detectable.

ANTIBIOTIC-RESISTANT MICROORGANISMS

One must decide which organisms pose potential adverse health effects as a first step in considerations of antibiotic-resistant microorganisms. Since transferable antibiotic resistance is known to occur only in Gram-negative organisms (Baldwin, 1970), we can narrow our considerations relatively safely to those Gram-negative organisms found most frequently in meats and meat products. Therefore, the group is narrowed to some species of salmonellae, *Shigella*, coliforms, *Vibrio*, *Campylobacter*, *Yersinia*, *Pasteurella*, *Brucella*, *Neisseria*, *Haemophilus*, *Pseudomonas*, *Achromobacter*, *Proteus*, *Flavobacterium*, and *Alcaligenes*. Since the latter five are not known to include pathogens, we can probably afford to omit them from further consideration. The shigellae are well known as enteric pathogens, while the involvement of Vibrio, Campylobacter, and Yersinia in gastrointestinal disturbance is becoming more apparent. Brucella in milk and dairy products must continue to be of concern because of brucellosis.

The salmonellae and the coliforms (especially Escherichia coli) deserve our greatest attention, the former because they are known animal and human pathogens that are transferred between the two and the latter because they are almost ubiquitous, are routinely used as indicators of inadequate hygienic practices, are routinely present in the human alimentary tract, can easily transfer drug resistances, and have an increasingly recognized role in outbreaks of gastrointestinal disorders in humans. Review articles and reports of original research (Groves et al., 1970; Gustafson, 1975; Howe et al., 1976; Kobland, 1975; Licciardello et al., 1968; Linton et al., 1977, in press; Newell and Williams, 1971; Patterson, 1969; Walton, 1970, 1971; Weissman and Carpenter, 1969) reveal an extremely wide variation in the reported incidence of salmonellae and E. coli on animal carcasses in slaughterhouses or the market. Figures for salmonellae incidence range from 34% for chickens (Licciardello et al., 1968) to 84% for pork carcasses (Kobland, 1975), and to 74% for beef carcasses (Weissman and Carpenter, 1969). One paper cites a rate of 9% for carcasses of ducks and turkeys (Patterson, 1969). Figures reported for the incidence of E. coli contamination range from 97% for pig carcasses (Walton, 1971), to 73% for beef carcasses (Walton, 1971), and to 81% for chicken carcasses (Linton et al., in press). These variations appear to be due to differing levels of sanitation in processing plants, to the use or nonuse of bactericidal preparations in rinse waters and in chill tanks, to variations in sampling procedures, and to differences in culture techniques. Several of these authors also reported antibiotic resistance in E. coli in up to 58.5% of the isolates from chickens (Linton et al., in press), up to 79% of those from pork (Walton, 1970), and up to 39% of those from cattle (Walton, 1970). Antibiotic resistance was also reported in up to 23% of the salmonellae isolated from pigs (Kobland, 1975). It is safe to conclude that both resistant E. coli and Salmonella can probably be found frequently in carcasses of all species of meat animals. There is little available data upon which to assess the level of contamination by these organisms.

SOURCES OF CONTAMINANTS

E. coli is routinely found in the gut of both domestic animals and humans. Even minor transgressions in proper sanitary practices in slaughterhouses readily result in contamination of carcasses, which most often results from spillage of intestinal contents during removal of the viscera. Salmonellae, while in no way "normal" inhabitants, are found in the intestinal tract of animals very frequently. Most authorities agree that the primary source of salmonellae in domestic animals is contaminated feed or contaminated protein supplements. Groves et al. (1970), in a study of salmonellae contamination of slaughter pigs, reported isolation of the organisms from feed on 33% of the farms surveyed and in pigs from 33.3% of the farms (correlation between the two was not specified). Conversely, work cited by Edel et al. (1974) indicated that pigs gained little or no salmonellae infection from pelletized feed. However, they also cited data showing that the use of pelletized feed alone did not prevent salmonellae infections and concluded that environmental influences must also play a major role.

Lapses in enforcement of proper hygienic practices rapidly lead from salmonellae and E. coli contamination of the gut to contamination of the carcasses, slaughter equipment, the slaughter environment, and the processing environment to the finished product and on to the kitchens in private homes and institutions. There, unknown to the preparer, cross-contamination to other foods occurs frequently.

The hide of cattle and the skin of hogs are routinely contaminated by intestinal contents. Jensen and Hess (1941) concluded that these constituted the main source of organisms for carcass contamination. Intestinal contents also readily contaminate transportation facilities and holding pens where other animals are subsequently contaminated, many of which are young animals later shipped to farms or to heavily concentrated populations in fattening pens. During transportation animals are subjected to major stress and may become sick. The therapeutic use of certain antibiotics in treating these sick animals could lead to rapid dissemination of resistant strains if the animals are not isolated during therapy. Threlfall et al. (1978) have proposed that similar circumstances might possibly have been involved in the recent outbreaks of salmonellosis in Britain involving the chloramphenicol-resistant strain of Salmonella phage type 204. Datta (1965) stated that some resistance factors carry resistance to as many as seven different drugs. Van Houweling (1967) noted that exposure to an antibiotic could result in transfer of resistance to other antibiotics as well because of the linkage of resistance genes.

As early as 1943, Stuart and McNally showed that eggs are not contaminated by the parent bird during egg formation or laying.

They confirmed that the egg, shell and all, is deposited in the nest in a sterile condition. Sound eggs from normal chickens are contaminated after laying by coming into contact with the external body or feet of birds or with the nest. Therefore, efforts to reduce contamination of shell eggs should be aimed at environmental factors rather than at the physiological processes of egg formation.

VALUE OF ANTIBIOTICS IN FOODS

Since there is no question regarding the potential dangers of antibiotic residues in foods, one must also ask whether such residues also have beneficial effects. Such effects have been clearly demonstrated. Chlortetracycline and oxytetracycline were formerly approved by the FDA in concentrations of 5 to 7 ppm for delaying microbial spoilage of fresh poultry, scallops, shrimp, and eviscerated fish. Approval for these uses was withdrawn in 1966 because small residues could sometimes be detected in the products after they were cooked. According to the Food, Drug, and Cosmetic Act, residues of any drug in tissues of animals receiving the products are considered as food additives, the same as when they are added directly. Furthermore, the use of any food additive in a manner other than that approved by the FDA is regarded as an adulteration and renders the food ineligible for interstate shipment. An FDA-approved use of antibiotics will not result in the presence of residues (or at least not after a specified withdrawal period has been observed).

CONTROLLING CONTAMINATION BY PATHOGENS

One might ask whether antibiotics might be used in animal feeds to reduce the incidence of pathogens in the gut of live animals, hence reducing the potential for carcass and environmental contamination leading ultimately to the consumer. Smith and Tucker (1978) recently commented that the administration of feed containing neomycin to broilers a few days prior to slaughter is being advocated and practiced in Britain as a means of reducing the proportion of birds shedding salmonellae. Their studies using 500 g/long ton (1,016 kg), i.e., 480 g/kg, for 9 days produced only a slight reduction. The use of 225 g/long ton (221 g/kg) for 2 days also produced only a slight reduction in the proportion of birds shedding salmonellae but resulted in the emergence of enormous populations of *E. coli* that possessed multiple, transmissible-type antibiotic resistance in the alimentary tract of the treated chickens. Childers *et al.* (1977) suggested very strongly that environmental controls within the slaughterhouse are the most appropriate, and possibly the safest and simplest, means of reducing contamination of carcasses by pathogenic organisms. Transporting and holding swine in sanitized surroundings prior to slaughter did not effectively reduce contamination of carcasses with either salmonellae or *E. coli*. However, several relatively minor modifications of the evisceration procedures were effective in reducing contamination levels to between 12% and 20% as opposed to between 50% and 63% in control carcasses. The significant changes were the instillation of greater care on the part of workers to avoid spillage of intestinal contents and to wash their hands and disinfect cutting knives in chlorine solutions before handling a new carcass. Studies by Mosley *et al.* (1976) had indicated that hypochlorites and iodophors were similar in effectiveness and that both were superior to quaternary ammonium compounds in reducing levels of Gram-negative organisms, including salmonellae, on stainless-steel surfaces.

INSPECTION OF FOREIGN-ORIGIN MEATS

All control activities mentioned so far have concerned products of U.S. origin. Since the volume of imported products is rather extensive, we should address this topic also. The responsibility for reviewing foreign programs regulating meat production and for inspecting imported meats, poultry, and products of meat and poultry is vested in the Foreign Programs Branch, Field Operations Division, Meat and Poultry Inspection Program, Food Safety and Quality Service of the USDA (McEnroe, 1971).

Review of foreign programs was initiated in 1966 to assess the effectiveness of meat and poultry inspection programs in those countries that desired to export their products to the United States. The Federal Meat Inspection Act of 1907, amended in 1938 and revised by the Wholesome Meat Act of 1967, requires that countries that export meats or meat products to the United States have facilities, sanitation standards, and inspection practices at least equal to our own. Section 20 of the Act also requires visits by U.S. experts to ensure compliance of foreign plants. In describing the program, Lyons (1971) stated that official certification by the USDA also requires the concurrence of the Department of State. Furthermore, foreign products are accepted only when the country's inspection program and the standards in the processing plant have been certified as meeting U.S. standards.

Most plants are visited at least annually. Those with minor problems are visited more frequently. Products originating from authorized plants in recognized countries must still be accompanied by a certificate signed by a qualified representative stating that the meat or meat product comes from animals that passed veterinary ante-mortem and post-mortem inspection, that it is wholesome and free of preservatives, and that it is otherwise in compliance with U.S. requirements. Meat products (but not fresh carcass meats) are then sampled at the port of entry by USDA officials and are subjected to incubation and to laboratory analyses for pesticides, antibiotics, and other chemical residues. Basically, the program relies on evaluation of the inspection program of the foreign country, inspection of the plants of origin, reliance on the validity of certification, and dependence on the quality control programs of the importing U.S. firms. Microbial analyses would be performed only as part of the sampling programs discussed above.

USDA officials do maintain close contact with their counterparts in foreign countries and are well aware of the animal husbandry and food preservation practices in these countries. In case there are significant variances from our own practices, the inspection program can be adjusted to focus on any specific problems that might be anticipated. The status of these programs was confirmed via personal communication (C. S. Johnson, Veterinary Staff Officer, Meat and Poultry Inspection Training Program, FSQS/USDA, Dinton, Texas, personal communication, 1979).

SUMMARY

There is no question that the use of subtherapeutic levels of antibiotics in animal feeds has resulted in increasing the amount of animal protein available to the world's consumers. This increase is due to increased growth rates and to the control of low grade infections which often reduce the efficiency of feed utilization. On the other hand, it becomes more and more apparent that sanitation is the ultimate key to controlling initial levels of carcass and product contamination and that proper refrigeration is the key to controlling multiplication of those few unavoidable microbial contaminants that will still continue to slip through. The use of antibiotics or other agents as preservatives or shelf-life extenders can be used too easily to cover up poor quality control or to compensate for inadequate or improper animal husbandry practices. This may not hold entirely true in some developing nations where refrigeration and rapid transportation are less than adequate. In those cases, benefits to be gained would have to be balanced against the degree of risk involved.

It appears that the primary need today is a vastly stepped-up educational program aimed at producers, processors, service personnel, and consumers. Such a program must stress the importance of sanitation and personal hygiene at every step, the essentiality of avoiding cross-contamination, and the fact that products of animal-origin are not (and are not intended to be) sterile and must be handled accordingly. The effectiveness of public health programs in the United States has contributed greatly to a healthier population with an enhanced nutritional status, but they have also produced a nation of consumers who take for granted the safety of the products they consume and who know little about what precautionary measures they should take or why. Because the government has helped to create this problem, it has a responsibility to continue to protect the consumers from themselves.

RECOMMENDATIONS

From the view of the food scientist, several recommendations are in order:

1. FDA's criteria for approval of NADA's should remain as they are.

2. Sampling for antibiotic residues in meats, poultry, and their products should be increased.

3. Sampling for pathogens and determination of their antibiotic resistance should be significantly increased, especially for items of foreign origin.

4. USDA's Meat and Poultry Inspection Programs should place increased emphasis on in-plant sanitation, especially on measures that might reduce carcass contamination.

5. The Center for Disease Control should determine the antibiotic resistance of cultures of all Gram-negative organisms involved in outbreaks of human illness (especially when food-borne transmission is known or suspected). When unusual resistance patterns are recognized, follow-up epidemiological studies should be initiated to

confirm or to rule out involvement of subtherapeutic use of antibiotics in animal feeds.

6. Intergovernmental exchange programs should be established to exchange data from studies recommended in 5. This is especially significant for countries that export or import foods for human consumption to or from the United States.

7. FDA and state animal regulatory officials should strongly encourage isolation of animals that are on antibiotic therapy.

8. Extensive educational programs such as those described in the summary should be initiated.

REFERENCES

Baldwin, R. A. 1970. The development of transferable drug resistance in *Salmonella* and its public health implications. J. Am. Vet. Med. Assoc. 157:1841-1853.

Childers, A. B., E. E. Keahey, and A. W. Kotula. 1977. Reduction of *Salmonella* and fecal contamination of pork during swine slaughter. J. Am. Vet. Med. Assoc. 171:1161-1164.

Datta, N. 1965. Infectious drug resistance. Br. Med. Bull. 21: 254-259.

Edel, W., M. van Schothorst, P. A. M. Guinée, and E. H. Kampelmacher. 1974. Preventive measures to obtain Salmonella-free slaughter pigs. Zentralbl. Bakteriol. Parasitenkd. Infektionskr. Hyg., I. Abt. Orig. Reihe B 158:568-577.

Groves, B. I., N. A. Fish, and D. A. Barnum. 1970. An epidemiological study of Salmonella infection in swine in Ontario. Can. J. Public Health 61:396-401.

Gustafson, R. H. 1975. Antibiotic sensitivity in Salmonella isolated from swine in a Pennsylvania slaughter house. Pp. 193-211 in Animal Industry Research Progress Report, AIR, Vol. 3. Project No. 3-721. American Cyanamid Company, Princeton, N.J.

Howe, K., A. H. Linton, and A. D. Osborne. 1976. An investigation of calf carcass contamination by *Escherichia coli* from the gut contents at slaughter. J. Appl. Bacteriol. 41:37-45.

Jensen, L. B., and W. R. Hess. 1941. A study of ham souring. Food Res. 6:273-326.

Kobland, J. D. 1975. Antibiotic sensitivity of salmonellae isolated from swine in an Iowa slaughter house. Pp. 291-321 in Animal Industry Research Progress Report, AIR, Vol. 3, Project No. 3-733. American Cyanamid Company, Princeton, N.J.

Licciardello, J. J., J. T. R. Nickerson, and S. A. Goldblith. 1968. The Effect of Repeated Treatment with Gamma Rays on the Radio-Resistance, Virulence, and Culture Characteristics of Certain Pathogenic Bacteria. Final Report. Prepared by the Massachusetts Institute of Technology for the U.S. Atomic

Energy Commission, Contract No. AT(30-1)-3325. NTIS No. MIT-3325-40. National Technical Information Service, Springfield, Va. 152 pp.

Linton, A. H., B. Handley, A. D. Osborne, B. G. Shaw, T. A. Roberts, and W. R. Hudson. 1977. Contamination of pig carcasses at two abattoirs by Escherichia coli with special reference to O-serotypes and antibiotic resistance. J. Appl. Bacteriol. 42:89-110.

Linton, A. H., K. Howe, C. L. Hartley, M. Clements, and A. D. Osborne. In press. Antibiotic resistance and sensitive Escherichia coli O-serotypes in the gut and on the carcass of commercially slaughtered broiler chickens and the potential public health implications. Dept. of Bacteriology, University of Bristol, and Dept. of Veterinary Medicine, Langford House, Langford, Bristol. 35 pp.

Lyons, J. P. 1971. U.S. Department of Agriculture controls over imported meats. J. Am. Vet. Med. Assoc. 159:1551-1555.

McEnroe, K. M. 1971. A changing meat and poultry inspection program. J. Am. Vet. Med. Assoc. 159:1546-1550.

Mercer, H. D. 1975. Antimicrobial drugs in food-producing animals. Control mechanisms of governmental agencies. Vet. Clin. N. Am. 5:3-34.

Morrison, A. B., and I. C. Munro. 1969. Appraisal of the significance to man of drug residues in edible animal products. Pp. 255-269 in The Use of Drugs in Animal Feeds. Proceedings of a Symposium. Publication No. 1679, National Academy of Sciences, Washington, D.C.

Mosley, E. B., P. R. Elliker, and H. Hays. 1976. Destruction of food spoilage, indicator and pathogenic organisms by various germicides in solution and on a stainless steel surface. J. Milk Food Technol. 39:830-836.

Mussman, H. C. 1973. The changing face of meat and poultry inspection. J. Am. Vet. Med. Assoc. 163:1061-1064.

Newell, K. W., and L. P. Williams, Jr. 1971. The control of salmonellae affecting swine and man. J. Am. Vet. Med. Assoc. 158:89-98.

Patterson, J. T. 1969. Salmonellae in meat and poultry, poultry plant cooling waters and effluents, and animal feedingstuffs. J. Appl. Bacteriol. 32:329-337.

Smith, H. W., and J. F. Tucker. 1978. Oral administration of neomycin to chickens experimentally infected with Salmonella typhimurium. Vet. Rec. 102:354-356.

Stuart, L. S., and E. H. McNally. 1943. Bacteriological studies on the egg shell. U.S. Egg Poult. Mag. 49:28-31, 45-47.

Threlfall, E. J., L. R. Ward, and B. Rowe. 1978. Epidemic spread of a chloramphenicol-resistant strain of Salmonella typhimurium phage type 204 in bovine animals in Britain. Vet. Rec. 103: 438-440.

Van Houweling, C. D. 1967. Drugs in animal feeds? A question without an answer. Food and Drug Administration Papers (September):11-15.

Walton, J. R. 1970. Contamination of meat carcasses by antibiotic-resistant coliform bacteria. Lancet 2:561-563.

Walton, J. R. 1971. Part VI. Antibiotics and drug resistance in animals. The public health implications of drug-resistant bacteria in farm animals. Ann. N. Y. Acad. Sci. 132:358-361.

Weissman, M. A., and J. A. Carpenter. 1969. Incidence of salmonellae in meat and meat products. Appl. Microbiol. 17:899-902.

APPENDIX I
INFECTIOUS DISEASE: EFFECT OF ANTIMICROBIALS ON BACTERIAL POPULATIONS

Thomas F. O'Brien[1]

EPIDEMIOLOGY OF ANTIBIOTIC RESISTANCE

We have known for a century that germs cause infection. For a third of a century we have had antibiotics to control infection and molecular biology to explain, ultimately, how the process works. We can now see each strain of bacteria as a specific collection of genes. Some specify the life cycle. Some code for markers we find convenient for speciation. Others code for virulence factors or for enzymes that inactivate antibiotics.

The specific linkage of genes in a bacterial strain is not fixed. We know increasingly more about the ways in which bacteria can lose, gain, or exchange genes in experiments and, presumably, in nature to fill virtually every habitat (Arber, 1979). However, there have been few measurements of actual rates of bacterial gene reassociation in natural environments (O'Brien *et al.*, 1977). Such measurements are of critical importance because "cost-benefit estimates" of the behavior of bacterial populations may depend ultimately on their rates of gene reassociation.

We know how most antibiotics work (Kucers and Bennett, 1975). Each binds to and inactivates a critical specific target site in the bacterial cell. The discovery of each new family of antibiotics--penicillins, streptomycin, tetracyclines, chloramphenicol, etc.--proved in retrospect, to have also been the discovery of a new target site. Unfortunately, few new classes of antibiotics are being discovered. The last discovery of an antibiotic with a truly new target site may have been rifampicin, which was first marketed 15 years ago (Hartmann *et al.*, 1967). Most of the newer antibiotics circumvent resistance mechanisms to reach old target sites (Christensen *et al.*, 1979). This declining rate of discovery of new target sites for antibiotics suggests that these sites are, like fossil fuels, another unreplenishable resource.

---

[1]Director, Microbiology Laboratory, Peter Bent Brigham Hospital, Boston, Mass.

Also, it costs increasingly more to reach those target sites. If it were not for the prevalence of intervening resistance mechanisms, the less expensive, older agents could continue to be used. These resistance mechanisms force us to use succeeding waves of newer antibiotics that are expensive to develop and promote. These costly products now account for most of the antibiotic dollar volume which is, in turn, a large part of the pharmaceutical dollar volume.

Mutational and "Gained" Resistance

Our understanding of bacterial resistance to antibiotics has improved over the past two decades. Early concepts were based on studies conducted with an *in-vitro* model of acquired resistance to streptomycin. These studies showed that a mutation altered the target site in such a way that it still functioned enzymatically, but that the antibiotic could no longer bind to it. Thus, susceptibility was lost. We now realize that it is far more common for resistance to be gained, i.e., the target site remains unchanged, as vulnerable as ever, but that the bacterial cell acquires something like an antibiotic-inactivating enzyme or a permeability barrier that prevents the antibiotic from getting near the target site (Davies, 1979).

We can imagine and have begun to observe the implications of "gained" resistance being more common than lost susceptibility. Mutational loss of susceptibility to an antibiotic might be expected to occur at a measurable rate. So should the subsequent overgrowth replacement of susceptible strains by the mutant-resistant clone in populations exposed to the antibiotic. Consequently, for the mutational loss-of-susceptibility model, the relationship between number of bacteria exposed to an antibiotic and the prevalence of antibiotic-resistant bacteria seems to be relatively simple with few intervening variables. It would also seem possible that this model could be used to estimate the prevalence of antibiotic resistance in one population of bacteria that is ascribable to the administration of antibiotics to another population, if the rate of interchange of bacteria between the two populations is known.

Gained resistance is more complex. Usually, one of two types of genes is acquired--a gene for an enzyme, which inactivates the antibiotic or bypasses a blocked enzyme, or a gene for a protein, which impairs the antibiotic's entry into the cell (Davies, 1979). These are large, specific molecules that are too big to arise often by chance mutation. Therefore, most strains of bacteria have to acquire such genes from other bacteria (Arber, 1979; Falkow, 1975).

Thus, when relating antibiotic usage to prevalence of resistance in a bacterial population one would first calculate the probability of the arrival of the resistance gene from another population instead of determining the mutation rate as with loss of susceptibility.

Antibiotic Resistance Genes

Origin and Evolution. The source of antibiotic resistance genes is not known. Some of them may have developed to protect antibiotic-producing organisms from their own products (Davies and Courvalin, 1977). The β-lactamases could have evolved if the active sites of transpeptidases of the bacterial cell wall, which selectively bind but do not hydrolyze penicillins, had begun to acquire a hydrolytic function (Crosa *et al.*, 1977; Tipper and Strominger, 1965). Techniques for characterizing products of resistance genes are so new, and surveillance so sketchy, that there has been little opportunity to distinguish evolution of a new gene from dissemination of a previously rare one. However, examples that must involve one or the other have been observed, e.g., the emergence of the newer aminoglycoside-inactivating enzymes (Davies and Courvalin, 1977; LeGoffic *et al.*, 1977).

There are also opportunities for evolution towards improved efficacy for existing antibiotic-inactivating enzymes. For example, a modification of active site configuration might permit binding of an increased range of substrate (antibiotic) analogs as new ones come onto the market (LeGoffic *et al.*, 1979). The R1818 β-lactamase, which produces only low-level resistance, could increase that resistance if it could evolve to have a higher substrate turnover number (Medeiros *et al.*, 1974). Evolution of an improved enzyme environment can also help. The TEM β-lactamase produces resistance to ampicillin that is much less dependent on inocula in *Escherichia coli* than in *Haemophilus influenzae* because the outer membrane of the latter is more permeable to ampicillin (Medeiros and O'Brien, 1975).

Dissemination. Whatever the origin and rates of evolution of antibiotic resistance genes, their transmission through bacterial populations is increasingly well understood. Clearly, there are multiple levels of genetic mobility and persistence. Many antibiotic resistance genes, e.g., a majority of the known β-lactamases of Gram-negative bacilli, have never been shown to be plasmid-borne and are presumably chromosomal (Sykes and Matthew, 1976). Essentially, they can go only where their fixed-host bacteria can go, which depends on the specific colonizing and competing capabilities that are built into the other genes on the chromosome.

An entirely different level of mobility is open to antibiotic resistance genes that become located on plasmids, but the extent of the mobility depends greatly on the plasmid on which the gene is carried. Many plasmids are nonconjugative. They can transfer between bacteria only if "rescued" by a conjugative plasmid (Mitsuhashi, 1979). Others are conjugative and self-transferable but only at a limited rate or to a limited number of host bacteria. If transferred, they become unstable in many bacteria and are readily segregated. Moreover, plasmids cannot transfer to bacteria that already contain plasmids of the same incompatibility group (Falkow, 1975). Thus, a resistance gene on a plasmid of a group already widely distributed in a bacterial population might achieve only limited dissemination in that population.

The ultimate dissemination and persistence of a plasmid-borne resistance gene also depends on the other types of genes that are on the same plasmid. Many of the plasmids bearing resistance genes are large and have space for many other genes. Some of these other genes code for resistance to other antibiotics. The prevalence of any one of these resistance genes, and of the plasmid itself, is amplified whenever the plasmid's hosts are exposed to one of the antibiotics to which any of the other genes code resistance. A plasmid is essentially a gene cooperative in which an advantage accruing to any member gene is shared by all. In this sense, plasmids can be looked upon as devices that cause an increased prevalence of resistance to several antibiotics to result from the use of one antibiotic.

Linkage to Genes for Other Characteristics. Some genes, which code for functions other than resistance to antibiotics, also amplify and sustain the prevalence of an antibiotic resistance gene that was associated with them on the same plasmid. Some plasmid-borne genes code for functions that permit host bacteria to survive in specific environments such as those containing specific metallic ions (McHugh _et al_., 1975; Pinney, 1977). Others code for colonization (Silver and Mercer, 1978) or for metabolic functions, e.g., lactose catabolism (Kopecko _et al_., 1979), on which host bacteria might depend either always or only under certain environmental conditions. The functions of these other genes, which occupy so large a part of so many plasmids bearing resistance genes, are just beginning to be elucidated. The glimpses of them to date, however, suggest that they may be major codeterminants of the ultimate distribution of resistance genes carried with them on the same plasmids (Novick, in press).

The closeness and stability of the linkages between a particular antibiotic resistance gene and other resistance or nonresistance genes on the same plasmid also influence the prevalence of that specific antibiotic resistance gene. The increasingly well understood mechanisms for genetic recombination serve not only to put genes together but also to disrupt and separate them, ultimately segregating genes that no longer provide a survival advantage. Conforming to the analogy of the cooperative venture, genes that never bring any advantage are eventually dismissed, but the time of dismissal varies greatly. A gene coding for resistance to a rarely used antibiotic could persist on a plasmid for long periods during which it offers no survival advantage if it is closely and stably linked to another gene that provides an advantage. The close linkage of genes coding for resistance to streptomycin and sulfonamide on a commonly encountered plasmid (van Treeck et al., 1979) could be part of the reason why the gene for resistance to streptomycin remains prevalent long after clinical usage of streptomycin in humans has declined.

Transposons. The recently discovered transposons provide yet another level of genetic mobility. Transposons are segments of a DNA chain flanked by special insertion sequences. These transposons and genes carried on them are able to transpose from one plasmid to another or from plasmid to chromosome and back (Heffron et al., 1975). Location on a transposon could greatly enhance the prevalence of any gene.

Genes coding for resistance to a number of commonly used antibiotics have been found on transposons (Campbell et al., 1977). A resistance gene can be limited in its distribution by its position on the chromosome of, or on a nonconjugative plasmid in, a poorly colonizing strain; on a plasmid of limited host range; or on a plasmid carrying few other genes with survival advantages. Such a gene could become more prevalent if it could be transposed to a more mobile plasmid carrying a more advantageous collection of genes, possibly including other resistance genes, or, better still, to a variety of such plasmids.

Implications of the Resistance Mechanism

The entire assemblage of these properties for any antibiotic resistance gene, including the substrate range and the efficiency of its gene product, and its genetic location and mobility, can be regarded as an antibiotic resistance mechanism. Defined in this way, the mechanism can be viewed as a major variable in determining the prevalence of resistance to antibiotics. When a population of bacteria is exposed to an antibiotic, the extent and distribution of the resulting antibiotic resistance will depend largely on the properties of the mechanisms of resistance to that antibiotic in that population.

This can be best illustrated by considering some examples. If no mechanism for resistance to the antibiotic is available to the exposed population of bacteria, there will be no resistance. This situation prevailed for a number of years in populations of Enterobacteriaceae exposed to gentamicin in the United States (O'Brien *et al.*, 1978). If the only mechanism available is a gene coding for an enzyme with a narrow specificity including only that antibiotic and if that gene is the only resistance gene on the chromosome of a bacterial species with poor colonizing and competing abilities, the ensuing resistance would be directed only against the antibiotic used and would be unlikely to persist. However, resistance would become widespread and persistent if the population contains a resistance mechanism consisting of a gene coding for an enzyme with a broad substrate range and if the gene is located on a transposon in a plasmid with a broad host range and is rich with closely linked genes for resistance to other antibiotics and for other survival advantages.

Consider a bacterial population in a chemostat or in nature that includes one cell with a resistance mechanism and a similar population that includes one cell with a different mechanism. Each population could be exposed for the same period to an antibiotic to which its mechanism produces resistance. Each population could then be scored for the total number of resistant cells times the total number of antibiotics to which each is resistant times the number of generations during which resistance persists. The values could differ greatly and would constitute for each mechanism an index of its efficiency at converting selection pressure into resistance prevalence.

A different kind of index could acknowledge the heterogeneity of bacterial populations in nature. Such populations contain many different strains and species of bacteria coexisting, competing, and cooperating to occupy all possible niches in the ecosystem. For a resistance mechanism introduced in one strain in such a population, it would be possible to score the number of different strains and specimens into which the mechanism became incorporated after a controlled period of antibiotic exposure. Some mechanisms could remain only in the strain in which they were introduced. Such a strain would presumably overgrow its susceptible neighbors during exposure to the antibiotic but might not by itself be able to occupy all of the niches very fully. After the exposure to the antibiotic, the strain might promptly be displaced and revert to its natural domain in the population, which could be nonexistent.

In the same population exposed for the same period to the same antibiotic, a different mechanism of resistance on a plasmid with a broad host range could be incorporated into many strains and species. Or a resistance gene on a transposon in a plasmid of limited host range might be transposed to one or more plasmids with a broader range of hosts and enter many strains and species by this route. In each strain and species the resistance gene would, in effect, be associated with a different assemblage of other genes. Therefore, this score would be an index of gene reassociation and, to the extent that the selection pressure promotes it, antibiotic-induced gene reassociation.

Two consequences of this process are worth examining. If many of the strains and species constituting the original bacterial population came to possess the resistance mechanism enabling them to survive exposure to an antibiotic, they would then presumably be better able to fill all niches during the exposure than would a single strain. They would also be less rapidly displaced by susceptible species after the exposure ended. In the hypothetically perfect situation, all strains and species in the original population would receive the resistance mechanism so that exposure to antibiotics would not alter their ecological balance. In such a case there would be no tendency after the exposure had ended for reemerging or reentering susceptible species to displace resistant strains in the process of regaining their old niches. In this population, the prevalence of resistance after exposure would be diminished primarily by the segregation rates of the resistance mechanism from each of the strains, which may also be a variable characteristic of the resistance mechanism (Levin, in press) or, possibly, the normal influx of new strains colonizing and displacing the older members, although these new strains could also be susceptible to infection by a mobile plasmid widely resident in the population.

Secondly, if a resistance mechanism has evolved to gain a great increment in prevalence per episode of exposure to antibiotics and to have a high degree of interspecies mobility, it has a greater chance of ultimately getting into a pathogen. The bacteria that actually infect humans or animals are only a miniscule part of the total bacterial flora of the world and, usually, of the infected individual as well. But they do all the damage. The arrival of a resistance mechanism in a pathogen can be a significant and tragic event. The recent arrival of the TEM β-lactamase (Medeiros and O'Brien, 1975) into group B *Haemophilus influenzae*, the commonest cause of bacterial meningitis in children, has led to treatment failure and to the need to treat all children thought to have the disease with a potentially toxic antibiotic, chloramphenicol (Howard *et al.*, 1978).

All of these considerations lead to one essential question: What is the source of the more efficient and more efficiently distributing resistance mechanisms? Everything suggests that the mechanisms themselves are the ultimate evolutionary products of the cumulative application of antibiotic selection pressures to bacterial populations. Exposure to antibiotics is the only imaginable stimulus that would provide evolutionary survival advantage to antibiotic-inactivating enzymes or to other resistance genes prevalent enough to overcome the odds against their forming favorable linkages with one another or with other advantageous genes or eventually becoming located on plasmids or transposons.

Summary

The antibiotic resistance observed in a population of bacteria after exposure to an antibiotic can be attributed to:

1. The net effect of all prior antibiotic exposure on the bacterial flora of this planet in shaping and delivering to this particular population the specific resistance mechanisms it has acquired.

2. The effect of those specific resistance mechanisms in determining the number and types of resistant bacteria that will be generated by the present episode of exposure to the antibiotic.

INTERCHANGE BETWEEN DIFFERENT BACTERIAL FLORAS

Compartmentalization of Floras

The preceding considerations have a very practical bearing on how we view the relationship of antibiotic usage in different compartments of the world's bacterial flora. These compartments could be defined as domains within which bacteria can be imagined to circulate more readily than they do between compartments. For example, the flora of each human being, the flora of an intensive care unit as opposed to the rest of the hospital, the flora of an entire hospital (O'Brien *et al.*, 1975) as opposed to the community, or, on a larger scale, the flora of humans in the United States as opposed to that in humans in some other part of the world. Although compartmentalized, the bacterial flora of the world undoubtedly circulates between all of compartments, but generally less than within them.

If the only concern with antibiotic resistance were quantitative, the resistance in compartment A would change the resistance in compartment B only to the extent that bacteria from A moved into B. If A had 100% resistance and B by itself would have had only 10% resistance, yet 1% of B's strains actually came from A, then they would add 1% resistance for a total of 11% resistance in B.

If there are qualitative differences among resistance mechanisms, as discussed in the preceding section, then the influence of resistance in one compartment on that of another may be quite out of proportion to the circulation between them. Suppose compartment A were to contain a mechanism of resistance still absent in B but ideally suited for circulation there because of its plasmid incompatibility grouping, its special ability to inactivate an antibiotic widely used there, or its linkage to some other genes admirably suited for survival in B. Even if there were very little circulation between the compartments, a few bacteria with the mechanism could transfer from A to B. Once there, the mechanisms could become prevalent.

Recent Observations

Recently, an apparent example of this has been observed with the use of gentamicin, which had been widely used since 1970 in the United States to treat hospitalized patients infected with Enterobacteriaceae. Through 1975, however, exceedingly few strains of Enterobacteriaceae isolated in the United States had any ability to resist that antibiotic (O'Brien *et al.*, 1978). For purposes of bacterial ecology, there was a great need for some mechanism of resistance, but apparently none, or none with appreciable genetic mobility, had become available to strains in the United States. In other parts of the world--in France, for example--there were genes for two aminoglycoside-inactivating enzymes (O'Brien *et al.*, 1978; Witchitz and Chabbert, 1972). The 2"-aminoglycoside nucleotidyl transferase (AAD 2") and the 3-aminoglycoside acetyl transferase (AAC-3) were known to be widely distributed in nosocomial strains.

In early 1976 a strain of *Klebsiella pneumoniae* of serotype 2 with an unusual biotype was isolated from a patient in one of the U.S. hospitals in our international collaborative study (O'Brien *et al.*, in press). This strain had a distinctive conjugative plasmid of 56 Mdal belonging to incompatibility group M, which carried genes for resistance to sulfonamides as well as to chloramphenicol acetyl transferase, the TEM 1 β-lactamase, and the AAD 2" enzyme, one of the two gentamicin resistance enzymes that are common in other parts of the world.

Over the next 4 months this distinctive strain of *K. pneumoniae* was isolated from 40 patients in the hospital. Thereafter, this strain was isolated only infrequently, but by then, the plasmid was being found in isolates of other strains of *K. penumoniae* and in other species of Enterobacteriaceae as well (O'Brien *et al.*, in press). Ultimately, this one plasmid was found in 49 different biotypes of six different bacterial strains. Restriction endonuclease digestion analyses conducted on plasmids from *Escherichia coli* K-12 transconjugants of eight different strains of six different species confirmed the identity of the plasmid throughout the outbreak (O'Brien *et al.*, in press).

In this instance, a restrictive mechanism not previously circulating in one compartment (the hospital flora) and probably not circulating in a much larger one (flora of humans in the United States), but which circulated widely in another compartment for several years (European hospital flora) appeared in one hospital compartment and rapidly became prevalent. An almost identical sequence in one other U.S. hospital has since been reported (Gerding *et al.*, 1979; Sadowski *et al.*, 1979). We are beginning to search files in microbiological laboratories in other U.S. hospitals for evidence of further spread.

There is no proof that the mechanism was imported from outside of the flora compartment of humans in the United States, although it had been prevalent there (O'Brien et al., 1978) and might have been expected to be imported if there had been any appreciable exchange between these compartments. Another item circumstantially suggesting such importation was the plasmid's carriage of the chloramphenicol resistance gene, which tends to be relatively rare in the flora of humans in the United States but common in flora outside that compartment. Proof of its genealogy will have to come from studies identifying plasmids on a larger scale, which are beginning to become practical.

This experience illustrates that if there are qualitative differences between resistance mechanisms, the influence of resistance in one bacterial flora compartment on that of another may be completely out of proportion to the rate of interchange between them. The compartment in which this particular complex mechanism had evolved could not have had great interchange with the compartment of flora in humans in the United States because only traces of it could be found there prior to the outbreak. Apparently, however, this particular mechanism was qualitatively so "fit" for this hospital flora compartment that once introduced it circulated widely and became prevalent.

The consequences of the entry and circulation of this one plasmid in a hospital where it had previously been absent were substantial. The resistance of all Gram-negative bacillary isolates at the hospital to a set of six antibacterial agents (APAR index) (O'Brien et al., 1978) increased approximately 50% because of this plasmid. The number of isolates with resistance to more than six antibiotics increased nearly 10-fold. A number of cases of Gram-negative sepsis were virtually untreatable. Most of the resistant isolates came, as usual, from patients being treated or having recently been treated with antibiotics. Yet the level of antibiotic usage had not appeared to change appreciably. As discussed previously, the entry and dissemination of a qualitatively different resistance mechanism had reset the equilibrium so that a given amount of antibiotic usage now generated a greater prevalence of resistance to antibiotics.

IMPLICATIONS TO HUMAN HEALTH FROM ANTIBIOTIC USE IN ANIMALS

Exchange Between Compartments

The considerations discussed in the preceding paragraphs generate concern about the veterinary use of antimicrobial agents.

The flora of animals, particularly animals raised as food sources in the United States, can be regarded as a compartment of the total bacterial flora subjected to its own selection pressure. Flora of animals is known to exchange with flora of humans (Levy, 1978; Shooter *et al.*, 1970) although the extent is disputed. Two major routes of exchange are envisioned. One is through farm workers or meat production workers who come into close contact with the animals or animal products. The other is through contamination of the uncooked meats, which are handled daily by anyone preparing meals. Better estimates of the overall rates at which bacteria flow from animals to humans would give us a better estimate of the potential quantitative transfer of antibiotic resistance from animals raised for food to humans.

There is probably also less compartmentation between floras of individual animals that have received an antibiotic than there is between individual, treated humans. Antibiotic-treated humans are a minority separated from each other at any time by untreated humans in the community and in hospitals, except for intensive care units (Shapiro *et al.*, 1979). Moreover, human hygienic practice, modern sewage systems, and procedures to control hospital infection, although imperfect, tend to minimize exchange of bacteria between humans including antibiotic-treated humans. The exchange of antibiotic-treated flora between animals in a feedlot, all of whom may be receiving antibiotics, would appear to be of great magnitude. Recycling of large numbers of the same strains of bacteria through successive rounds of exposure to antibiotics would also seem to favor reassociation of antibiotic resistance genes and other genes towards the development of more efficient resistance mechanisms and more efficient distribution (Threlfall *et al.*, 1978).

Effects of Dose on Selection Pressure

Of even greater concern, however, are the qualitative aspects of the transfer of resistance mechanisms between compartments of bacterial flora. The total weight of antibiotics used in food animals in this country approximates that used in humans. Since much of this is administered at a subtherapeutic level, the amount may exert a greater selection pressure overall, i.e., in the flora of animals the number of bacteria that encounter antibiotic molecules probably exceed the number that do in the flora of humans. The reported prevalence of antibiotic resistance in the flora of animals (Babcock *et al.*, 1973) suggests that the concentrations of antibiotic encountered in a great many of these instances must still be high enough to inhibit susceptible species and favor overgrowth by resistant isolates, i.e., high enough to exert selection pressure.

Discussion

Consideration of these very general characteristics of the use of antibiotics in animals indicates that the flora compartment of animals in the United States could be a development ground--by analogy, a vast recombinant DNA laboratory--for the evolution of efficient antibiotic resistance mechanisms. Moreover, it could have an output even greater than that of the flora compartment of humans in the United States.

Note, for example, that the TEM β-lactamase, as identified presumptively by small inhibition zone diameters for carbenicillin but not for cephalothin (Medeiros *et al.*, 1974) in Figure 1, is relatively common in veterinary isolates of salmonellae. If this prevalence is representative of that in other animal isolates of Enterobacteriaceae, the total number of individual TEM β-lactamase genes in all animal flora may exceed that in all flora in humans in the United States. If this were true, then some or all of the evolutionary developments that eventually enabled the TEM β-lactamase to gain entry into strains of *Haemophilus influenzae* type b after 30 years of penicillin usage (Elwell *et al.*, 1975) would probably have occurred in the flora of antibiotic-treated animals. This illustrates the potential importance of qualitative differences in resistance mechanisms. The occurrence of one or more such events once somewhere in the flora of animals could conceivably have been a decisive step in the ultimate emergence of a major medical problem for humans.

OBSERVING THE ANTIBIOTIC RESISTANCE SYSTEM

The foregoing discussions have emphasized dissemination and entrenchment of antibiotic resistance in bacterial populations as implied by studies of the resistance mechanisms themselves. For more than a decade, understanding developed in laboratory studies of how resistance mechanisms can spread has provided the most compelling reasons for concern about how they may actually be spreading in the world. Those who have been conducting the experiments have generally been the most concerned.

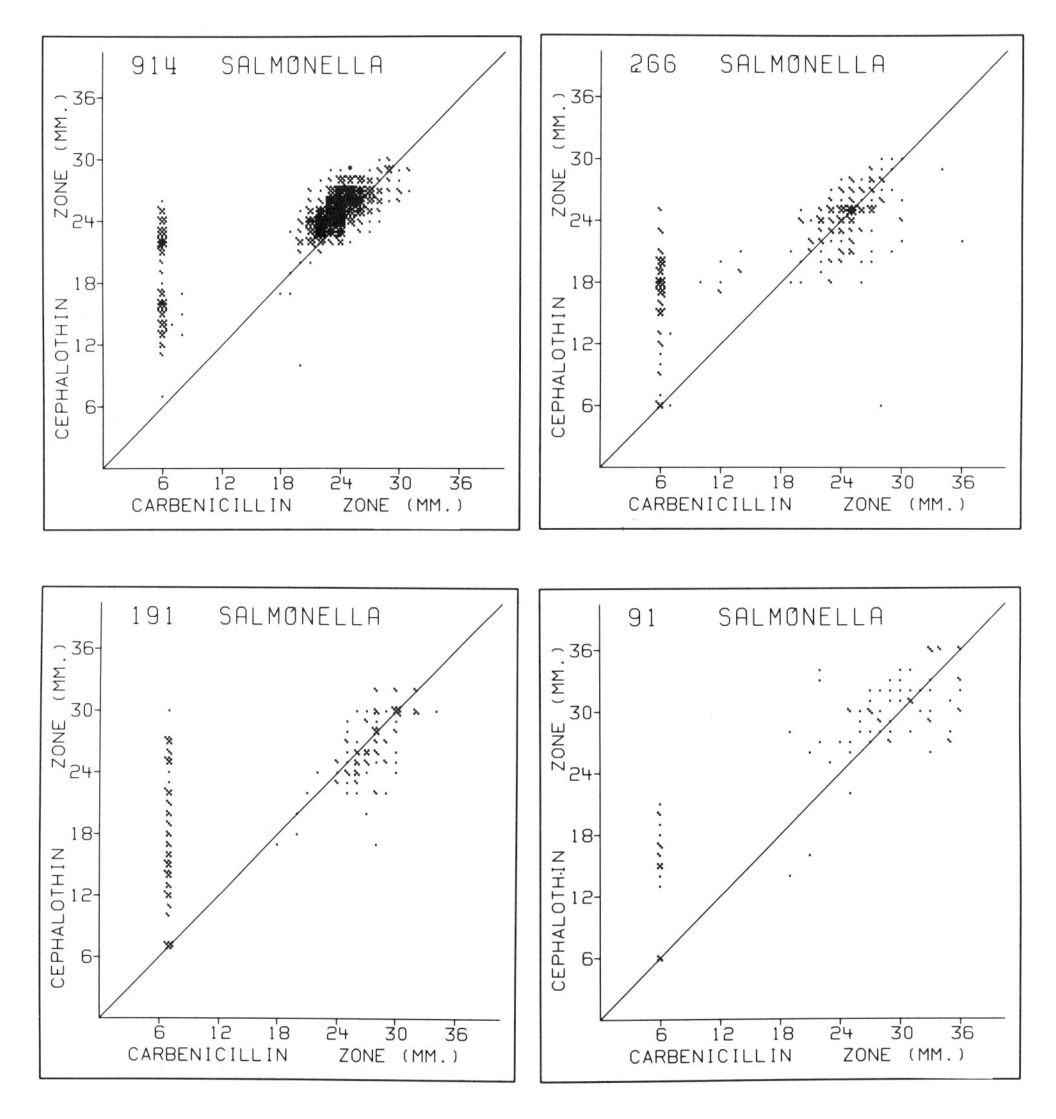

FIGURE 1. Computer-generated plots of diameters of zones of inhibition around the carbenicillin and cephalothin disks for four of the Salmonella collections in Figure 2. Upper left is the collection of veterinary isolates, upper right those from a hospital in the United States, and the lower two are from hospitals outside the United States. Figure provided by the International Survey of Antibiotic Resistance Group.

The general conclusion provided by the evidence from molecular biologists is that antibiotic resistance throughout the world is probably an interrelated system. Antibiotic resistance genes are the ultimate indivisible units of that system. They may transpose from one plasmid to another within a bacterial cell, transfer on a plasmid from one bacterial cell to another, or be carried in a bacterial cell that leaves one patient or animal and colonizes another. Antibiotic usage exerts selection pressure at each level, concentrating resistance genes on transposons, transposons on plasmids, plasmids in bacterial cells, and resistant cells at the expense of their susceptible counterparts.

Although experiments have improved understanding of the system, the operation of the system has not yet been completely observed. Evidence concerning the actual spread of resistance is fragmentary. There is no comprehensive overview of the distribution of antibiotic resistance mechanisms in the bacterial flora of the world or its compartments or of the manner in which the distribution is shifting over time.

It is within the framework of this incomplete surveillance that we have to examine the effect of the use of antibacterial agents in livestock upon resistance to antimicrobial agents in flora of humans in the United States.

There are other obstacles besides incomplete surveillance. One is the above-mentioned inherent difficulty in detecting the possible occurrence in the flora of animals of rare qualitative alterations in resistance mechanisms that might have epidemic potential in the flora of humans. Another is that phentoypic antibiotic resistance, as commonly measured by susceptibility testing, does not discriminate between different mechanisms that confer resistance to the same antibiotic. Since it usually scores only resistance or nonresistance to each agent, and since the same agents-- β-lactams, tetracyclines, and streptomycin-- have been commonly used in both animals and humans, the same combinations of resistance may be displayed in both floras and are thus less useful as markers of resistance flow between them.

Another way of visualizing this would be to suppose that incursions of resistant flora from animals had come to account for most of the resistance in the flora of humans. Resistance patterns might then be so similar in both floras that they would be useless for tracing exchange between them. The success of the incursion would have obliterated the possibility of detecting it.

This problem is a very general obstacle to tracing the spread of resistance mechanisms in naturally occurring bacterial populations. Most common phenotypic resistance markers have been so widely distributed in most bacterial populations that their further exchange is extremely difficult to detect, let alone measure overall. Generally, we are able to detect and measure exchange only when a new marker enters a population as it did in the previously mentioned outbreaks, which involved a previously rare aminoglycoside-inactivating enzyme (O'Brien *et al.*, in press). Similarly, incursions of resistance without gene exchange is usually observed only when a previously rare type of resistance is involved, as with penicillinase-producing gonococci, ampicillin-resistant *Haemophilus influenzae*, methicillin-resistant staphylococci, and penicillin-resistant pneumococci. With regard to the dissemination of antibiotic resistance, it seems likely that only the tip of the iceberg has been observed.

A corrolary to this is that improved discrimination of any component in this system--levels of antibiotic resistance, identification of inactivating enzymes, identification of specific transposons or plasmids, or identification of specific biotypes or serotypes of host bacteria--will greatly increase our ability to find distinctive combinations that can be traced through bacterial populations. Every strain of bacteria would be distinctive and traceable if we knew enough about it.

Despite these obstacles, some investigators have observed the spread of antibiotic resistance from the flora of animals to the flora of humans. For example, farm workers who work with antibiotic-fed animals have in their flora a higher prevalence of antibiotic-resistant, plasmid-containing bacteria than do other humans (Levy, 1978; Wiedemann and Knothe, 1971). Moreover, multiresistant strains of salmonellae have been traced from infected animals to humans on many occasions (Anderson, 1968; Anonymous, 1979; Center for Disease Control, 1977).

These documented episodes of the flow of antibiotic resistance from the flora of animals to the flora of humans are important because they confirm, in spite of the obstacles, what molecular biologists have implied.

In the near future, it should be possible to overcome some of these obstacles and to improve our ability to observe the spread of resistance, including that between compartments of flora, e.g., between animals and humans. Two new techniques should enable us to observe antibiotic resistance as an interrelated system throughout the world.

One technique is computerized analysis of results of tests for antibiotic susceptibility. Every day, thousands of laboratories in all parts of the world test the susceptibility of tens of thousands of clinical bacterial isolates. In the aggregate, these data, which have already been paid for, represent the workings of the antibiotic resistance exchange system. The problems of quality control, accurate sampling, data management, and analytic methods have been examined (O'Brien *et al.*, 1977, 1978), and an international collaborating group now representing 30 centers is pooling these types of data for continuing analysis (International Antibiotic Resistance Survey Group and O'Brien, 1978 and in press). In addition, other sets of susceptibility testing results, such as data observed from isolates of salmonellae from humans and animals (Figure 2) and a collection of test files from several hundred U.S. hospitals are being put into computers and similarly analyzed.

These analyses provide a detailed view of the distribution of antibiotic resistance and its trends in time. Much of the controversy over any aspect of antibiotic use concerns the magnitude of the resistance problem and the direction it is taking. Information on both of these issues should be extractable from the data in the computer files and could be observed continually thereafter if monitoring is maintained. Moreover, this type of reconnaissance might serve as a starting point in the development of strategies to minimize resistance resulting from the use of antibiotics in humans or animals.

Furthermore, these analyses should also provide unprecedented detail about the distribution of resistance mechanisms in the flora of humans in the United States. This is extremely important to this report because it should enhance the detection of the incursion of individual or a combination of resistance mechanisms into the flora of humans in the United States from another compartment. Previously noted incursions of this kind, e.g., penicillinase-producing gonococci from the Far East, have been observed, usually because they were extremely conspicuous. The more sensitive and selective are one's techniques for identifying resistance mechanisms, the greater is one's ability to detect incursion of more subtly distinctive groups from the flora of humans in the United States or from the flora of animals. For example, it was possible to trace the entry and dissemination in the flora of a patient in a U.S. hospital of the AAD 2" resistance gene, previously more common in isolates from humans in other countries, because in its early circulation it was linked with a grouping of other resistance genes virtually unique for that hospital (O'Brien *et al.*, in press).

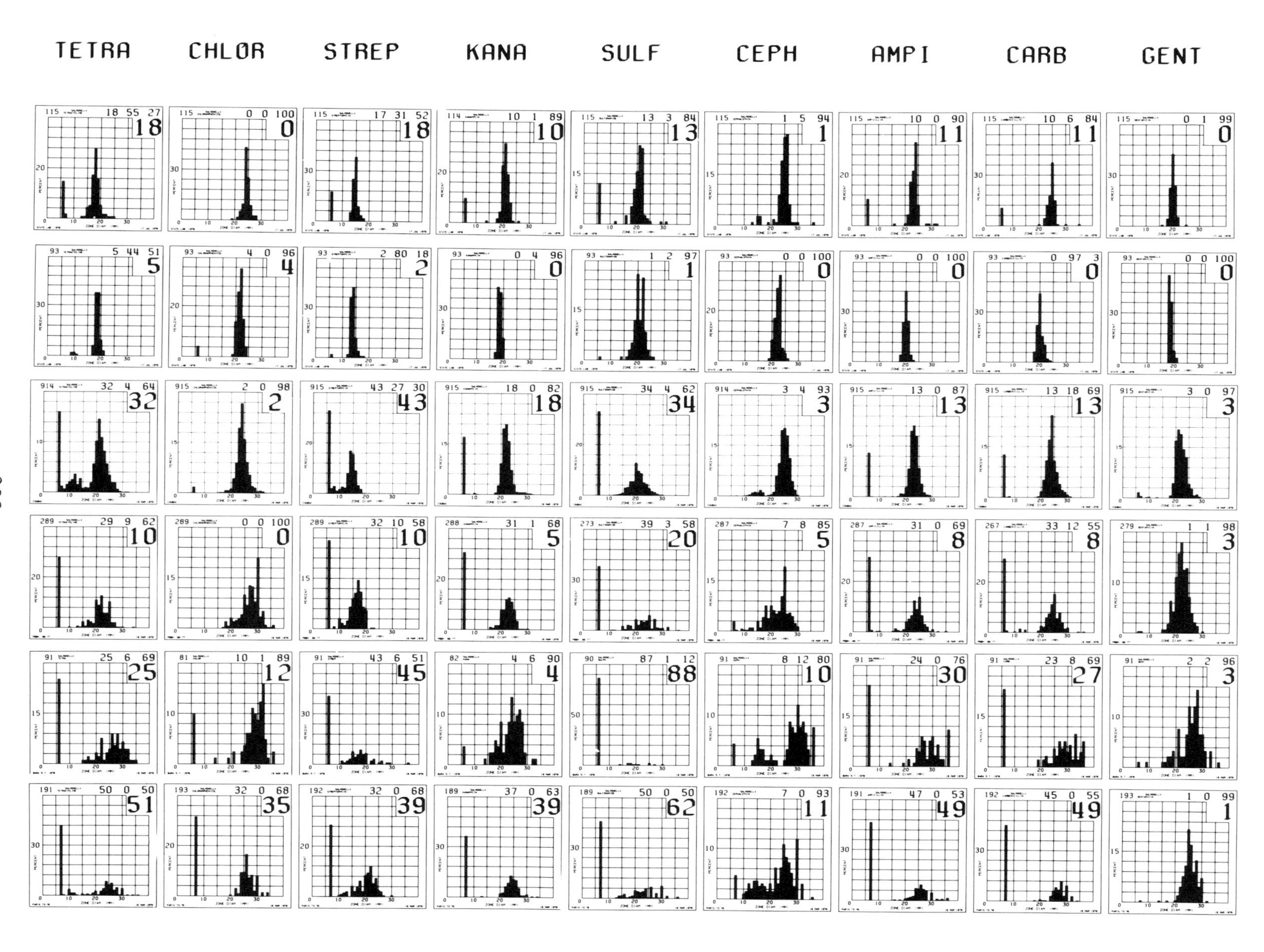
TETRA
CHLØR
STREP
KANA
SULF
CEPH
AMPI
CARB
GENT

FIGURE 2. Computer-plotted frequency distribution of zone diameters around antibiotic disks for collections of *Salmonella* isolates. Vertical lines represent 5-mm increments in zone diameter. The number at upper left is the total number of isolates tested. Numbers at upper right are, from left to right, percent of all isolates classified as resistant, intermediate, and susceptible. The large number, also upper right, is the percentage of isolates showing resistance, excluding repeated isolates obtained from one patient. Vertical scales (percentage) shift to accommodate data.

The top two rows of charts are reference laboratory collections of isolates obtained from humans between 1976 and 1979. The third row is a collection of veterinary isolates from various parts of the United States. The fourth row contains charts of human isolates from a U.S. hospital laboratory and the fifth and sixth rows from foreign hospital laboratories.

TETRA, tetracycline; CHLOR, chloramphenicol; STREP, streptomycin, KANA, kanamycin, SULF, sulfonamide; CEPH, cephalothin; AMPI, ampicillin, CARB, carbenicillin, GENT, gentamicin.

Figure provided by the International Survey of Antibiotic Resistance Group.

Surveillance of the prevalence of antibiotic resistance mechanisms in the compartment of flora of humans outside of the United States will continue to have an important bearing upon the issue surrounding the use of antibiotics in animal feed for two reasons. First, this is the major source other than animal flora of the importation of distinctive resistance mechanism-host combinations into flora of humans in the United States, and it has thus far provided the most conspicuous examples of such importation, including penicillin-resistant gonococci, penicillin-resistant pneumococci, chloramphenicol-resistant typhoid, methicillin-resistant staphylococci, etc. Therefore, knowledge of what is prevalent in human flora abroad could help greatly in deciding the likelihood that a particular mechanism observed in the flora of humans came from animals, rather than from humans from another country.

Figure 2 shows that resistance to sulfonamide in salmonella isolates from humans in the United States could have come from animal sources or from foreign human sources, in both of which it appears to be highly prevalent. Examination of the serotype distribution of sulfonamide resistance in the three compartments might provide further evidence for exchange. In contrast, the low-level resistance to tetracycline (zone diameters of approximately 10 mm) observed in several of the isolates of salmonella from humans in the United States appears more likely to be related to strains from animals, which have a high proportion of this type of resistance, than to isolates of salmonella from humans outside the United States, in which only a very small fraction of resistant isolates appear to be of this type.

The second reason for the pertinence of foreign data is that different countries, in effect, have been testing grounds for a variety of antibiotic uses and food procurement and distribution practices, which have developed in them. The prevalence of various resistance mechanisms in the flora of humans from these different countries are presumably largely the consequences of these practices. Observation of these results could, therefore, be an indispensable guide to the development of optimal antibiotic usage policy. For example, the prevalence of resistance to chloramphenicol, presumably due to the chloramphenicol acetyl transferase gene, was found to be more than 10 times more prevalent among isolates from humans in France than in the United States (O'Brien _et al_., 1978). The French investigator collaborating in this study believes that the use of chloramphenicol in humans is not excessive in France but that chloramphenicol is the antibiotic most widely used in food-source animals in that country. If this could be shown to be true, it could constitute a powerful argument for the influence of antibiotic use in food animals on the prevalence of antibiotic resistance in human flora.

Similarly, resistance to streptomycin remains relatively common in isolates of Enterobacteriaceae from humans in the United States long after its use in treating humans has declined. This could represent fortuitous linkages of the streptomycin resistance gene, as discussed previously, but it might also reflect continuing use of streptomycin in livestock in the United States.

The second resource for improved future observation of the antibiotic resistance system is the newer techniques for characterizing resistance mechanisms, ranging from the detailed characterization of inactivating enzymes to analyses conducted by incubating the plasmid(s) with restriction endonucleases to establish the identity, diversity of, or to map, plasmids. The increasing availability of these methods should improve discrimination of resistance mechanisms, which, as mentioned previously, should greatly enhance our ability to trace their spread in bacterial populations. These techniques may be particularly useful when coupled with computer survey of the large data bases. Discriminant analysis of these data bases may result in the identification of specific antibiotic-inactivating enzymes (Guzman, and O'Brien, 1978; Kent *et al*., in press). The computer analyses could indicate isolates of special interest for these laboratory studies and then project the results of the studies back to a large population.

REFERENCES

Anderson, E. S. 1968. The ecology of transferable drug resistance in the enterobacteria. Ann. Rev. Microbiol. 22:131-180.

Anonymous. 1979. Salmonellosis--an unhappy turn of events. Lancet 1:1009-1010 (Editorial).

Arber, W. 1979. Promotion and limitation of genetic exchange. Science 205:361-365.

Babcock, G. F., D. L. Berryhill, and D. H. Marsh. 1973. R-factors of *Escherichia coli* from dressed beef and humans. Appl. Microbiol. 25:21-23.

Campbell, A., D. Berg, E. Lederberg, P. Starlinger, D. Botstein, R. Novick, and W. Szyblaski. 1977. Nomenclature of transposable elements in prokaryotes. Pp. 15-22 in A. I. Bukhari, J. A. Shapiro, and S. L. Adhya, eds. DNA Insertion Elements, Plasmids, and Episomes. Cold Spring Harbor Laboratory, Cold Spring Harbor, N.Y.

Center for Disease Control. 1977. An Outbreak of Multiple-Drug Resistant *Salmonella heidelberg*, Connecticut. Reported by M. L. Cohen, J. G. Wells, C. L. Samples, P. A. Blake, J. L. Conrad, and E. J. Gangarosa. Report Number EPI-77-13-2. Center for Disease Control, Atlanta, Ga. 8 pp.

Christensen, B. G., L. J. Ruswinkle, and L. D. Cama. 1979. The design of new drugs that resist microbial inactivation. Rev. Infect. Dis. 1:64-72.

Crosa, J. H., J. Olarte, L. J. Mata, L. K. Luttropp, and M. E. Penaranda. 1977. Characterization of an R-plasmid associated with ampicillin resistance in *Shigella dysenteriae* type 1 isolated from epidemics. Antimicrob. Agents Chemother. 11:553-558.

Davies, J. 1979. General mechanisms of antimicrobial resistance. Rev. Infect. Dis. 1:23-27.

Davies, J., and P. Courvalin. 1977. Mechanisms of resistance to aminoglycosides. Am. J. Med. 62:868-872.

Elwell, L. P., J. De Graaff, D. Seibert, and S. Falkow. 1975. Plasmid-linked ampicillin resistance in Haemophilus influenzae type b. Infect. Immun. 12:404-410.

Falkow, S. 1975. Infectious Multiple Drug Resistance. Pion Limited, London, England. 300 pp.

Gerding, D. N., A. E. Buxton, R. A. Hughes, P. P. Cleary, J. Arbaczawski, and W. E. Stamm. 1979. Nosocomial multiply resistant Klebsiella pneumoniae: Epidemiology of an outbreak of apparent index case origin. Antimicrob. Agents Chemother. 15:608-615.

Guzman, M. A., and T. F. O'Brien. 1978. Mechanisms of resistance to aminoglycoside antibiotics in clinical isolates of Serratia marcescens. Abstract 288 in Program and Abstracts. Eighteenth Interscience Conference on Antimicrobial Agents and Chemotherapy. Sponsored by the American Society for Microbiology, Washington, D.C., 1-4 October 1979, The Atlanta Hilton, Atlanta, Ga.

Hartmann, G., K. O. Honikel, F. Knüsel, and J. Nüesch. 1967. The specific inhibition of the DNA-directed RNA synthesis by rifamycin. Biochem. Biophys. Act. 145:843-844.

Heffron, F., C. Rubens, and S. Falkow. 1975. Translocation of a plasmid DNA sequence which mediates ampicillin resistance: Molecular nature and specificity of insertion. Proc. Nat. Acad. Sci. (USA) 72:3623-3627.

Howard, A. J., C. J. Hince, and J. D. Williams. 1978. Antibiotic resistance in Streptococcus pneumoniae and Haemophilus influenzae. Br. Med. J. 1:1657-1660.

International Antibiotic Resistance Survey Group and T. F. O'Brien. 1978. Multicenter sensitivity studies. International collaborative antibiotic resistance survey. Pp. 534-536 in W. Siegenthal and R. Luthy, eds. Current Chemotherapy. Proceedings of the 10th International Congress of Chemotherapy, Volume 1, Zurich/Switzerland, 18-23 September 1977.

International Survey of Antibiotic Resistance Group and T. F. O'Brien (coordinator). In press. Average percent antibiotic resistance in isolates from multiple centers. In J. D. Nelson and C. Grassi, eds. Current Chemotherapy and Infectious Disease. American Society for Microbiology, Washington, D.C.

Kent, R. L., T. F. O'Brien, A. A. Medeiros, J. J. Farrell, and M. A. Guzman. In press. Identification of antibiotic-inactivating enzymes by stepwise discriminant analysis of susceptibility test results. In J. D. Nelson and C. Grassi, eds. Current Chemotherapy and Infectious Disease. American Society for Microbiology, Washington, D.C.

Kopecko, D. J., J. Vickroy, E. M. Johnson, J. A. Wohlhieter, and L. S. Baron. 1979. Molecular and genetic analyses of plasmids responsible for lactose catabolism in salmonellae isolated from diseased humans. In Collected Abstracts from the IV Symposium on Antibiotic Resistance, Smolenice, Czechoslovakia.

Kucers, A., and N. McK. Bennett. 1975. The Use of Antibiotics. A Comprehensive Review with Clinical Emphasis. Second Edition. J. B. Lippincott Company, Philadelphia, Pa. 679 pp.

Le Goffic, F., M. L. Capmau, D. Bonnet, C. Cerceau, C. Soussy, A. Doblanchet, and J. Duval. 1977. Plasmid-mediated pristinamycin resistance PAC IIA: A new enzyme which modifies pristinamycin IIA. J. Antibiot. (Tokyo) 30:665-669.

Le Goffic, F., N. Moreau, A. Martel, and M. Masson. 1979. Could a single enzyme inactivate aminoglycoside antibiotics by two different mechanisms? In Collected Abstracts from the IV Symposium on Antibiotic Resistance, Smolenice, Czechoslovakia.

Levin, B. R. 1979. The conditions for the existence of plasmids in bacterial populations. In Collected Abstracts from the IV Symposium on Antibiotic Resistance, Smolenice, Czechoslovakia.

Levy, S. B. 1978. Emergence of antibiotic-resistant bacteria in the intestinal flora of farm inhabitants. J. Infect. Dis. 137:688-690.

McHugh, G. L., C. C. Hopkins, R. C. Moellering, and M. N. Swartz. 1975. Salmonella typhimurium resistant to silver nitrate, chloramphenicol, and ampicillin. A new threat in burn units? Lancet 1:236-239.

Medeiros, A. A., and T. F. O'Brien. 1975. Ampicillin-resistant Haemophilus influenzae type B possessing a TEM-type β-lactamase but little permeability barrier to ampicillin. Lancet 1:716-718.

Medeiros, A. A., R. L. Kent, and T. F. O'Brien. 1974. Characterization and prevalence of the different mechanisms of resistance to beta-lactam antibiotics in clinical isolates of Escherichia coli. Antimicrob. Agents Chemother. 6:791-801.

Mitsuhashi, S. 1979. Nonconjugative resistance plasmids. In Collected Abstracts from the IV Symposium on Antibiotic Resistance, Smolenice, Czechoslovakia.

Novick, R. In press. The development and spread of antibiotic resistant bacteria as a consequence of feeding antibiotics to livestock. Ann. N.Y. Acad. Sci.

O'Brien, T. F., R. L. Kent, and A. A. Medeiros. 1975. Computer surveillance of shifts in the gross patient flora during hospitalization. J. Infect. Dis. 131:88-96.

O'Brien, T. F., R. A. Norton, R. L. Kent, and A. A. Medeiros. 1977. International surveillance of prevalence of antibiotic resistance. J. Antimicrob. Chemother. 3(suppl C):59-66.

O'Brien, T. F., J. F. Acar, A. A. Medeiros, R. A. Norton, F. Goldstein, and R. L. Kent. 1978. International comparison of prevalence of resistance to antibiotics. J. Am. Med. Assoc. 239:1518-1523.

O'Brien, T. F., D. G. Ross, M. A. Guzman, A. A. Medeiros, R. W. Hedges, and D. Botstein. In press. Dissemination of an antibiotic resistance plasmid in hospital patient flora. Antimicrob. Agents Chemother.

Petrocheilou, V., M. H. Richmond, and P. M. Bennett. 1979. Persistence of plasmid-carrying tetracycline-resistant Escherichia coli in a married couple, one of whom was receiving antibiotics. Antimicrob. Agents Chemother. 16: 225-230.

Pinney, R. J. 1977. Pharmaceutical significance of plasmid-mediated mercury resistance. J. Pharm. Pharmacol. 29 (suppl.):70P.

Riley, M., and A. Anilionis. 1978. Evolution of the bacterial genome. Annu. Rev. Microbiol. 32:519-560.

Sadowski, P. L., B. C. Peterson, D. N. Gerding, and P. P. Cleary. 1979. Physical characterization of ten R plasmids obtained from an outbreak of nosocomial Klebsiella pneumoniae infections. Antimicrob. Agents Chemother. 15:616-624.

Shapiro, M., T. R. Townsend, B. Rosner, and E. H. Kass. 1979. Use of antimicrobial drugs in general hospitals. II. Analysis of patterns of use. J. Infect. Dis. 139:698-706.

Shooter, R. A., S. A. Rousseau, E. M. Cooke, and A. L. Breaden. 1970. Animal sources of common serotypes of Escherichia coli in the food of hospital patients. Lancet 2:226-228.

Silver, R. P., and H. D. Mercer. 1978. Antibiotics in animal feeds: An assessment of the animal and public health aspects. Pp. 649-664 in J. N. Hathcock and J. Coon, eds. Nutrition and Drug Interrelations. Academic Press, New York, San Francisco, London.

Sykes, R. B., and M. Matthew. 1976. The β-lactamases of Gram-negative bacteria and their role in resistance to β-lactam antibiotics. J. Antimicrob. Chemother. 2:115-157.

Threlfall, E. J., L. R. Ward, and B. Rowe. 1978. Spread of multiresistant strains of Salmonella typhimurium phage types 204 and 193 in Britain. Br. Med. J. 2:997.

Tipper, D. J., and J. L. Strominger. 1965. Mechanism of action of penicilllins: A proposal based on their structural similarity to acyld-alanyl-d-alanine. Proc. Nat. Acad. Sci. (USA) 54:1133-1141.

van Treeck, U., B. Wiedemann, and W. Kalthofen. 1979. Characterization of a frequently occurring plasmid/rPB1/ in clinical isolates of E. coli. In Collected Abstracts from the IV Symposium on Antibiotic Resistance, Smolenice, Czechoslovakia.

Wiedemann, B., and H. Knothe. 1971. Epidemiological investigations of R factor-bearing enterobacteria in man and animal in Germany. Ann. N.Y. Acad. Sci. 182:380-382.

Witchitz, J. L., and Y. A. Chabbert. 1972. Résistance transférable a la gentamicine. II. Transmission et liaisons du caractère de résistance. Ann. de L'Institut Pasteur 122:24, 368-378.

APPENDIX J
IMMUNOLOGICAL CONSEQUENCES OF ANTIMICROBIALS IN ANIMAL FEEDS

N. Franklin Adkinson, Jr.[1]

This paper addresses the issue of whether antibiotic residues consumed in edible animal tissues sensitize and/or elicit allergic reactions in humans. Although many antibiotics are potentially sensitizing in susceptible individuals, the focus of this paper is upon the penicillins and tetracyclines. Of these, the penicillins have far greater allergenic potential.

The allergenicity of penicillins has been studied extensively (Levine, 1966; Stewart, 1973). Because the penicillin group of drugs is considered the prototype for allergic reactions to drugs (Parker, 1975), much of the following commentary is derived from knowledge of hypersensitivity to penicillin. The principles involved, however, should apply to less allergenic antibiotics including the tetracyclines and aminoglycosides.

There are three basic questions concerning this issue:

1. Is there a potential for allergic reactions in humans either directly or indirectly attributable to antibiotics in foodstuffs?

2. Are there documented cases of such allergic reactions to antibiotic residues, and, if so, what is the magnitude of the problem?

3. What studies could be conducted to document further the extent of the problem, both actual and potential?

PREVALENCE OF ALLERGIC SENSITIVITY TO PENICILLINS AND TETRACYCLINES

Penicillins display remarkably little toxicity even in high doses. Most adverse reactions are attributed to "allergy." Allergic reactions to penicillin range from anaphylactic shock, which can be life-threatening and even fatal, to mild evanescent skin rashes of little clinical consequence. These allergic reactions have differing immunological mechanisms (Table 1). When

[1]Division of Clinical Immunology, Department of Medicine, Johns Hopkins University School of Medicine at the Good Samaritan Hospital, Baltimore, Md.

TABLE 1

Immunopathological Reactions to Penicillin

Gell and Coombs Type	Description	Examples of Adverse Penicillin Reaction
I	Anaphylactic (IgE-mediated injury)	Acute anaphylaxis Urticaria
II	C'-dependent cytolysis	Hemolytic anemias Thrombocytopenia Interstitial nephritis
III	Immune complex damage	Serum sickness Drug fever Cutaneous eruptions[a]
IV	"Delayed" or cellular hypersensitivity	Contact dermatitis

[a]Immunopathogenesis of cutaneous eruptions is not clear.

penicillins are given in therapeutic doses, the incidence of severe life-threatening reactions is small, probably less than 1 in 50,000 courses of treatment (Idsøe et al., 1968). However, because of the huge quantities of penicillin drugs administered yearly in the United States, there are an estimated 300 to 500 deaths from anaphylactic reactions to therapeutic penicillin each year (Feinberg, 1961). On the other hand, mild reactions to penicillin, principally skin eruptions resembling those of measles, are common, and, at least for one semisynthetic penicillin (ampicillin), may afflict 10% to 12% of treated patients (Almeyda and Levantine, 1972).

Between 1% and 10% of the general population will relate a history of some adverse experience associated with penicillin therapy. The lower prevalence figure (1%) is probably more applicable to children and young healthy adults, while the higher prevalence figure (10%) reflects the frequency with which medical charts are likely to be marked "allergic to penicillin" among older patients hospitalized for serious medical problems. More recent studies of the most serious forms of allergy to peniicillin (type I in Table 1: IgE-mediated, or reagenic, allergy) have shown that some patients spontaneously lose allergic sensitivity with time (Adkinson et al., 1971; Green et al., 1977; Levine and Zolov, 1969). This spontaneous loss of allergic sensitivity is likely to occur for other less serious types of allergic reactions as well, judging from the fact that it is often possible to treat previously allergic individuals safely (Bierman et al., 1972; Levine, 1972).

Tetracyclines are infrequently implicated in allergic reactions. Allergic reactions of the type I variety (anaphylactic shock and urticaria) have occasionally been documented in the literature (Schindel, 1965) but are extraordinarily rare. Tetracycline-induced skin rashes, including phototoxic dermatitis, are the most common adverse reactions that are generally considered "allergic," although there is no clear evidence of an immunological basis for these reactions (Dewdney, 1977).

CONDITIONS FOR SENSITIZATION

Some of the factors that influence the development of allergic hypersensitivity to penicillin are: chemical structure and reactivity of the drug; cross-reactivity with other sensitizers; dosage, duration of therapy, number of courses of therapy; mode of administration of the drug; use of additives and solvents; and patient factors, including history of drug sensitivity, atopy,[1] age, genetic factors controlling drug metabolism or immune response, and underlying disease affecting metabolism of excretion of the drug.

Three factors deserve mention in the present context: protein reactivity, individual susceptibility, and dose requirements.

Protein Reactivity

Drugs, like all small molecular weight chemicals, cannot stimulate an immune response in animals or humans unless they possess the capacity to "haptenize," i.e., interact irreversibly with larger molecules, usually proteins, thereby forming an immunogenic multivalent drug-protein complex. The immunochemistry of such interactions between penicillin and native proteins has been studied in detail (Stewart, 1967). The principal pathways involved are schematized in Figure 1.

The major antigenic determinant for penicillin is the penicilloyl moiety of the complex, formed by covalent linkage of the beta lactam ring of penicillin to epsilon amino groups of lysine residues in native proteins. This antigenic complex is formed naturally and spontaneously under physiological conditions without known participation of enzymes or catalysts. This penicilloyl-protein complex stimulates the host immune system to produce antibodies and immunoreactive cells that are capable of inflicting immunopathological damage. It is now well established that preformed penicilloyl-protein complexes are much more efficient than the unconjugated penicillin molecule at both stimulating an immune response and eliciting an allergic reaction in a previously sensitized individual (Siegel, 1959; Stewart, 1967). Immunologically, the antibiotic "residue" of prime importance is the penicilloyl-protein complex rather than the free penicillin molecules. As is discussed further below, no analyses of penicilloyl residues in foodstuffs obtained from penicillin-treated animals have ever been undertaken.

---

[1]The relationship of the atopic status to various types of reactions to penicillin is uncertain except for fatal anaphylactic reactions, which occur more frequently among atopic persons.

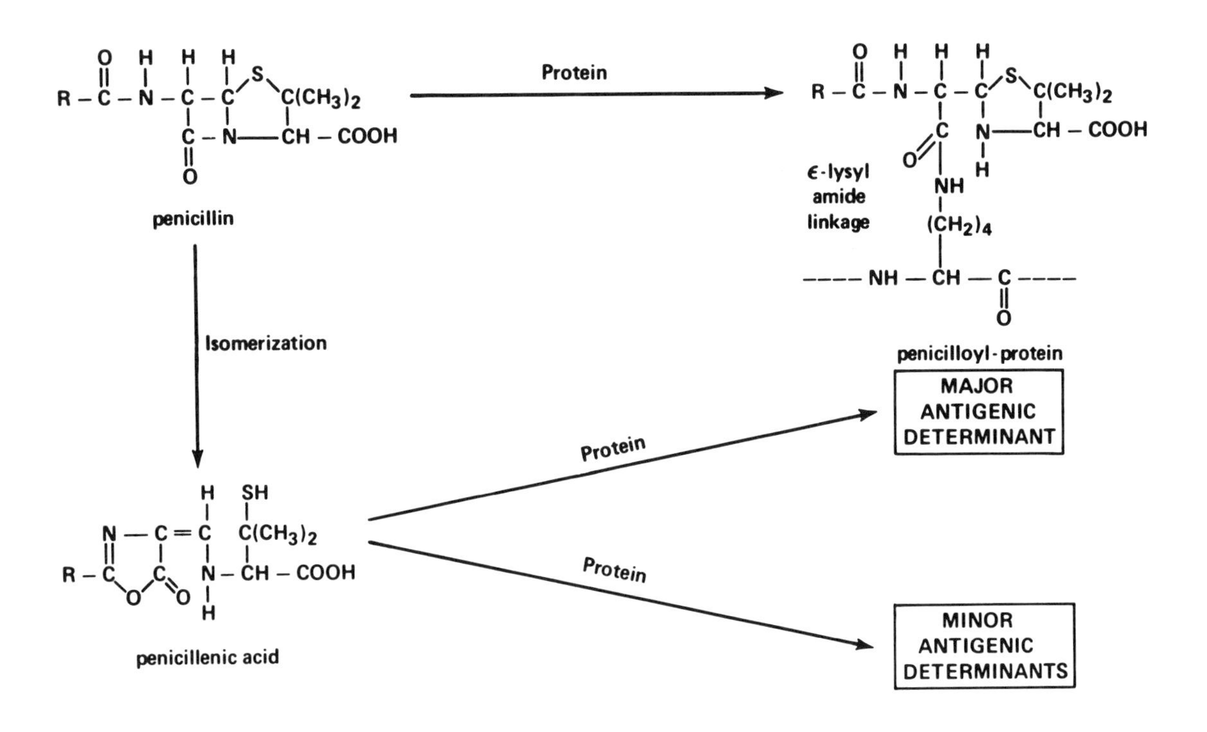

FIGURE 1. Major pathways of penicillin-protein interactions.

There have been no detailed immunochemical studies of interactions of tetracycline with host proteins (Dewdney, 1977). The protein reactivity of tetracyclines is generally considered to be quite small. This fact alone is thought to account for the rarity of hypersensitivity reactions to this class of antibiotics.

Individual Susceptibility

Recent studies by my laboratory have indicated that not all individuals possess the capacity to respond immunologically to therapeutically administered penicillin, even if treated with prolonged high dose therapy (Adkinson, 1977). This suggests that there may be genetic and/or metabolic restrictions on the ability to develop hypersensitivity reactions to penicillin. The proportion of the general population that may be susceptible to the development of allergy to penicillin remains to be determined.

Dosage Requirements for Sensitization

From immunological studies of laboratory animals and humans, it is clear that the dose of any immunogenic substance required for initiating an immune response is appreciably greater than that required to elicit an allergic reaction of the type I variety. The optimal immunizing dose and the minimal dose for eliciting an acute allergic reaction may differ by several orders of magnitude. Furthermore, evidence from studies of both laboratory animals and humans suggests that low-dose immunization favors the production of IgE antibody over IgG antibody in animals that are genetically capable of mounting an IgE antibody response (Marsh, 1975). Thus, there is reason to suspect that there may be a potential for the development of IgE-mediated hypersensitivity by chronic low dose antigenic exposure. However, for ingested antigens (as opposed to inhaled, airborne antigens) this potential risk has not been explored by studies in either laboratory animals or humans. Thus, there are no data to indicate whether penicillin administered to humans chronically at residue-level doses can elicit a penicillin-specific immune response in a susceptible individual. Likewise, data concerning the threshold sensitizing dose for orally administered penicilloyl-protein complexes are not available either for laboratory animals or humans.

CONDITIONS FOR PROVOCATION OF ALLERGY SYMPTOMS

In an individual who has been rendered allergic to penicillin by prior therapeutic administration, what is the risk of provoking allergic symptoms by penicillin residues in ingested foodstuffs? As discussed above, the dose required to elicit an allergic reaction would be expected to be considerably below that required to initiate an immune response. The threshold dose for provoking an allergic reaction depends upon the degree of allergic sensitivity of the individual ingesting the antibiotic residues.

Clinical observations were made by Walzer and Siegel in 1956 (Siegel, 1959). They passively sensitized skin sites on normal subjects with serum drawn from patients with high reagin (IgE) titers to penicillin. All serum donors had previously experienced immediate allergic reactions following treatment with penicillin. Seventy-two hours later the recipient subjects were fed measured amounts of crystalline penicillin G, and the sensitized sites were observed for the appearance of wheal and flare signs, which are indicative of IgE-mediated skin reactions. In those studies, which were positive, the oral threshold dose of penicillin required to produce a positive skin test was 40 to 50 units. Administered intravenously, doses of 12.5 to 25 units were sufficient to produce a positive skin response.

Siegel (1959) and Bierlein (1956) have provided evidence that the oral dose of penicillin required to activate a passively sensitized skin site in a normal recipient is from 100 to 10,000 times larger than that needed to induce a clinical reaction in the allergic patient from whom the reaginic serum was drawn. If one assumes a conservative ratio of 100:1, then the oral administration of as little as 0.4 units of penicillin would be sufficient to elicit allergic reactions in patients with severe IgE-mediated penicillin allergy.

A number of reports document systemic reactions in sensitive individuals who were skin-tested with less than 1 unit of penicillin G, including one patient who developed systemic symptoms following an intradermal test with 3×10^{-7} units of penicillin (Bierlein, 1956). It is therefore clear that very small doses of penicillin, administered orally or through the skin, are capable of eliciting allergic reactions in some exquisitely sensitive patients. It is doubtful that such small doses could elicit clinical symptoms in a majority of penicillin-allergic patients. Whether chronic ingestion of subthreshold doses can eventually result in symptoms is likewise unknown.

EVIDENCE OF ALLERGIC REACTIONS TO ANTIBIOTIC RESIDUES

Milk

The literature yields only a few documented cases of allergic symptoms that are clearly related to the presence of antibiotic residues in animal foodstuffs. Almost all of these reports deal with penicillin-contaminated milk. In 1959 Siegel carefully reviewed the data on allergic reactions to penicillin in milk. He noted that in a 1956 Food and Drug Administration (FDA) nationwide survey of penicillin contamination of milk, 5.9% of the samples were found to be contaminated with penicillin. The degree of contamination ranged from 0.003 to 0.55 units/ml of milk, averaging 0.032 units/ml (D. C. Grove, personal communication; Welch, 1957). Zimmerman (1957-1958) reported that urticaria following ingestion of milk was a common occurrence among 52 penicillin-sensitive patients. Unfortunately, these patients were not studied immunologically, nor were the implicated milk samples analyzed for penicillin content.

The best studied case of allergic reaction from penicillin in milk was reported by Borrie and Barrett (1961) in Great Britain. A 25-year-old woman suffered a moderately severe subacute eczematous eruption, which was traceable to penicillin-contaminated milk. Analysis revealed that some milk samples that did not contain penicillin were still capable of provoking allergic symptoms. The patient's symptoms were relieved, however, by addition of penicillinase to the milk she consumed at home. Attempts at desensitization by the oral route were undertaken starting at 1 unit of penicillin per day. Desensitization had to be abandoned because of recurrent symptoms of allergy. For this patient, who possessed an intense IgE-mediated allergy to penicillin, less than 1 unit (<0.6 g) of penicillin per day was sufficient to provoke allergic symptoms. The elimination of her symptoms by the addition of penicillinase to her milk may be taken as evidence that preformed penicilloyl-milk protein complexes were not a major contributor to the elicitation of her allergic reactions.

Stricter governmental enforcement of FDA regulations concerning penicillin-contaminated milk has reduced considerably the occult intake of penicillin by the general population over the past two decades. By the mid-1960's the prevalence of penicillin-adulterated milk in the United States had dropped to 0.5% (Huber, 1971b). As recently as 1969, Wicher *et al.* reported an acute allergic reaction in a highly penicillin-sensitive patient who had ingested commercially available milk containing penicillin at approximately 10 units/ml.

Current FDA regulations prohibit measurable penicillin residues in milk offered for sale in the United States. Virtually all penicillin contamination of milk products can be traced to the therapeutic use of antibiotics in livestock and not to the use of animal feeds containing subtherapeutic doses of penicillin. Thus, the existence of allergies in humans that are attributable to penicillin-contaminated milk can be considered irrelevant to the substantive issue before the committee, namely, the health hazards of subtherapeutic doses of antibiotics. However, these cases of allergy induced by penicillin-contaminated milk provide useful information regarding minimal threshold doses required for provoking allergic symptoms in highly sensitive patients.

Nonmilk Foodstuffs

A single case report from the Federal Republic of Germany (Tscheuschner, 1972) documents acute angioedema and pruritus in a penicillin-allergic patient who ingested freshly processed meat from a pig that had been given a therapeutic injection of penicillin 3 days prior to slaughter. Analysis of the ground pork revealed a penicillin content of between 0.3 and 0.45 units/g of meat. Since the patient noted symptoms after the first bite of the ground pork, the minimum allergenic dose for this patient was likely to have been less than 10 units of penicillin.

In France, Cany (1977) reported five cases of urticarial reactions apparently induced by ingestion of food contaminated with antibiotics. Unfortunately, the antibiotic residue contained in the foodstuffs was not determined nor was the antibiotic sensitivity of the patients confirmed immunologically. Nevertheless, taken together, these descriptive case summaries raise the possibility that antibiotic-contaminated foodstuffs may be responsible for triggering allergic reactions more frequently than is generally appreciated. Additional study of antibiotic residues in meat products produced in France would be helpful in further evaluations.

The literature contains no other documented cases of allergic reactions attributable to residual antibiotics in animal tissues other than milk.

LEVEL OF ANTIBIOTIC RESIDUES IN NONMILK FOODSTUFFS

Penicillins have a relatively short half-life and are rapidly eliminated from mammalian tissues after discontinuation of therapy.

Tetracyclines are excreted fairly rapidly in urine but may require 4 to 5 days to disappear from soft tissues. Moreover, they have a high affinity for bones and teeth. Messersmith *et al.* (1967) demonstrated that pigs fed up to five times the usual recommended concentration of penicillin in their feed (50 g of penicillin/ton) continuously for 14 weeks had undetectable (<0.025 units penicillin/g) penicillin residues in edible tissues within 0, 5, and 7 days after withdrawal. In the same study, residues in pigs fed up to 500 g of chlortetracycline/ton continuously for 14 weeks were less than 1 ppm in all tissues in all sampling periods.

In 1970 Huber (1971b) studied the prevalence of antibacterial drug residues in more than 5,000 animals at the time of slaughter. Tissues, urine, and/or feces were collected from swine, sheep, cattle, and poultry. Antibiotic residues ranged from a low of 9% in beef cattle to a high of 27% in swine. Tetracycline residues were found more frequently than were penicillin residues. This and similar surveys (Dean *et al.*, 1964) indicate that exposure to antibiotic residues in foodstuffs by the general public has been appreciable.

In view of the elimination studies by Messersmith *et al.* (1967) and others (Huber, 1971a), the widespread antibiotic residues in edible meats as late as 1970 suggest that antibiotics were used frequently in therapeutic doses and/or that required periods for withdrawal from antibiotic-enriched feeds were being widely ignored. More recent surveys have reported that penicillin residues were found infrequently in edible meats except when the animals had received injections of penicillins (Food and Drug Administration, 1978). No tetracycline residues were detected among thousands of meat samples analyzed in 1976 (Food and Drug Administration, 1978).

In the United States the impact of these tissue residues on human allergy may be mitigated somewhat by the fact that most edible meats are cooked prior to consumption. Chlortetracycline is changed by cooking into isochlortetracycline, a compound without known biological activity (Shirk *et al.*, 1956-1957). Similarly, the antibacterial activity of penicillin (and presumably its allergenic potential) is significantly reduced by heating (Shahani *et al.*, 1956).

RISK ASSESSMENT

In view of the paucity of clinical, experimental, and epidemiological data, precise estimates of the risk of acquiring or manifesting allergic disease as a result of antibiotic residues in human foodstuffs are impossible to derive. Nevertheless, several observations can be made in an attempt to set the potential human health risks in perspective.

First, it seems highly unlikely that a sizable proportion of those individuals ingesting foodstuffs containing trace quantities of antibiotic residues will become sensitized to a clinically significant degree. This assertion is based on three facts:

- There is no evidence that such primary sensitization occurred, even after ingestion of penicillin-contaminated milk. Of course this does not prove that sensitization does not or cannot occur, but merely that clinically apparent cases are very rare or nonexistent.

- In this age of antibiotics, exposure to penicillin (and other antibiotics) in therapeutic doses is very common, and the prevalence of prior therapeutic exposure to antibiotics among the adult population is appreciable. Thus, an individual is at many orders of magnitude greater risk of becoming sensitized to penicillin after treatment with a prescribed course of antibiotic than after ingestion of antibiotic residues in food. This supposition reflects the frequency of antibiotic prescription.

- Moreover, a greater rate of sensitization is to be expected from high (therapeutic) doses of antibiotics than from the low-level exposures from foodstuffs. However, we know virtually nothing about the immunogenicity of chronic low-dose administration of penicillins and tetracyclines in human populations. Clearly, such studies would be useful in defining further the risk potential for antibiotic sensitization by low level exposure.

Of greater potential concern for human health is the potential provocation of an allergic reaction in a previously sensitized individual by ingestion of antibiotic residues. Here again the literature contains only a sparse number of references to allergic reactions that are traceable to antibiotic residues in foods. Almost all of the cases reported have to do with penicillin-contaminated milk, a moot issue from a regulatory point of view, although there is certainly reason to continue monitoring compliance to existing regulations.

The case reports dealing with sensitivity reactions to penicillin-contaminated milk have led us to appreciate that very small quantities of antibiotics are required to elicit clinically significant allergic reactions in very sensitive individuals. Apparently, some exquisitely sensitive individuals can experience adverse reactions to levels of penicillin that are undetectable with standard assay methods. Judging from the rarity of such cases, however, it is not unreasonable to conclude that either most penicillin-allergic patients are not adversely affected by penicillin residues in contaminated milk and/or milk supplies are not frequently contaminated with penicillin residues. The second conclusion is demonstratably true. The first conclusion is also likely to be correct since there has been little evidence that widespread contamination has resulted in a flurry of allergic problems, even during the early 1950's when the prevalence of contamination of milk by penicillin was 7% to 15% in the United States.

Using the conservative estimate that the incidence of penicilloyl IgE antibody in the general population is 1 in 50,000 and the assumption that 1% of penicillin-sensitive patients may have ingested penicillin-contaminated milk over 1 year in the early 1950's, one could expect an appreciable number of milk-induced allergic reactions if the contaminated milk supplies were capable of eliciting allergic reactions in an appreciable number of sensitive individuals.

This analytical approach leads one to the tentative conclusion that antibiotic-contaminated foodstuffs can provoke allergic reactions in highly sensitive individuals, but these reactions appear to occur only rarely.

Thus, the admittedly sparse data indicate that there appears to be no reason to implicate antibiotic residues in animal foods as a significant source of allergic disease, either potential or actual, for the public at large.

CONCLUSIONS AND RECOMMENDATIONS

Based upon the above analysis, the following conclusions appear warranted.

(1) There is little reason to believe that foodstuffs obtained from animals fattened with antibiotic-supplemented feeds impose a significant risk to human health by contributing to antibiotic-induced allergic reactions.

(2) Data are currently lacking with regard to the clinical consequences of oral administration of antibiotic residues to patients with various degrees of provable allergic sensitivity and the capacity of antibiotic residues to engender a specific immune response in a genetically susceptible individual who ingests them chronically in low doses.

The following investigations could be undertaken to provide more definitive information on this question:

- A study of the content of penicilloyl-protein complex in edible tissues from animals who have been fed subtherapeutic amounts of penicillin in their feed. Since the penicilloyl-protein complex may have a much longer half-life than does the free penicillin molecule and since penicilloyl protein conjugates are much more immunogenic than free penicillin, such a study would provide needed information on the presence or absence of a potentially important immunogenic residue, which until now has been ignored.

- Epidemiological studies of the incidence of penicillin antibodies among populations frequently ingesting foods with penicillin residues versus similar populations not regularly consuming such antibiotic residues. Careful attention would have to be given to matching the exposure to therapeutically administered penicillin in both groups. Ideally, this study might be best conducted among individuals who can provide documentation that they have never received penicillin therapeutically.

REFERENCES

Adkinson, N. F., Jr. 1977. Quantitative studies of the IgE and IgG immune response to penicillin administration in man. Ann. Allergy 39:73 (Abstract).

Adkinson, N. F., Jr., W. L. Thompson, W. C. Maddrey, and L. M. Lichtenstein. 1971. Routine use of penicillin skin testing on an inpatient service. N. Engl. J. Med. 285:22-24.

Almeyda, J., and A. Levantine. 1972. Drug reactions XIX. Adverse cutaneous reactions to the penicillins--ampicillin rashes. Br. J. Dermatol. 87:293-297.

Bierlein, K. J. 1956. Repeated anaphylactic reactions in a patient highly sensitized to penicillin. A case report. Ann. Allergy 14:35-40.

Bierman, C. W., W. E. Pierson, S. J. Zeitz, L. S. Hoffman, and P. P. VanArsdel, Jr. 1972. Reactions associated with ampicillin therapy. J. Am. Med. Assoc. 220:1098-1100.

Borrie, P., and J. Barrett. 1961. Dermatitis caused by penicillin in bulked milk supplies. Br. Med. J. 2:1267.

Cany, J. 1977. [In French; English summary.] Une source clandestine de réactions allergiques par sensibilisation a la pénicilline: La pollution des aliments. Rev. Fr. Allergol. 17:133-136.

Dean, D., J. K. Bennett, and E. L. Breazeale. 1964. Residual antibiotics found in food products. Southwestern Med. 45:352-353.

Dewdney, J. M. 1977. Immunology of the antibiotics. Pp. 74-225 in M. Sela, ed. The Antigens. Volume IV. Academic Press, New York, San Francisco, and London.

Feinberg, S. M. 1961. Allergy from therapeutic products. Incidence, importance, recognition, and prevention. J. Am. Med. Assoc. 178:815-818.

Food and Drug Administration. 1978. Pp. A5, A33 in Draft Environmental Impact Statement--Subtherapeutic Antibacterial Agents in Animal Feeds. Bureau of Veterinary Medicine, Food and Drug Administration, Department of Health, Education, and Welfare, Rockville, Md.

Green, G. R., A. H. Rosenblum, and L. C. Sweet. 1977. Evaluation of penicillin hypersensitivity: Value of clinical history and skin testing with penicilloyl-polylysine and penicillin G. A cooperative prospective study of the penicillin study group of the American Academy of Allergy. J. Allergy Clin. Immunol. 60:339-345.

Huber, W. G. 1971a. The impact of antibiotic drugs and their residues. Adv. Vet. Sci. Comp. Med. 15:101-132.

Huber, W. G. 1971b. The public health hazards associated with the nonmedical and animal health usage of antimicrobial drugs. Pure Appl. Chem. 21:377-388.

Idsøe, O., T. Guthe, R. R. Willcox, and A. L. De Weck. 1968. Nature and extent of penicillin side-reactions, with particular reference to fatalities from anaphylactic shock. Bull. W. H. O. 38: 159-188.

Levine, B. B. 1966. Immunochemical mechanisms of drug allergy. Annu. Rev. Med. 17:23-38.

Levine, B. B. 1972. Skin rashes with penicillin therapy: Current management. N. Engl. J. Med. 286:42-43.

Levine, B. B., and D. M. Zolov. 1969. Prediction of penicillin allergy by immunological tests. J. Allergy 43:231-244.

Marsh, D. G. 1975. Allergens and the genetics of allergy. Pp. 271-361 in M. Sela, ed. The Antigens. Volume III. Academic Press, New York, San Francisco, and London.

Messersmith, R. E., B. Sass, H. Berger, and G. O. Gale. 1967. Safety and tissue residue evaluations in swine fed rations containing chlortetracycline, sulfamethazine, and penicillin. J. Am. Vet. Med. Assoc. 151:719-724.

Parker, C. W. 1975. Drug therapy. Drug allergy (first of three parts). N. Engl. J. Med. 292:511-514.

Schindel, L. E. 1965. Clinical side-effects of the tetracyclines. Antibiot. Chemother. 13:300-316.

Shahani, K. M., I. A. Gould, H. H. Weiser, and W. L. Slatter. 1956. Stability of small concentrations of penicillin in milk as affected by heat treatment and storage. J. Dairy Sci. 39:971-977.

Shirk, R. J., A. R. Whitehall, and L. R. Hines. 1956-1957. A degradation product in cooked chlortetracycline-treated poultry. Antibiot. Annu. 843-848.

Siegel, B. B. 1959. Hidden contacts with penicillin. Bull. W. H. O. 21:703-713.

Stewart, G. T. 1967. Allergenic residues in penicillins. Lancet 1: 1177-1183.

Stewart, G. T. 1973. Allergy to penicillin and related antibiotics: Antigenic and immunochemical mechanism. Annu. Rev. Pharmacol. 13:309-324.

Tscheuschner, I. 1972. [English translation from German.] Anaphylactic reaction to penicillin after ingestion of pork. Z. Haut Geschlechtskr. 47:591-592.

Welch, H. 1957. Problems of antibiotics in food as the Food and Drug Administration sees them. Am. J. Public Health 47:701-705.

Wicher, K., R. E. Reisman, and C. E. Arbesman. 1969. Allergic reaction to penicillin present in milk. J. Am. Med. Assoc. 208: 143-145.

Zimmerman, M. C. 1957-1958. Penicillinase treatment of fifty-two patients with allergic reactions to penicillin. Antibiot. Annu. 312-326.

APPENDIX K

ANTIBIOTICS IN ANIMAL FEEDS

Committee on Animal Health and the
Committee on Animal Nutrition

Board on Agriculture and Renewable Resources
National Research Council

CONTENTS

EXECUTIVE SUMMARY

The food-producing animal and poultry industries have undergone a dramatic change that began around 1950. What was an extensive industry became extremely intensive: units increased in animal concentration, both physically and numerically. Utilization of the beneficial responses of feed-additive antibiotics in improved growth and feed efficiency developed concurrently with the intensification of the animal industry. It has been proposed that feed-additive antibiotic usage was an integral part of this revolution in animal-production technology. It is estimated, at present, that 40 percent of the antibiotics produced are used for feed additives. Estimates allocate 0.5 million kg to the cattle industry, 1.0 million kg to poultry, 1.4 million kg to swine, and 0.4 million kg to other animals such as companion animals.

The animal producer can obtain antibiotics in the form of balanced supplements and premixes that are processed and sold by the feed-manufacturing industry. The producer also has access to and can purchase antibiotic products from farm and veterinary supply centers. Administration of antibiotics in the drinking water is becoming increasingly important in both poultry and swine production.

Feedlot systems for beef cattle and sheep would not change if low-level antibiotic feedings were not permitted, but it is likely that disease problems and therapeutic use of antibiotics would increase.

The discontinuance of low-level (5 to 10 g/ton) usage of penicillin and tetracyclines would have little effect on the poultry industry. However, the elimination of higher levels (100 to 200 g/ton) would make it very difficult to control bacterial disease in young chickens and turkeys. If all tetracyclines and penicillin were banned as feed additives for poultry, the effective alternative antibiotics and sulfa drugs would likely maintain present production and efficiency standards. However, the problem of selective pressure for some multiple antibiotic resistance mediated by plasmids may still persist with alternative antimicrobials.

If only tetracyclines and penicillin were banned as feed-additive antibiotics for swine, there would be little if any effect on swine productivity or efficiency. There are other promising antibacterial agents that could serve the industry well.

If subtherapeutic use of feed additive antibiotics is banned, future changes in disease control will include preventing exposure to infectious agents, treatment of disease after an outbreak has occurred, and control of infectious disease by immunological means. Preventing exposure to infectious agents will be extremely difficult and will result in a slowing down of animal production. Post-outbreak treatment has had variable effectiveness, but would certainly be less effective than the present use of subtherapeutic levels of antibiotics. The control of infectious disease by immunological means would be an ideal way to safeguard against subclinical infection. However, thus far there has been limited success in protecting animals against bacterial pathogens that affect the intestinal and respiratory tracts.

Antibiotics have been effective in improving the rate and efficiency of gain in swine, cattle, and poultry. The responses in poultry and swine are generally greater in younger animals than in those reaching the end of the growing-finishing period. There is some evidence that the improved farrowing rate of swine is associated with the use of antibiotics. Responses in cattle have not been as great as those in swine and poultry. Improvement in rate of gain and feed efficiency in cattle has averaged about 5 percent. Evidence indicates that the effectiveness of antibiotics has not decreased over time.

Antibiotics in feed have also been used in animal production in Europe since 1953. The British have monitored microbial resistance to antibiotics and have conducted some basic and applied research concerning this aspect. Although the use of antibiotics in the United Kingdom has been restricted as a result of the *Report of the Joint Committee on the Use of Antibiotics in Animal Husbandary and Veterinary Medicine* (referred to in this report as the Swann Report; Swann et al. 1969), the total tonnage used in animal production in 1975 was at an all-time high. Although the amount used in animals was only about 15 percent of the total usage, the ratio of the human population to the livestock population receiving antibiotics is substantially higher than in the United States.

Ingestion of antibiotics results in the development of resistance in bacteria such as in the *E. coli* and *Salmonella* species. The resistance appears to be related to usage patterns. British research has shown that resistance persists longer following long-term use, compared to short-term use. There is strong evidence that development of resistant strains of bacteria in humans is closely related to antibiotics used in humans. No concrete evidence has been reported in the United Kingdom showing that antibiotic resistance has decreased since the Swann Report, or that antibiotic use has decreased.

The wise use of antibiotics is not a substitute for, but a complement to, good sanitation and husbandry practices. Extensive use of low-level antibiotics in feeds has brought about concern for potential harmful effects due to development of resistant strains of organisms in host animals that might compromise animal as well as human health. Drug resistance in bacteria was observed soon after the introduction of antibiotics. Antibiotics have been used extensively in animal feeds for nearly 30 years. Questions and discussions concerned with the potential human health hazards from subtherapeutic antibiotic feeding to animals have been aired for nearly 30 years. Yet, it is difficult to cite human health problems that can be attributed specifically to meat animals fed antibiotics or that can be associated with contact with animals fed low levels of antibiotics. There have been incidents of salmonellosis in humans involving antibiotic-resistant strains of animal origin but there is no evidence of any relation to low-level antibiotic feeding.

Surveys of the use of drugs for therapeutic purposes indicate that antibacterial agents account for almost 50 percent of drugs used by practicing veterinarians. *In vitro* testing has sometimes been questioned in that infections associated with organisms that seem to be resistant *in vitro* are quite responsive to antibacterial therapy *in vivo* in clinical use.

Scattered reports, published and unpublished, attribute failure in drug therapy to low-level antibiotic feeding. Others claim continued effectiveness of drugs previously fed for long periods at subtherapeutic levels. Carefully controlled studies exploring possible relationships between antibiotic feeding and subsequent drug effectiveness are needed.

Critical experimental studies on the effect of low-level antibiotic feeding on animal therapy and human health are definitely needed. It is proposed that studies be conducted in the following areas:

1. Does the Feeding of Tetracycline and Penicillin Compromise Animal Therapy?--This research should be done with swine, poultry, and cattle. In swine and poultry, conditions should be closely controlled. In cattle it would seem essential that research be conducted in commercial-type feedlots.

2. The Relationship of Antibiotic Feeding to Human Health--Although these studies are very complex and time-consuming, it is important that some effort be started in this direction. The incidence of disease-resistant organisms could be determined in humans in industries in which the workers have close contact with animals and animal products and with people who work in industries that have no contact with animals or animal products. Also the incidence of disease and the effectiveness of therapy should be studied. Some information might be obtained by surveys of existing information.

3. Mechanisms of Action of Antibiotics in Growth Promotion--Current evidence strongly suggests that the growth-promoting effect from low-level feeding of antibacterial compounds is not solely related to disease prevention. Knowledge of the mechanisms involved is a vital missing link. If known, the study of other means of eliciting a similar response would become feasible. Thus, such new knowledge would offer the potential for eliminating some or all of the current reasons for using feeding levels of antibacterial drugs.

CHAPTER 1

INTRODUCTION

The use of subtherapeutic levels of penicillin and the tetracyclines in animal feeds has raised the question of the effects of such practices on human health. The Food and Drug Administration (FDA) has proposed a ban on certain antibiotics at subtherapeutic levels in feed because of the potential for compromising the health of humans. A large segment of the regulated industry, including farmers and ranchers, has contended that in nearly 30 years of use, antibiotics at subtherapeutic levels in animals have not compromised human or animal health or influenced the therapy of human disease.

The FDA has contracted with the Assembly of Life Sciences, National Academy of Sciences, for a review and evaluation of human health effects of antibiotics in animal feeds. The Committee to Study Human Health Effects of Subtherapeutic Antibiotic Use in Animal Feeds has been appointed to:

1. study the human health effects of subtherapeutic use of penicillin and tetracyclines (chlortetracycline and oxytetracycline) in animal feeds;

2. review and analyze published and unpublished epidemiological and other data as necessary to assess the human health consequences of the subtherapeutic use of penicillin and tetracyclines in animal feeds; and

3. assess the scientific feasibility of additional epidemiological studies, and, if needed, to make recommendations about the kind of research necessary, its estimated cost and time requirements, and possible mechanisms to be used to conduct such studies.

Under the terms of the contract, subtherapeutic levels are defined as use of the agent at levels of 200 g/ton or less, and/or use of the agent for 2 weeks or longer. Animal feeds include milk replacers, medicated blocks, and liquid feeds.

The Committee has requested the Board on Agriculture and Renewable Resources (BARR) to prepare a critical review/position paper on certain aspects of the problem. The following list of questions to be answered was submitted to the BARR (the Chapter numbers after each question refer to the chapter in this report that discusses the question):

1. How effective are antibiotics--especially penicillin and tetracycline--in animal feeds? (Chapter 3)

2. Would animal husbandry methods change if antibiotics were eliminated, or if penicillin and tetracyclines were removed? (Chapter 2)

3. Does animal disease decrease as a result of use of antibiotics and would there be an increase in therapeutic use of antibiotics if subtherapeutic use was discontinued? (Chapter 2)

4. What do the data from European countries show with respect to animal health and nutrition where antibiotics have been restricted? Has the restriction of subtherapeutic use led to increased therapeutic use, thus cancelling the benefits of restriction? (Chapter 4)

5. Is it likely that there would be a black market? (Chapter 2)

6. How much therapeutic use is there and has it caused resistance problems? What is the evidence that therapeutic use of penicillin and tetracyclines contributes to resistance and possible health effects? (Chapter 6)

7. What epidemiological studies exist that would be valuable for the committee to consider? Are there epidemiological studies that should be carried out? (Chapter 6)

8. What amounts of penicillin and tetracyclines are used subtherapeutically? (Chapter 2)

9. What amounts of penicillin and tetracyclines are used therapeutically? (Chapter 6)

10. How are animal feeds prepared and how are the antibiotics used in animal feeds mixed and used by farmers or feedlot operators? (Chapter 2)

11. How are antibiotics for therapeutic use in animals regulated? Do veterinarians have guidelines or antibiotic audits? (Chapter 6)

12. Has therapeutic efficacy been compromised by the use of subtherapeutic levels of antibiotics in animal feeds? Are resistant infections more prevalent in animals? (Chapters 5, 6)

13. Critically review the documentation for increase in resistance, pathogenicity, and increase in numbers of pathogens after use of subtherapeutic antibiotics. (Chapters 5, 6)

BARR asked its Committees on Animal Nutrition and Animal Health to set up a panel of their members and outside consultants to address these questions. The Panel met on June 11 and July 2 to 3, 1979, and prepared the statement that follows that addresses the 13 questions.

The panel is indebted to Enriqueta C. Bond and Roy Widdus, of the Division of Medical Sciences, for providing published research documents on the subject, and to Philip Ross and Selma P. Baron for their advice and guidance in the preparation of the report.

CHAPTER 2

SUBTHERAPEUTIC USE OF ANTIBIOTICS

ANIMAL MANAGEMENT

Swine

Pig production in the United States is more diverse geographically than broiler, turkey, and feedlot cattle production. About 90 percent of the nation's pork supply is produced in the 12 north central states plus Georgia, Kentucky, North Carolina, and Texas. The number of pigs slaughtered in the United States has varied from about 73 to 95 million head per year and yielded about 25 to 36 kg (carcass basis) annual per capita consumption for the U.S. citizen during the last 15 years.

The swine industry has changed from an enterprise that historically employed pasture to one that predominantly employs confinement buildings and concrete lots. The swine industry differs from the broiler industry, however, since nearly all the production is by private producers rather than by industrial entities. An appreciation of the change to intensive swine production is evident in Table 2.1. There has been a dramatic decrease in the number of farms which produce pigs, both nationwide and in Iowa, the largest producing state. The total production trend has changed little, except year-to-year responses to feed cost and pig selling price relationships.

Evidence of the continuing intensification since the 1974 census in the swine industry is provided by survey information obtained in 1975 and 1978 from large producers in the United States (Stemme et al. 1978, 1979). The number of producers that market 5,000 head or more and those producing from 2,500 to 4,999 head has increased during the 3-year period (Table 2.2). The annual production of this group of producers would account for more than 20 percent of the total U.S. production. Over 70 percent of the producers in this group have confinement housing facilities. Their worst problem in their farrowing facilities was reported to be *E. coli* scours.

A new organizational form in pork production, the subsidiary sow-farrowing firm or sow-farrowing cooperative, has come into existence since 1970. These firms are organized generally by a group of producers as subchapter S corporations or cooperatives.

TABLE 2.1 Number of Farms with Pigs in the United States and Iowa and Total U.S. Production

Year	Number of Farms with Pigs, United States	Number of Farms with Pigs, Iowa	Total U.S. Carcass Weight Produced (million pounds)
1954	1,424,000	136,800	12,002
1964	743,000	108,900	14,598
1974	450,000	66,300	14,331

SOURCE: U.S. Bureau of the Census (1974).

TABLE 2.2 Number of Large-Volume Producers and Size of Operation[a]

Year	Number of Operations Producing 2,500 to 4,999 Head/Year	Average Size of Operation	Number of Operations Producing 5,000 Head or More/Year	Average Size of Operation
1975	1,567	2,418[a]	1,168	7,053
1978	1,661	3,196	1,340	10,192

[a] A producer was included in this category if production was 2,500 head or more in any year included in the survey.

SOURCE: Stemme et al. (1978, 1979).

The purpose of the organization and production unit is to produce feeder pigs (40 lbs) for the members or shareholders who do not want to farrow pigs, but do want to finish them (40 lbs to 220 lbs) on their farms (Hepp 1977, Paulsen and Rahm 1979). In Iowa 63 such firms were identified that began operation since 1974. The breeding herd size of those firms in the second year of production averaged 537 sows with an annual production capability of more than 8,000 feeder pigs each (Paulsen and Rahm 1979).

With intensification the disease problems have also changed. Historically, hog cholera, swine erysipelas, tuberculosis and brucellosis were the disease problems most troublesome. These have largely disappeared due to eradication programs. With concentration and confinement production the enteric diseases and respiratory diseases are the most prevalent problems reported.

As a group, both the large producers and the organized sow-farrowing firms employ an early weaning management system whereby the nursing pigs are weaned at 3 to 4 weeks of age. In 1976 an average investment of $1,176 per sow in the unit was reported (Paulsen and Rahm 1979). Because of the high fixed costs, the management places a high priority on total production. With early weaning the sow can be re-bred within a few days after her pigs are weaned and thereby increase the number of pigs produced per sow per year. Historically nursing pigs were weaned at 8 to 10 weeks of age and the sows were not re-bred until their farrowing date fit expected mild weather and/or the other activities associated with the farm enterprise, such as corn planting or harvesting. In the process of early weaning, natural protection from enteric disease problems in young pigs has been diminished (IgA immune globulins in sow's milk).

It is interesting to note that the introduction and use of feed-additive antibiotics has been concurrent with change in production technology in the swine industry. It is likely that the use of antimicrobial agents has facilitated the development of the concentrated operations.

Poultry

As part of the effort to produce poultry meat and eggs as economically as possible, it is common practice in the United States to maintain broilers, turkeys, and laying hens in large flocks in one location. From 10,000 to 20,000 broilers are typically raised in one house and some operations have as many as a million laying hens in one location. With such a concentration of birds it is essential to have disease control programs that will prevent disastrous losses to the poultry industry. Drugs, including the antibiotics, have played a major role in maintaining the health of poultry flocks since the 1950s.

The management procedures used in today's poultry production have made it possible to provide poultry meat and eggs for consumers very economically. In fact, until very recently the prices of broilers and eggs were similar to those 25 years ago despite a decrease in the value of the dollar through inflation. It is unlikely that future changes in management will result in any reduction in the concentration of poultry. Changes will probably involve upgrading of physical facilities for maintaining the birds, including environmentally controlled housing and the adoption of more automated equipment in the feeding and management of the birds.

Cattle and Sheep

In 1962 feedlots with a capacity of 1,000 head or more accounted for 40 percent of fed cattle marketings, while in 1978 lots of this size marketed 68 percent of the fed cattle (USDA 1979a). Due to the economics of feeding, increases in concentrations can be expected, but at a slower rate. As concentrations of feedlot cattle have increased, there has been increasing need for improved management and management systems.

Penicillin is not used in cattle feeding in the United States. However, the continuous low-level use of other antibiotics in cattle feeding is regional. In the more arid areas of the Southwest, there is no response to antibiotics as growth promotants, and therefore, they are not continuously fed. This lack of response appears to be related to climate. In the remainder of the feeding areas, low-level continuous feeding of antibiotics is routine. An estimated 50 to 60 percent of feedlot cattle are fed low-level antibiotics during the feeding period and a total of 40 percent of the total beef supply has been fed low-level antibiotics (USDA 1979b).

AMOUNT USED AND FEED PREPARATION

Swine

Feed requirement for swine is estimated at about 4.40 kg of feed per kilogram of liveweight sold at market (Van Arsdall

1978). In 1978 about 88 million head were slaughtered in the United States with an estimated average liveweight of 250 lbs. So in total, about 44 billion kg of feed were consumed by swine. The FDA (U.S. DHEW/FDA 1978) from the U.S. International Trade Commission (1974) data estimated the production of feed-additive antibiotics at 3,350,000 kg. About 10,000 feed mills manufacture or mix feeds containing drugs and they supplied about 12 million tons of feed to the swine industry. Several types of products are sold to farmers. Most of the feed-manufacturer tonnage is sold as supplements (protein, minerals, vitamins, and feed additives) to be further mixed or diluted with grain for feeding as a complete balanced diet by the swine producer.

A more concentrated form manufactured is a premix (vitamins, minerals, and feed additives). The premix is further mixed by an intermediate or secondary feed mill or mixed by the producer using grain and generally soybean meal as a protein source. Most pig starter diets used by the producers are purchased from a feed manufacturer as a complete feed. The purchase of complete mixed diets for the other stages of production is not as prevalent. The market structure of the feed industry is presented in Figure 2.1. Antibiotic usage by the feed industry is controlled by periodic inspections and sampling by representatives of the FDA and state feed-control inspectors. Such things as drug inventory control, approved levels of incorporation, product claims, and assay of finished product are monitored.

The consumption of feed-additive antibiotics per market pig is estimated in Table 2.3. It is estimated that in 1978, the 88 million pigs marketed consumed 1,408,000 kg of antibiotics or about 40 percent of the feed-additive antibiotics produced.

Poultry

Very little use is made of penicillin and the tetracyclines for low-level feeding (5 to 10 g/ton) for stimulating growth in poultry production. A major reason for this is that these antibiotics are not approved by the FDA for use in combination with monensin ("Coban," an anticoccidial drug). Monensin is used in about 85 percent of the broiler feed prepared in this country. Only the antibiotics lincomycin, bacitracin, and the bambermycins can be used at low levels in combination with this anticoccidial drug (Anonymous 1979c).

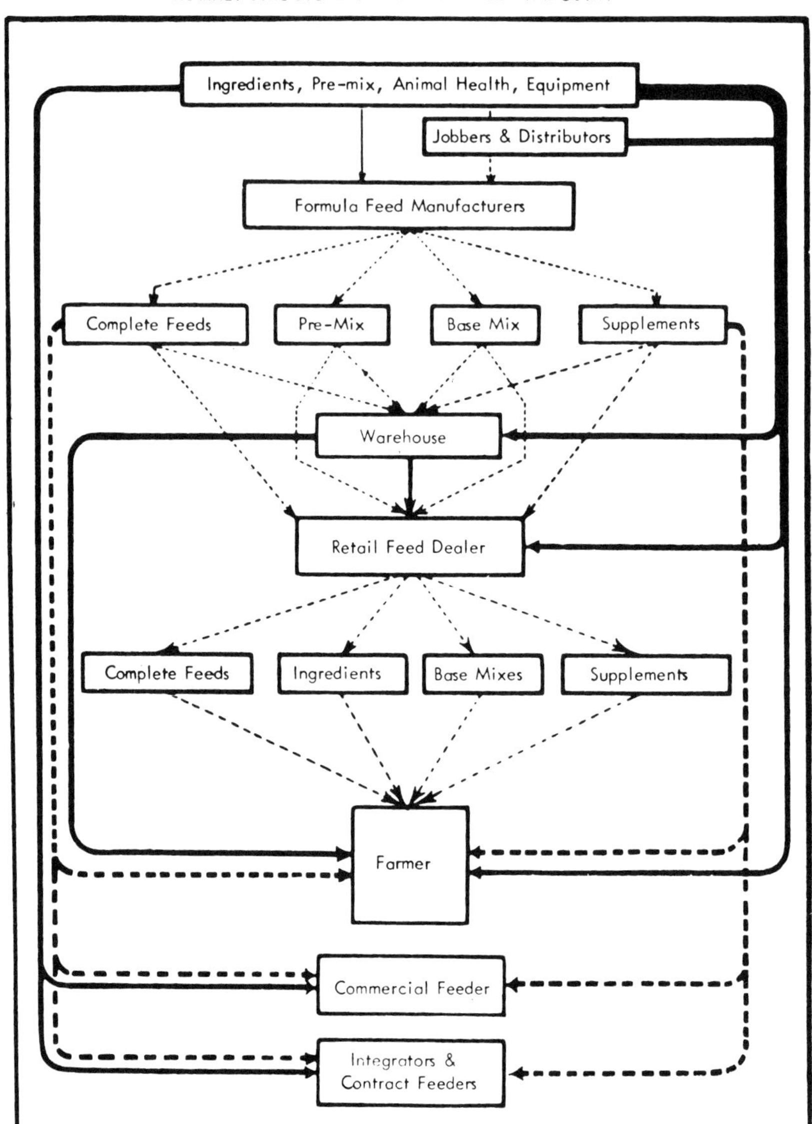

SOURCE: Anonymous (1978).

FIGURE 2.1 Market structure of formula feed industry.

TABLE 2.3 Feed Required to Produce a 250-lb Pig, Recommended Antibiotic Levels, and Consumption of Antibiotics per Pig (estimates)

Stage of Production	Pounds of Feed Required per 250-lb Pig	Recommended Antibiotic Level (mg/lb diet)	Estimated Use (mg/lb diet)	Grams per Pig
Breeding Boar	15	---	Trace	---
Breeding Sow				
Pregnancy	150	---[a]	5.0	0.75
Lactation	60	50[b]	25.0	1.50
Starter	25	100-125	100.0	2.50
Grower	50	50	25.0	1.25
Finisher	800	1-25	12.5	10.00
Total	1,100			16.00

[a] For pregnancy, recommendations would include an antibiotic at a high level (1.0 g/day) during the breeding period, about 20-25 days. Not all sows would be fed an antibiotic.

[b] Since response to antibiotics fed to the lactating sow are not consistent, no general recommendation is made for their inclusion by experiment stations.

SOURCE: V. C. Speer, Iowa State University, personal communication, 1979.

Very little penicillin is used in poultry production either for subtherapeutic or therapeutic purposes. Some penicillin is used in the diluent for Marek's disease vaccine, which is injected into day-old chicks. It is also used as a treatment for erysipelas in turkeys at a level of 100 g/ton plus a level injected to provide approximately 5 mg/kg body weight. Apparently little or no penicillin is used for treatment of diseases in chickens.

The tetracycline drugs are used quite extensively for treatment of diseases and for improving suboptimal performance of birds. Frequently, tetracycline (200 g/ton) or a combination of oxytetracycline (50 to 100 g/ton) and neomycin (35 to 140 g/ton) is used in the starter feeds for both turkeys and broilers. These are used in the first 0.23 kg of feed for each bird. In the case of broilers, the anticoccidial drug is removed since the combinations are not permitted by FDA regulations. The antibiotic drugs during this period of time are used to control several bacterial diseases and to get the birds off to a good start. Considerable amounts of tetracyclines are also used in laying hen diets at various times. From 50 to 100 g/ton are used for a 2-to-3-week period to improve shell quality and egg production in laying hens, particularly during the latter part of the laying cycle.

Most of the feed mixed for poultry production in the United States is made by large integrated companies and in large feed mills where careful control of the inclusion of the drugs and other feed ingredients is maintained on inventories. The feed manufacturers, in using drugs in poultry rations, must follow regulations of the FDA and be inspected periodically by this agency and state feed control officials.

A point that should be emphasized is that poultry producers do not indiscriminately use antibiotics in poultry feeds. Poultry operations only use antibiotics when their cost will be more than covered by the improved performance of the birds.

Ruminants

Based on approved claims, tetracyclines serve four purposes in cattle rations: (1) control of liver abscesses; (2) control of respiratory disease related to shipping fever; (3) control of foot rot; and (4) improved gains and feed efficiency (Anonymous 1979c). Cattle finishing diets contain high levels of grain and the incidence of liver abscesses increases as the level of grain feeding increases. Low-level feeding of the tetracyclines may reduce the incidence of liver abscesses by as much as 50 percent (Foster and Woods 1970, Woods 1970, Davis 1978). Daily gains in steers with liver abscesses may be depressed by 5 to 10 percent. No doubt a portion of the increased gain noted because of low-level feeding of the tetracyclines is due to the reduction of liver abscesses. On the basis of 1970 cattle and feed prices, Foster and Woods (1970) estimated a $9.30 loss for each animal with an abscessed liver. This value considered both feed cost and liver loss due to condemnation.

Subtherapeutic use of tetracyclines in cattle feeding may be divided into two categories (Woods 1970, Anonymous 1979c).

1. Incoming cattle may be fed 250 to 1,000 mg/day for a 7- to 28-day period after receipt for control of shipping fever. The highest feeding level would be equivalent to 200 g antibiotic per ton of feed. For incoming cattle, administration of antibiotics via water may also be used. During the feeding period, levels of 250 to 1,000 mg/day may be fed for short periods during outbreaks of respiratory problems. After recovery from shipping fever, the level is reduced to 70 to 80 mg/day for the remainder of the feeding period in areas where continuous feeding of low-level antibiotics is practiced.

2. For growth promotion and improvement of feed efficiency, the recommended levels of feeding are 70 to 80 mg/day (Anonymous 1979c). This may be included in the total feed or the daily supplement in areas where the ration is fed as grain, roughage, and supplement. The combination of chlortetracycline and sulfamethazine has been shown to be effective for control of the shipping-fever complex in cattle (Woods 1970).

The tetracyclines have been used primarily for disease treatment with lambs, although continuous feeding at 20 to 50 g per ton of feed has been shown to be beneficial for growth and aid in reduction of enterotoxemia. However, effective vaccines are available for enterotoxemia. Improvement of growth of suckling lambs occurs when the tetracyclines are included in the creep ration at 20 to 50 g per ton of feed (Beeson 1978).

The tetracyclines up to levels of 100 g per ton in milk replacer and starters for baby calves are effective in growth promotion and control of bacterial scours (Warner 1972).

EFFECTS OF RESTRICTIONS

Swine

The removal of antibiotics as feed additives, while continuing their therapeutic or prescription usage, would not necessarily reduce the total quantity used.

If antibiotics were eliminated as feed additives, it is questionable whether production in confinement swine operations could be maintained at an intensive level. It is likely that weaning age would be increased. Inventory would be reduced, more labor and time would be required to thoroughly clean and disinfect between groups of pigs, and the breeding herd efficiency would be reduced to conform to calendarized farrowings. In the long run, because of the increased cost of operating confinement units, a reversion to extensive or pasture production could take place. The seasonal nature of extensive production would mean large month to month variability in marketings reminiscent of historical patterns and would be disruptive for today's packing industry.

Poultry

The discontinuance of the use of penicillin in poultry feeds would have little effect, since this antibiotic is not used extensively at the present time. The only major problem would be in the treatment of erysipelas in turkeys since this antibiotic seems to be particularly effective against this disease. The complete removal of the tetracyclines, however, would have a much greater impact on the industry. Restriction of the use of these at low levels (5 to 10 g/ton) for growth stimulation would have little effect since they are not used now to any extent for this purpose. The elimination of the use of higher levels of tetracyclines, however, would create problems in the control of bacterial diseases in young chickens and turkeys and in maintaining optimum performance of laying hens. What undoubtedly would happen with the restriction of use of tetracyclines in feeds is a much greater use of these antibiotics in the water. This would lead to increased cost of medication and probably would result in no general reduction in the use of total quantities of tetracyclines in poultry production.

Ruminants

Unless the tetracyclines are completely restricted for use as a subtherapeutic low-level feeding, the resident veterinarian might prescribe them for low-level feeding to prevent certain disease problems.

Feedlot systems for beef cattle and sheep would not change if low-level feedings were not permitted. Disease problems and carcass condemnations would increase, and therapeutic use of antibiotics would increase.

ECONOMIC EFFECTS OF A BAN ON THE USE OF ANTIBIOTICS

Potential economic effects of a ban on antibiotic feed additives for 1973 livestock output, price, and cost conditions were examined by Gilliam and Martin (1975). They considered two hypothetical ways in which producers might react to such a ban: (1) by feeding additional numbers of beef cattle, veal calves, and hogs to achieve pre-ban output levels; and (2) by feeding the same number of animals on the same schedule, with the result of reduced output.

In situation (1), increased costs of production would be $801.7 million, assuming no change in mortality and no change in the cost of feeder cattle and pigs. If the costs were borne by consumers, annual per capita red meat costs would increase $3.85.

In situation (2), the annual expenditures for red meat would increase $2,134.5 million annually or $10.26 per capita.

If mortality increased in either situation, costs would be estimated to increase $0.36 to $1.25 per capita for each 1-percent increase in death rates.

A U.S. Department of Agriculture study (USDA 1978) considered the effects of a total ban on feed-additive antibiotics for each species of food-producing animals, assuming moderate drug efficiency and high drug efficiency. They considered the impact on total farm income and changes in consumer food costs during the first year of a total ban, and then the adjustments that would occur in 5 years. Their conclusions are summarized in Table 2.4. It is interesting to note that total farm income is projected to rise the first year. This is because of the inelastic relationships between price and supply for meat products.

TABLE 2.4 Summary of Changes in Net Farm Income and USDA Food Market Basket from Banning All Subtherapeutic Use of Animal Drugs, First and Fifth Year after Ban

	First Year	Fifth Year
Farm Income		5
Moderate Drug Efficacy		
Change in billion dollar	+ 1.2	- 0.5
Change in percent	+ 4.7	- 2.1
High Drug Efficacy		
Change in billion dollars	+ 2.8	- 0.9
Change in percent	+10.8	- 3.81
Food Market Basket:[a]		
Base (dollars)	2,132	2,530
Moderate Drug Efficacy		
Change in dollars	+32.0	+ 5.0
Percent change from base	+ 1.5	+ 0.2
High Drug Efficacy		
Change in dollars	+99.0	+16.0
Percent change from base	+ 4.6	+ 0.7

[a]The market basket is the average quantities of domestic farm-origin foods purchased annually in retail food stores per urban household.

SOURCE: USDA (1978).

Headley (1978) reported the results of an econometric analysis on the meat-animal industry as a result of banning different drug combinations. The consumer and national costs are presented in Table 2.5. The estimates of the economic impact to the industry and consumers appear to be realistic.

FUTURE CHANGES IN ANTIBIOTIC USE

As research in the control of diseases and the maintenance of optimum health continues, the use of antibiotics in the future will undoubtedly change. Producers will use the most economical means of preventing diseases to attain the lowest cost of production per unit of meat or eggs. If new vaccines, alternative drugs, and total eradication programs become more effective and/or more economical than the use of tetracyclines, these methods will replace the use of tetracyclines.

The concentrated raising of cattle, swine, and poultry has brought about new problems in control of infectious disease. Conditions have changed: the number of farms raising livestock has decreased 80 percent since 1940, and yet the number of animal units has doubled. The control of infectious disease has been responsible for the success of these concentrated enterprises. Such control is particularly important for young susceptible animals during the rapid growth phase. The main methods of controlling infectious disease are:

1. Preventing Exposure to Infectious Agents--Attempts to raise swine under specific pathogen-free conditions in strict isolation have been tried, but found to be expensive and impractical. Cattle can be raised successfully and disease controlled through range-type rearing. However, this system would result in reducing total beef production by approximately 50 percent as feedlot production would be lost. Isolation of dairy animals has been partially successful where calves are fed ample levels of colostrum and herds are confined. Some success has been achieved at raising poultry in isolation, but this is not a practical procedure by itself.

2. Subtherapeutic Use of Antibiotics--This approach has made possible the disease control and production gains known today. However, it has created an antibiotic-resistant bacteria problem that may affect the use of these drugs in both man and animals.

TABLE 2.5 Effects of Banning Selected Antibiotic and Drug Feed Additives on Annual Consumer Expenditures for Meat

Option	Estimated Annual Consumer Costs	
	Per Capita ($)	Nationally (billion $)
Ban tetracyclines and penicillin[a]	5.70	1.2
Ban nitrofurans and sulfa	12.00	2.6
Ban all of above	19.00	4.1

[a]It is assumed that substitute antibiotics will be available, mainly tylosin and bacitracin.

SOURCE: Headley (1978).

3. Treatment of Disease After Outbreak has Occurred--This technique is difficult and impractical especially in young stock because losses occur rapidly and morbidity and mortality during the growing period have major unrecoverable effects on production.

4. Control of Infectious Disease by Immunological Means--The main concerns in controlling infectious diseases in cattle, swine, and poultry are immunizing young animals and protecting the portals of entry, such as the respiratory and intestinal tracts. Under the present conditions of concentrated production, the natural protection afforded by maternal antibodies should be utilized by allowing the young to suckle for as long as possible.

There has been little success thus far in protecting animals against bacterial respiratory and intestinal pathogens. Certainly strides are being made in developing immunogens for certain coliform organisms, but solid long-term protection against pathogens of the respiratory and intestinal tracts may be difficult to produce. The immunological approach to disease control will not replace the use of antibiotics in the near future.

ALTERNATIVES

Resistance characteristics similar to those from tetracyclines and penicillin evolve when most other approved feed-additive antibiotics for swine are fed (Fagerberg and Quarles 1979). Certain sulfa drugs may be eliminated as feed additives because of residue problems, and carbadox and furazolidone are possible carcinogens. Bacitracin and Flavomycin (bambermycins) are not viable alternative feed additives, since they lack efficacy for the young pig (Hays 1978). Virginiamycin is the only approved feed-additive antibiotic that would then remain that would be efficacious for the young pig and growing-finishing pigs. Similar microbial defense mechanisms are likely to emerge against virginiamycin or against new antibiotics developed specifically for animal use.

In some situations, antibiotics other than the tetracyclines or penicillin could be used for the treatment of diseases in poultry. With few exceptions penicillin could be replaced by other antibiotics presently available. Elimination of tetracyclines would create more of a problem because these appear to be the most economical and effective for certain purposes in poultry production.

A detailed description of the approved subtherapeutic use and levels of the tetracyclines for cattle is given in the Feed Additive Compendium (Anonymous 1979c). At the present time, besides the tetracyclines, only three antibiotics (tylosin, bacitracin, and erythromycin) are available for subtherapeutic use in feedlot cattle. The only approved claim for tylosin is as an aid in reducing liver abscesses. Tylosin costs three times as much as the tetracyclines. While there is an approved claim for erythromycin for growth promotion and feed efficiency, it has not been used in the field. Very little field information has been developed for the use of bacitracin in cattle feeds. There is no approved substitute for chlortetracycline-sulfamethazine combination used for control of the shipping-fever complex.

If feed-additive drugs were available therapeutically via prescription, there probably would be little or no reduction in usage in swine, poultry, and ruminants.

If feed additives were not available through approved channels, violations by segments of the industry would be likely. Examples would include the use of chloramphenicol, dimetridazole, and high levels of copper sulfate.

Alternatives to feed-additive drug usage, discussed in more detail below, might include the following: (a) environmental and management changes, (b) selection for genetic resistance, (c) development of vaccines, (d) adoption of minimal disease programs, and (e) development of new feed additives that do not promote bacterial resistance relevant to human and animal health.

Environmental and Management Changes

Reducing the production intensity of facilities would reduce the enteric problems commonly encountered in farrowing and baby pig facilities, and would reduce respiratory problems in cattle feedlots. A time lapse between groups would allow adequate time for more thorough cleaning and sanitation of the facilities. As new facilities are constructed for swine, knowledgeable producers are building modified isolation rooms with reduced capacity to allow the opportunity for better sanitation between farrowings. In the case of broilers the use of cages would also allow for improved sanitation. A recent innovation has been the use of small wire-penned enclosures for young pigs which reduces the chance of contamination from one pig to another.

Progressive swine producers are becoming more appreciative of herd isolation to reduce disease problems. Many of the more intense units are applying artificial insemination as a means of introducing new blood lines into the herds. By raising their own boars and gilts for breeding herd replacements, producers avoid the risk of introducing new animals, possibly bearing new diseases, into the herds.

Selection for Genetic Resistance in Natural Immunity

Although information on this topic is limited, there are indications that older animals are more resistant to respiratory problems than younger ones. Usually, older, lactating sows confer an immunity to their offspring not present in pigs from young sows. Also some strains or breeds of animals may be more susceptible to respiratory and enteric problems.

Development of Vaccines

The need for disease control by antibiotics could be reduced by vaccinating animals for certain disease conditions, commonly the most troublesome in production. A bacterin was recently developed to control atrophic rhinitis in swine, and was successfully demonstrated in the field. Research is in progress on similar approaches for control of mycoplasma and *E. coli* organisms and the agent for porcine pleuropneumonia.

Adaptation of Minimal Disease Programs

Swine herds free of respiratory problems can be maintained in that condition for some reasonable period of time. This state can be attained by hysterectomizing pregnant sows and raising the young pigs in isolation in the first generation. Subsequent generations are obtained naturally. The largest problem has been the accidental reintroduction of respiratory diseases. For this approach to be successful over long periods of time, complete isolation from man, pets, birds, and rodents is essential, which would be impractical.

Development of New Antibiotics

There are new experimental antibiotics effective for swine that are not being used in human medicine. Whether they have all the desirable attributes by present-day standards is not known. The goal of research should be the development of such compounds that avoid the characteristics that are thought to pose health hazards of men and animals as recognized by today's standards.

CHAPTER 3

EFFICACY OF ANTIBIOTICS IN ANIMAL FEEDS

SWINE

Several compilations of the average weight gain and feed efficiency improvements from feed-additive antibiotic additions to swine diets have been reported since the discovery of antibiotic growth stimulation (see Table 3.1). These reports represent mainly research or experiment-station trials, and it has been suggested that the improved performance observed in research facilities because of better sanitation and disease control is a conservative estimate of the response of animals fed in commercial production facilities. The percentage of responses in the young animal are great, but decrease as the animal nears market weight (Hays 1978). This is explained by the performance of the control animals and their increasing daily gain as they mature.

Hays (1978) compared present-day efficacy of antibiotics to their past effectiveness. The liveweight gain response of young pigs fed tetracyclines during the 1967 to 1977 period was greater than during the 1950 to 1956 period. Feed efficiency response was not as great, but the initial weights of the experimental pigs used in the 1967 to 1977 comparison was considerably greater (7 vs. 11 kg liveweight). The percentage of responses during the growing and finishing phases of production were not as great, but the liveweight gains of the growing pigs fed tetracyclines were essentially the same, while the rate of gain of the controls in the 1967 to 1977 group improved more than 11 percent for growing pigs and 3 percent for growing-finishing pigs compared to groups of animals used in the 1950 to 1956 comparison groups.

Beneficial effects of antibiotics on farrowing rates of sows have been summarized (Speer 1979c) in Table 3.2. In most cases the antibiotic or chemotherapeutic was fed at the rate of 1.0 g/sow/day for a short time before and after mating (about 20 days). Sows fed the control diets averaged 68.4 percent and sows fed the control diets plus drug averaged 77.4 percent farrowing rate.

An increase in the number of pigs farrowed by sows fed antibiotics before mating has been reported in a few experiments, but there is not enough evidence on this production trait to demonstrate that it has had a real effect.

TABLE 3.1 Experimental Antibiotic Responses for Swine

Years	Number of Experiments	Feeding Period	Percent Improvement Rate of Gain	Percent Improvement Feed/Gain	Author
1960-1967	8	Baby pigs (<100 g/ton antibiotic)	36.0	13.5	Zimmerman (1965)
1960-1967	7	Baby pigs (>100 g/ton antibiotic)	49.5	13.2	Zimmerman (1968)
1965-1970	20	Baby pigs (8-20 lbs)	35.7	15.6	Teague (1971)
1965-1970	6	Young pigs (22-42 lbs)	5.1	9.0	Teague (1971)
1950-1977	378	Young pigs (<35-80 lbs)	16.1	6.9	Hays (1978)
1950-1953	165	Growing pigs (30-50 lbs)	8.7-15.0	2.6-7.8	Braude et al. (1953)
1965-1970	7	Growing pigs	9.0	1.4	Teague (1971)
		Finishing pigs (same pigs)	6.7	0.1	
1950-1977	276	Growing pigs (35-80 lbs)	10.8	4.5	Hays (1978)
1950-1963	9	Growing-finishing	9.0	2.9	Melliere and Waitt (1971)
		Growing-finishing (no antibiotic during finishing)	6.2	1.2	
1950-1977	279	Growing-finishing (32-207 lbs)	4.0	2.1	Hays (1978)

TABLE 3.2 Effect of Antibiotics on Farrowing Rate

Drug	Number of Sows	Farrowing Rate (%)	
		Control	Treated
Chlortetracycline	179	62	79
Chlortetracycline	198	74	86
Aureo SP-250	96	81	96
Aureo SP-250	126	53	56
Aureo SP-250	79	30	36
Tylosin	192	75	77
Tylosin	143	81	84
Tylosin-Sulfamethazine	197	70	83
Furazolidone	87	63	93
Chlortetracycline	249	67	75
Chlortetracycline	239	71	72
Aureo SP-250	184	61	70
Chlortetracycline	101	90	94

SOURCE: V. C. Speer, Iowa State University, personal communication, 1979.

POULTRY

It is generally conceded that management, housing, disease elimination, disease control, isolation, and genetic improvement is far more sophisticated in the poultry industry than any of the other industries. Poultry production facilities can be completely vacated between groups of birds, the facilities thoroughly cleaned, and then the whole production unit filled with birds of the same age and at the same time. Yet, improvements in production traits as a result of antibiotic administration are clearly evident from the summary data presented in Table 3.3. The only production criterion that was not improved was percent hatchability for turkey breeders. A comparison of the responses to antibiotics reported in the literature since 1970 compared to the period 1950 to 1977 was examined by Hays (1978). It can be concluded that the antibiotics continue to be as effective as they were originally.

CATTLE AND SHEEP

Feedlot cattle rate of gain and feed efficiency responses to antibiotics are both improved about 5 percent (Table 3.4). The tetracyclines have been the most widely used antibiotics in the beef cattle industry. (Recently monensin has been approved for use for improved feed efficiency in feedlot cattle. General use by the industry has been rapid. Only tylosin in combination with monensin has been approved for use at this time.) The response seems to be greater on high-roughage rations than low-roughage rations. A marked reduction in the incidence of liver abscesses in feedlot cattle fed antibiotics, particularly the tetracyclines or tylosin, is economically significant both from improved performance in the feedlot and increased carcass value. Responses in calves, both dairy and veal, are greater than with older cattle (Table 3.5). Feed-additive antibiotics have no recognized beneficial effects for the milking dairy cow.

Like other farm species, the young lamb responds to low levels of antibiotics (10 to 25 g per ton of diet). The response of western feeder lambs seems to be more variable. The tetracycline antibiotics are more commonly used in feeder lamb diets. Low levels of these antibiotics reduce the incidence of enterotoxemia in feedlot lambs.

TABLE 3.3 Experimental Antibiotic Responses for Poultry

Species or Type of Bird	State of Growth or Production	Number of Comparisons	Comparison: Control	Comparison: Antibiotic	Percent Improvement	Number of Comparisons	Comparison: Control	Comparison: Antibiotic	Percent Improvement
			Weight (grams)				Feed/Gain		
Chick	Hatch to about 4 weeks	565	382.0	407.7	6.72	313	2.03	1.94	4.43
Chick	Hatch to about 8 weeks	286	1,313.0	1,351.6	2.94	219	2.42	2.36	2.48
			Egg Production (%)				Feed/Dozen Eggs (lbs)		
Hens	Egg production	244	59.9	62.3	4.01	122	5.30	5.05	4.72
			Hatchability (%)						
Hens	Breeders	69	76.2	78.8	3.41				
			Weight (grams)				Feed/Gain		
Turkeys	Hatch to about 4 weeks	166	489.0	554.0	13.29	76	1.86	1.73	6.98
Turkeys	Hatch to about 8 weeks	126	1,963.0	2,101.0	7.03	100	2.08	2.00	3.85
			Weight (lbs)						
Turkeys	Hatch to market weight	85	19.80	21.22	7.17	77	3.18	3.12	1.89
			Egg Production (%)				Feed/Egg (grams)		
Turkeys	Breeders	15	44.2	44.8	1.36	9	516.00	483.00	6.40
			Hatchability (%)						
Turkeys	Breeders	16	70.0	70.0					

SOURCE: Adopted from Hays (1978).

TABLE 3.4 Cattle Feeding Trials with Chlortetracycline

Number of Trials	Comparisons: Control	Comparisons: Antibiotic	Percent Improvement	Source
	Daily Gain (lbs)[1]			
16	2.17	2.29	5.82	U.S. DHEW/FDA (1972)
	Feed/Gain[1]			
21	10.2	9.7	4.22	U.S. DHEW/FDA (1972)
	Liver Abscess Incidence (%)[1]			
8	41.5	15.9	-61.8[2]	U.S. DHEW/FDA (1972)
	Daily Gain (lbs)			
34	2.33	2.43	4.3 Rapid gaining animals	Burroughs et al. (1959)
31	1.42	1.50	5.6 Slower gaining animals	Burroughs et al. (1959)
	Feed/Gain			
34	10.34	9.96	3.7 Rapid gaining animals	Burroughs et al. (1959)
31	12.31	11.45	7.0 Slower gaining animals	Burroughs et al. (1959)

[1]Only trials in which <100 mg CTC/head/day was fed.
[2]Reduction

TABLE 3.5 Calf Feeding Trials with Chlortetracycline[a]

Number of Trials	Comparison: Control	Comparison: Antibiotic	Percent Improvement
	Daily Gain (lbs)		
16	1.16	1.38	19.0
	TDN/Gain (lbs)		
10	2.16	1.96	9.3

[a]Only trials in which <100 mg CTC/head/day was fed.

SOURCE: U.S. DHEW/FDA (1972).

CHAPTER 4

RESTRICTIONS ON ANTIBIOTICS IN EUROPE

BACKGROUND

Most of the activities concerning restriction of antibiotic use were initiated in the United Kingdom following the Swann Report (1969). Action in other European countries followed that of the United Kingdom. The British were among the first in Europe to use antibiotics extensively as growth promotants.

In 1947 a Penicillin Act was passed by the British Parliament prohibiting the sale of antibiotics except for medical and veterinary use (Braude 1978). In 1953 the Therapeutic Substances Act was passed following research in the United States and the United Kingdom showing substantial economic advantages from including penicillin or chlortetracycline in the diets of young animals, and advice from the Medical Research Council that no adverse effects were observed in humans eating meat from antibiotic-fed animals. The regulation allowed inclusion of penicillin or chlortetracycline at a maximum of 100 g/ton to diets of growing pigs and poultry. Later, oxytetracycline was approved. Use of antibiotics in ruminant feeds was not approved.

In 1956 workers convened by the Agricultural Research Council concluded that the only potential danger from feeding antibiotics was the possible establishment of resistant strains of pathogenic microorganisms. In 1960 a Joint Committee was appointed by the Agricultural and Medical Research Councils, under the chairmanship of Lord Netherthorpe. In the first report this committee recognized that continued exposure of a bacterial population to an antibiotic leads to a progressive reduction in sensitivity to that antibiotic. They indicated that there was firm evidence that antibiotic-resistant strains of certain microorganisms such as *E. coli* and *Salmonella* species became established in animals that had received antibiotics as feed additives or therapeutically. However, there were no substantial indications that bacterial resistance had interfered with therapy by a particular antibiotic.

Following agitation in the popular press and media, the Netherthorpe Committee met in January of 1966 and recommended that "an appropriate body with sufficiently wide terms of reference should consider the evidence about the use of antibiotics in both animal husbandry and veterinary medicine and its implications in the field of public health" (Braude 1978). In July 1968 the Ministers of Health and Agriculture, Fisheries, and Food appointed a joint committee on the Use of Antibiotics in Animal Husbandry and Veterinary Medicine under the chairmanship of Professor M. M. Swann. In November 1969 the Swann Report was published. The main recommendations were that:

1. the supply of penicillin, chlortetracycline, and oxytetracycline without prescription should be revoked, and that of tylosin, nitrofuran, and sulfonamides should be available only on prescrip tion;

2. "feed" antibiotics as defined by the Netherthorpe Committee should be available without prescription for pigs and poultry, and for calves up to 3 months of age, but not to laying poultry and adult breeding stock (the latter restriction was subsequently removed); and

3. "therapeutic" antibiotics should be available for use in animals only if prescribed by a member of the veterinary profession who has the animals under his care.

ANTIBIOTIC USE

The Swann Report noted that in 1967, 240 tons of antibiotics were used in the United Kingdom for medical use and 168 tons for veterinary use, a 6:4 ratio (Braude 1978). If penicillin and tetracyclines were removed, the ratio was 8:2. In an independent survey the same year a ratio of 8.5:1.5 was obtained (Braude 1978). In the latter survey two-thirds of the 15 percent used by veterinarians was for therapeutic purposes (10 percent of the total) and one-third for growth promotion (5 percent of total). The ratio between medical and other uses of antibiotics was about 7.5:2.5 in 1975 (Braude 1978). The 25 percent used for nonmedical purposes was divided 70:30 for veterinary and growth promotion, respectively.

There is little indication that overall sales of antibiotics for veterinary use has decreased as a result of the Swann Report (Linton 1977a). The total usage of antibiotics in the United Kingdom has increased since the Swann Report (Table 4.1). There was no substantial increase from 1963 to 1967, but the amount essentially doubled (penicillins, tetracyclines, and feed antibiotics) by 1975 (Braude 1978). "Feed" antibiotics include those that are allowed to be used in the feed and include flavomycin (bambermycins), virginiamycin, and zinc bacitracin. In a recent controversial BBC

TABLE 4.1 Usage of Antibiotics as Feed Additives (kg of active ingredients)

Year	Penicillins and Tetracyclines	"Feed" Antibiotics
1963	40,983	
1964	37,188	
1965	35,205	
1966	36,460	
1967	41,680	
1971		20,000
1973	19,000	
1974	22,000	
1975	26,500	55,000

SOURCE: Braude, R. (1978) Antibiotics in Animal feeds in Great Britain. Reprinted by permission of Journal of Animal Science 46:1425.

program, "Brass Tacks," misuse of antibiotics by farmers was alleged (Anonymous 1979a). It was suggested that veterinary surgeons may over-prescribe.

PERFORMANCE

There is no evidence that performance has been decreased as a result of the implementation of the recommendations of the Swann Report. However, antibiotics are still used in large amounts (Table 4.1) and substitutes such as copper sulfate have been introduced.

RESISTANCE

Low-level antibiotic feeding has resulted in bacterial resistance (Linton 1977 a,b; Smith 1977a; Braude 1978; Richmond and Linton 1980). Large differences have been found in drug resistance of *E. coli* between animals fed and those not fed antibiotics. The resistance to antibiotics is transmissible. In many instances the resistance is due to the presence of R-plasmids. These R-plasmids are able to mediate their own conjugal transfer in addition to specifying resistance to certain antibiotics.

An outbreak of *Salmonella typhimurium* phage type 29 occurred in calves in Britain from 1963 to 1969 (Linton 1977b). Evidence was obtained indicating that the emergence of resistant *S. typhimurium* correlated closely with the increasing range of antibiotics used, and that resistant strains also caused infections in man. The evidence concerning antibiotic-resistant *E. coli* of animal origin reaching man is not complete. It was concluded that antibiotic-resistant *E. coli* in animals cannot be distinguished from those found in man. Transferable drug resistance was demonstrated in chickens and calves, but not in pigs, by feeding large numbers of donor strains to these animals. Transfer of drug resistance to humans by feeding donor cells from animals or humans has not been substantiated.

Persistence of drug resistance has been related to the usage pattern of antibiotics (Linton 1977 a,b). Use of antibiotics in dairy herds for treating mastitis or as a prophylactic at the end of lactation had little or no effect on drug resistance in *E. coli*. In pigs, calves, and poultry, administration of antibiotics by the oral route for short periods resulted in high levels of drug resistance which soon decreased. Conversely, when antibiotics were fed continuously at subtherapeutic levels incidence of drug resistance was greater and persisted for a long period after the drug was discontinued. Continuous exposure appears to stabilize the resistant organisms, which become part of the flora of the gut.

Richmond and Linton (1980) recently conducted studies to determine if the animal or human use of tetracyclines was quantitatively the more important source of resistant *E. coli* for man. They studied the amount of tetracycline prescribed in the County of Avon, England. By extrapolation they found that 3 percent of all prescriptions were for tetracyclines. They found that in hospitals tetracycline was used in 26 percent of all acute beds and 55 percent of all long-stay beds. It was concluded that at any one time 0.75 percent of the county's approximately 1 million inhabitants will be excreting tetracycline-resistant organisms as a direct result of tetracycline treatment. This figure compares favorably with the value of 3 percent of the coliforms in Bristol sewage found to be resistant to tetracycline. Furthermore, sewage from hospitals was found to contain a higher proportion of resistant R-factor-carrying strains of *E. coli* with multiple resistance than did domestic sewage (Linton 1977b). Richmond and Linton also obtained evidence that use of other antimicrobial agents such as sulfonamide may select indirectly for tetracycline resistance.

Richmond and Linton (1980) stated "overall, therefore, it seems as though we must look to the medical, as opposed to the veterinary, use of tetracycline as the main selective pressure for the high incidence of tetracycline-resistant organisms in the human population, and the source of such organisms in human beings not receiving antibiotics is more likely to lie in human beings who are being treated than in the farm animal population." It has been suggested that "those doctors who criticize their veterinary colleagues for the indiscriminate and inappropriate use of antimicrobial agents in animals should pause awhile before casting their stones" (Anonymous 1979b).

It has been reported that tetracycline-resistant *Salmonella* species in swine and humans have decreased in the Netherlands since 1973 (van Leeuwen et al., National Institute for Public Health, Bilthoven, the Netherlands, personal communication, 1979). This decrease coincides with the discontinued use of tetracycline as a feed antibiotic. However, in calves the number of type 505 isolates of *S. typhimurium* has remained constant and the number of multiple resistant phage type 201 has increased.

In the United Kingdom there has been no change in the incidence of pigs excreting tetracycline-resistant *E. coli* (Braude 1978). No decrease in oxytetracycline-resistant *E. coli* in pigs was found in the United Kingdom from 1956 to 1975 (Smith 1977a). M. R. Richmond (University of Bristol, personal communication, 1979) stated that no reduction had occurred in the incidence of antibiotic-resistant *E. coli* in Europe following the implementation of regulations recommended in the Swann Report.

The Scientific Committee for Animal Nutrition was set up by the Commission of the European Communities to provide informed opinions on matters pertaining to animal nutrition and effects of production methods on food quality and the environment. A series of reports was prepared by the Scientific Committee for Animal Nutrition (1978) related to antimicrobials. Three of the reports concerned antibiotics. The reports covered (1) The Use of Macrolides and Related Products in Feedingstuffs, (2) The Conditions of Use of Certain Antibiotics in Feedingstuffs, and (3) Use of Zinc Bacitracin and Flavophospholipol and Feedingstuffs for Laying Hens. The antibiotics covered in the reports were: oleandomycin, spiramycin, erythromycin, tylosin, lincomycin, virginiamycin, zinc bacitracin, and flavophospholipol. Use of penicillin and tetracyclines was not addressed.

CHAPTER 5

EFFECTS ON ANIMAL DISEASE OF SUBTHERAPEUTIC USE OF ANTIBIOTICS

During the last 30 years, subtherapeutic levels of antibacterial drugs have been fed extensively in every major livestock and poultry producing country. The wide acceptance of antibiotics in low levels is attributed to their established benefits of improving feed conversion and growth rate and reducing the morbidity and mortality from subclinical and clinical diseases. During this same period, the poultry, swine, and beef cattle industries were able to develop large, highly intense production units by the use of antibiotics to control disease problems or to increase performance.

Subtherapeutic levels of antibiotics have been defined by the FDA as lower than the therapeutic levels needed to cure disease. This has arbitrarily been set at 200 g per ton of feed for chickens and/or swine and 11 mg/kg bodyweight per day for cattle (U.S. DHEW/FDA 1978).

It is unknown whether the activity of antibiotics used in low levels in animal feeds exerts its influence by: (a) metabolic effect, (b) nutrient sparing or increased absorption and utilization of nutrients, (c) activity against microorganisms, or (d) a combination of these activities.

Data presented by Hays (1978) indicated that the wise use of antibiotics is not a substitute for, but a complement to, good sanitation and husbandry for disease control.

Soon after the introduction of antibiotic agents, drug resistance in bacteria was observed. This phenomenon was also observed to occur spontaneously and in other stress situations. Under continuous antibacterial pressure such resistant organisms will become predominant (Smith 1967).

After 30 years of extensive use of antibiotics in animal feeds, discussions still deal with potential public health hazards. It is difficult to cite human health problems that can be attributed specifically to meat from animals fed antibiotics or that can be associated with direct or indirect contact with animals fed low levels of antibiotics. The evidence that resistant organisms in animals compromise the treatment of diseases in man or animals is sparse, indirect and difficult to evaluate.

A general decrease in the cost of antibiotics has encouraged the use of higher levels than were commonly used several years after the growth promoting effects of antibiotics were first discovered. The levels selected at that time were not levels that elicit maximum response. Generally they were compromised levels based upon a cost/benefit ratio.

The possible hazards to animal health from using antibiotics in low levels are: (1) adverse or toxic reactions in the animal, (2) development of resistant strains of pathogenic organisms, and (3) increased susceptibility to some infections through immunosuppression or alteration in the microflora.

Toxicity is usually not a problem in food animals from the use of antibiotics. When such problems occur, they are usually traced to human error, i.e., the misuse of the drug for purposes not included on the label or mixing errors.

There is likelihood that antibiotic utilization has been abused both in animal and human medicine. It has been shown that the use of subtherapeutic and therapeutic levels of antibiotics does in fact cause resistant strains of organisms to emerge. This may make it necessary to change drugs when treatment is not effective for the first drug of choice. As in man, there is no way to know what role the use of antibiotics in animal feeds at the subtherapeutic level has on the establishment of resistant populations of bacteria when compared to the therapeutic use of antibiotics.

Salmonella species are widespread in nature and frequently cause food poisoning in humans. Epidemiological studies show that foods of animal origin are frequently involved. Salmonellosis in humans involving antibiotic-resistant strains of bovine origin has occurred (Anderson 1968, Threlfall et al. 1978). Although the disturbances occurred under conditions of widespread antibiotic use, there is no evidence of any relationship to subtherapeutic feeding. These studies are not generally complete enough to determine the source of contamination. It is difficult to determine whether or not these foods were contaminated before or after slaughter or if the last vector was a food handler. It is doubtful that restricting antibiotic levels in animal feeds will cause a reduction in food-borne infections of humans.

Up to the mid-1960s, before antimicrobial resistance became recognized as a result of widespread use of antibiotics, the compromising effect of subtherapeutic antibiotic administration was repeatedly registered. Smith (1967) wrote "it is becoming increasingly apparent that the frequent prophylactic and therapeutic use in a pig herd of any of the available antibacterial drugs eventually results in penicillin drugs becoming largely ineffective in the treatment of *E. coli* infections." He also documented the development of penicillin resistance in 60 percent of staphylococcal strains in arthritis in chickens on diets containing penicillin and tetracyclines. Arthritis outbreaks in years prior to antibiotic feeding yielded strains susceptible to penicillin. More recently, Hjerpe (1976) reported a decline in response to tetracycline therapy by pneumonic cattle simultaneous with a rise in prevalence of tetracycline, penicillin, and sulfonamide-resistant strains of *Pasteurella* species after feeding of subtherapeutic levels (100 g/ton) of chlortetracycline was initiated in a feedlot.

The general rise in antibiotic resistance among bacteria during the past 30 years of intensive antibiotic use has undoubtedly curtailed the usefulness of some previously effective drugs. Documentation concerning this development is scarce, and the extent of it ascribable to subtherapeutic use of antibiotics is impossible to determine.

CHAPTER 6

THERAPEUTIC USE OF ANTIBIOTICS

BACKGROUND

Infectious diseases constitute the largest single category of medical problems in the several species of domestic animals. As a result, veterinarians have had a critical need for the anti-infective drugs in the course of everyday practice. Prior to the introduction of modern antibiotics, metallo-organic compounds, various antibacterial dyes, and other chemotherapeutic agents were employed. Shortly after sulfonamides were introduced in the late 1930s, they were recognized as being effective against bovine mastitis, and soon after against a wide spectrum of other bacterial infections of animals. Similarly, introduction of the various forms of penicillin soon led to their broad application in all species of domesticated and zoo animals. As the antibiotic era developed, each new addition to the antibiotic roster, such as the tetracyclines, chloramphenicol, bacitracin, streptomycins, neomycin, kanamycin, gentamicin, polymyxin, griseofulvin, nystatin, amphotericin B, erythromycin, tylosin, lincomycin, clindamycin, cephalosporins, and the semisynthetic penicillins soon found a valued position in veterinary medicine.

In-depth surveys (1967, 1972 to 1975) of the therapeutic usage of various classes of drugs in veterinary medicine have been reported from the University of Minnesota College of Veterinary Medicine. There, workers have, over the past years, surveyed the frequency of total drug usage in both large and small animals, including the categories of companion, zoo, and food-producing species (Stowe 1975). These studies clearly revealed that antibiotic drugs were the most frequently used agents in the treatment of animal disease. The studies involved the sampling of 5 percent of the clinical cases that were presented to the Veterinary Teaching Hospitals, including the out-patient and in-patient Large and Small Animal Hospitals and a rural outlying food-animal practice. In terms of the total number of drug treatments (many animals received more than one drug) the most frequently employed classes of drugs were as follows: antibiotic agents, 48 percent; anthelmintics, 15 percent; corticosteroids and other endocrine agents (exclusive of diethylstilbestrol), 12 percent; fluids and electrolytes, 7 percent; analgesics, anesthetics, and tranquilizers, 6 percent; and gastrointestinal agents, 5 percent; with the remainder scattered among the autonomic, cardiac, antihistamine, topical, and miscellaneous categories. While this survey dealt only with one large teaching hospital in the upper Midwest, frequent contacts with comparable institutions elsewhere and with both large and small animal practitioners leaves little doubt that infectious diseases constitute the largest single category of disease problems, and that antibiotic drugs are the most frequently employed agents.

Within the category of antibiotic agents, the most frequently employed drugs are the penicillins (including the broad spectrum derivatives such as ampicillin and the penicillinase-resistant penicillins such as cloxacillin, dicloxacillin, etc.) and the tetracyclines, particularly oxytetracycline. In addition to these "mainstays" which continue to be effective and serviceable in the majority of cases, the sulfonamides continue to be heavily used because of their efficacy in the frequently encountered pasteurellosis infections in cattle and sheep. Tylosin, a nonhuman antibiotic, is also very heavily employed. In general, the economics of livestock production is a significant determinant in deciding which antibiotic agent to employ: the newer antibiotics tend to be more costly, a fact that makes their routine use in food animals uneconomical. In companion animals, on the other hand, including horses, the cost of medication is often not a major consideration, and thus erythromycins, cephalosporins, gentamicin, and sulfonamide-trimethoprim combinations are more frequently employed.

In terms of efficacy and safety, there can be little doubt that the antibiotic drugs are essential therapeutic agents in the diseases of domestic animals.

The widespread usage of veterinary services in the livestock industry points to a very real economic gain to the producer when veterinary services are utilized. In a series of studies sponsored by the Minnesota Agricultural Experiment Station, the World Bank, and the U.S. Department of Agriculture, it was found that there is a strong positive correlation between the use of veterinary services, the health of livestock, and the net income from the farm operation (McCauley 1974 a,b). In view of the major use of antibiotic drugs in veterinary practice, it would seem reasonable to infer that these drugs constitute a significant contribution to livestock production and economics.

From time to time, infectious diseases do not seem to respond to treatment with a particular antibiotic drug. In such instances either the dosage is increased, or another antibiotic agent is selected. In most cases, when therapy with an appropriate drug is initiated early in the course of the disease, the outcome is ultimately successful. However, when faced with therapeutic failure, some veterinarians conclude that their initial selection was unsuccessful because of prior use of low-level feeding of antibiotic substances to a herd or flock. A few practitioners declare that the problems they perceive as drug failures can be attributed to low-level antibiotic feeding. When queried in detail about their justification for such statements, proof is lacking. Carefully controlled studies regarding the cause-and-effect relationships between antibiotic feeding and subsequent therapeutic failures are lacking. Certainly veterinary practitioners, whether rural or urban, are not equipped to undertake the in-depth studies required to establish or refute the point at issue and consequently their opinions, no matter how firmly expressed, have to be rejected due to lack of scientific evidence. It is self-evident that perceived therapeutic failures could be due to factors such as misdiagnosis, inadequate dosages, antibiotic drug antagonisms, and others.

In some of the larger group practices and at the veterinary teaching institutions, antibiotic drug sensitivity tests are employed quite routinely. Lack of susceptibility or resistance to standard concentrations of various antibiotic drugs is encountered to a varied degree with all drugs, including those that have not been used at all, or used only to a minimal extent for low-level antibiotic feeding (i.e., cephalosporins, chloramphenicol, gentamicin, kanamycin). Moreover, the validity of *in vitro* sensitivity testing has sometimes been questioned. Clinicians have reported therapeutic successes in treating infections due to agents shown to be resistant by laboratory tests (C. M. Stowe, University of Minnesota, College of Veterinary Medicine, personal communication, 1979). This general observation is further buttressed by comparing the apparent frequency of *in vitro* nonresponsiveness in the hospital-clinic setting to that which one obtains in the farm setting, where the frequency of nonresponsive organisms seems to be lower despite the juxtaposition in the latter case to low-level antibiotic feeding.

The use of data gathered from veterinary teaching hospitals and clinics regarding the frequency of resistance among pathogens may not be an accurate reflection of the true level of resistance in specific regions of the country or in the nation at large. Before any inferences are drawn regarding the degree or frequency of resistant animal pathogens, we need to have more in-depth knowledge of the spectrum, scope, and degree of antibiotic resistance that is representative at least in the domestic animal population. At present there simply is no body of incontrovertible evidence regarding the relative importance of the human as a source of resistant organisms in animals or of animals as a source of resistant organisms in man. Furthermore, it would be impossible at the present time to say whether the resistant organisms arose as a result of subtherapeutic antibiotic feeding, prophylactic use, or therapeutic use for the treatment of a specific disease outbreak.

CONTROL AND REGULATION

Control and regulation of the therapeutic use of antibiotic drugs is under the purview of the FDA, particularly the Bureau of Veterinary Medicine and the Bureau of Foods. Control is exercised through the mechanism of the New Animal Drug Application (NADA). Once approval is granted and the drug is marketed, therapeutic use by veterinarians and in some cases by livestock producers follows. Such usage is based on the indications of the drug; the experience of the practitioner; and the inherent constraints of the dosage, route of administration, and the residue or withdrawal times. In the overwhelming majority of cases care is taken to observe the requirements of proper withdrawal times for either milk or meat.

From time to time, the question of auditing antibiotic drug usage arises, primarily within the setting of human hospitals. Other than in an institutional setting, the auditing of drug usage would be very time consuming, costly, and difficult to control.

EPIDEMIOLOGICAL CONSIDERATIONS

There is general agreement that the use of antibiotics in both animals and humans leads to increased frequency of antibiotic resistance. Furthermore, there is little doubt that resistance can be transferred through plasmids from certain resistant microorganisms to others that were originally sensitive. These in turn have been shown to be transmissible to other animals and, in isolated cases, to humans (Levy et al. 1976 a,b; Hirsh 1977). This resistance transfer or "infectious drug resistance" has led on the part of some individuals, to the fear that resistant strains could be transferred to other animals and humans, thereby creating a reservoir of pathogens, which when involved in clinical infections, would be unresponsive to antibiotic treatment. While such fears may seem to be a logical extension of current knowledge regarding resistance, there is practically no information on the extent to which this is happening, nor is it clear in the case of the few such instances known whether they were due to low-level antibiotic feeding, therapeutic use of antibiotics in domestic animals (including companion and pet animals), or therapeutic or prophylactic use of antibiotic drugs in human beings. These vexing questions are not easily resolved, particularly in view of the fact that both humans and animals often share the same pathogens.

CHAPTER 7

VOIDS IN KNOWLEDGE AND SUGGESTED RESEARCH

Although voluminous research has been conducted regarding the effects of feeding antibiotics on performance, research has been very limited in certain other areas. Research results have shown that resistance of microorganisms exists in animals fed antibiotics and that this resistance can be transferred (Linton 1977 a,b; Smith 1977a). However, there is inconclusive evidence that the use of antibiotics as growth promotants compromises therapy of humans and animals. Few well-designed experiments have been reported, and clearly there is a need for well-designed intensive investigations of this important issue.

The main objectives of the proposed research to fill in the primary voids concerning antibiotics are to determine: (a) if the feeding of tetracyclines and penicillin compromise animal therapy, (b) the relation of antibiotic feeding to human health, and (c) the mechanism of action of antibiotics in growth promotion.

It is suggested that the research described in the following pages be undertaken.

EFFECT OF TETRACYCLINE FEEDING ON ANIMAL THERAPY

Poultry and Swine

The possibility that administration of subtherapeutic levels of antibiotics may compromise therapy has not been adequately investigated. Most previous studies have given negative results with respect to this question, but according to the FDA (U.S. DHEW/FDA 1978) experiments generally were poorly designed. Carefully planned and controlled experiments conducted with poultry and swine should be conducted to attempt to answer this question with organisms such as *Salmonella typhimurium*. This organism should be used in these animals to determine whether development of resistant organisms will compromise treatment of a severe infection in the species. Chicks and swine should be inoculated with *S. typhimurium* to induce a low-level, nonlethal infection, and be fed diets with and without tetracycline. After a few weeks the animals will be challenged with an inoculum calculated to cause a severe infection resulting in considerable mortality. This inoculum should be isolated from animals fed antibiotic and should be documented to contain antibiotic-resistant organisms. The effectiveness of therapeutic levels of tetracyclines and other antibiotics against this infection should be determined. To avoid the problem of possible development of immunity, animals unexposed to the organism should also be inoculated with the dose to cause a severe infection, and the effectiveness of antibiotic therapy in these animals should also be investigated. Careful laboratory work to monitor development of antibiotic-resistant organisms in the animals and immunity development would be needed.

Cattle

Cattle in commercial feedlots should be studied that (a) have not received antibiotics; (b) have received a high level of antibiotic during the first 3 to 4 weeks, followed by a low level during the remainder of the period on feed; and (c) have received a high level of antibiotic during the first 3 to 4 weeks, followed by withdrawal of the drug. Comparisons should be made of tetracycline therapy on sick animals from the lots on the various treatments. Response to therapy should also be monitored by the number of animals treated, the length of stay in the sick pens, and mortality. Measurements should also include antibiotic susceptibility of organisms in treated animals and samples of healthy animals from all lots at periodic intervals.

This type of experiment will need to be performed in cooperation with university or USDA scientists and feedlots. It would be ideal for most of the feedlots to be in the California and Arizona area where antibiotics are not normally used. However, it would be important that some feedlots, at least those that are treated, be located in the Colorado or Kansas area, where a continuous level of feeding of tetracyclines is routinely practiced. It will be essential that the cooperating feedlots use only tetracycline as the subtherapeutic and therapeutic drug. It will be essential to reimburse the feedlots for death losses above the normal mortality rate caused by the experimental treatments. Also, some compensation will have to be made for the extra labor involved in handling the cattle, such as monitoring the normal animals for antibiotic-resistant organisms. The organisms used to monitor resistance will likely be a common species of *Salmonella* and *E. coli*.

RELATION OF ANTIBIOTIC FEEDING TO HUMAN HEALTH

The information which would be required to answer the controversial question will necessitate investigations of staggering complexity and cost. It is likely that broad-based studies will involve monitoring of health-related problems among human populations involved in and isolated from low-level antibiotic feed programs. Of course, when studying people involved with animals and animal products, animal health should also be monitored. Baselines must also be established by determining the history of the subjects with regard to antibiotic exposure and the susceptibility of the microflora species to antibiotics.

Recent experiments with animals have shown that randomly selected individuals already carry some resistant enteric microorganisms. It may be necessary to study respiratory bacterial flora instead of, or in addition to, the changes or lack of changes in susceptibility by species over a period of time and the nature of any disease episode particularly if suggestive of microbial etiology. The susceptibility of any agent thought to be involved would have to be established and the success of antimicrobial therapy determined clinically and microbiologically. The logistics and mechanics of this type of study will be extremely demanding in time and labor. Some aspects, especially those involving humans, would require several years, a large population, or both, for the collection of adequate data. If the microflora present at the onset is already predominantly resistant to the antimicrobials of interest, this study would be pointless.

MECHANISMS OF ACTION OF ANTIBIOTICS IN GROWTH PROMOTION

"Growth promotion" from the low-level feeding of antibiotics refers to an improvement in both rate of gain and efficiency of feed conversion. Improvement normally occurs in both measures of performance but not necessarily to the same degree. In view of known factors that influence rate and efficiency of gain, antibiotic action affecting each measure of performance should prove to be, at least in some respects, different.

The different chemical nature, absorbability, and bacterial spectrum of growth promoting antibiotics suggest that the mode of action in growth promotion cannot be the same for all of the antibiotics that have proven efficacious. There is also good evidence that antibiotic action affecting growth in the different species is not entirely from the same mode of action. Factors involved are the complex mechanisms related to disease, feed intake, digestion, absorption, and metabolism of nutrients, as well as antibiotic effects on enteric flora and the systemic bacterial population.

In swine, frequent measurement of rate and efficiency of gain in control and antibiotic-fed animals reveals that a response to the antibiotic is not consistent but occurs only occasionally, and for what is usually a short period of time. Such an effect over an extended period promotes "average" performance above controls.

In view of this important temporary effect, studies are suggested in which short-term performance measurements (feed intake and rate of gain) are correlated with similar short-term measurements related to the microbiology and biochemistry of the different physiological systems in control versus responding animals. Intestinal cannulation to permit sampling of ingesta at different points in the tract, together with simultaneous blood measurements, are needed for such an approach.

Experiments designed to uncover mechanisms related to the growth-promotant effect might provide a means of exploiting these mechanisms other than by the use of feeding levels of antibacterial compounds.

REFERENCES

Anderson, E. S. (1968) The ecology of transferable drug resistance in the enterobacteria. Annual Review of Microbiology 22:131.

Anonymous (1978) Feed marketing and distribution. Reference issue. Feedstuffs 50(30):6.

Anonymous (1979a) Animal production and public health: TV programme looks at "risks." Veterinary Record 104:443.

Anonymous (1979b) Salmonellosis: An unhappy turn of events. Lancet 1:1009.

Anonymous (1979c) Feed Additive Compendium. Minneapolis, Minn.: Miller Publishing Co.

Beeson, W. M. (1978) Use of drugs and chemicals as feed additives to increase the productivity of sheep. Paper prepared for the Office of Technology Assessment, U.S. Congress. Washington, D.C.: U.S. Government Printing Office.

Braude, R. (1978) Antibiotics in animal feeds in Great Britain. Journal of Animal Science 46:1425.

Braude, R., H. D. Wallace, and T. J. Cunha (1953) The value of antibiotics in the nutrition of swine: A review. Antibiotics and Chemotherapy 3:271.

Burroughs, W., C. E. Summers, W. Woods, and W. Zmolek (1959) Feed additives in beef cattle rations. Animal Science Leaflet, AH 805. Ames, Iowa: Iowa State University.

Davis, G. K. (1978) Drugs and chemicals in livestock feeding. Paper prepared for the Office of Technology Assessment, U.S. Congress. Washington, D.C.: U.S. Government Printing Office.

Fagerberg, D. J. and C. L. Quarles (1979) Antibiotic Feeding, Antibiotic Resistance and Alternatives. Somerville, N.J.: American Hoechst Corporation.

Foster, L. and W. Woods (1970) Liver losses in finishing cattle. EC 70-218:1, University of Nebraska Beef Cattle Report. Lincoln, Nebr.: University of Nebraska.

Gilliam, H. C., Jr. and J. R. Martin (1975) Economic importance of antibiotics in feeds to producers and consumers of pork, beef and veal. Journal of Animal Science 40:1241.

Hays, V. W. (1978) Effectiveness of feed additive usage of antibacterial agents in swine and poultry production. Paper prepared for Office of Technology Assessment, U.S. Congress. Washington, D.C.: U.S. Government Printing Office.

Headley, J. C. (1978) Economic aspects of drug and chemical feed additives. Paper prepared for the Office of Technology Assessment, U.S. Congress. Washington, D.C.: U.S. Government Printing Office.

Hepp, R. E. (1977) Swine Farrowing Cooperatives. Cooperative Extension Service Bullet E-1056. East Lansing, Mich.: Michigan State University.

Hirsh, D. and N. Wiger (1977) Effect of tetracycline upon transfer of an R-plasmid from calves to human beings. American Journal of Veterinary Research 38:1137-1138.

Hjerpe, C. A. (1976) Treatment of bacterial pneumonia in feedlot cattle. Page 33, Proceedings of the 8th Annual Convention of the Association of Bovine Practitioners, Atlanta, Georgia.

Levy, S. B., G. B. Fitzgerald, and A. B. Macone (1976a) Changes in intestinal flora of farm personnel after introduction of a tetracycline-supplemented feed on a farm. New England Journal of Medicine 295:583-588.

Levy, S. B., G. B. Fitzgerald, and A. B. Macone (1976b) Spread of antibiotic-resistant plasmids from chicken to chicken and from chicken to man. Nature 260:40-42.

Linton, A. H. (1977a) Antibiotic resistance: The present situation reviewed. Veterinary Record 100:354.

Linton, A. H. (1977b) Antibiotics, animals and man: An appraisal of a contentious subject. Pages 315-343, Antibiotics and Antibiosis in Agriculture with Special Reference to Synergism, edited by M. Woodbine. Boston, Mass.: Butterworths.

McCauley, E. H. (1974a) The contribution of veterinary service to the dairy enterprise income of Minnesota farmers: Farm production equation analysis. Journal of the American Veterinary Medical Association 165:1094.

McCauley, E. H. (1974b) Economics and diseases of farm livestock. Canadian Veterinary Journal 15:213.

McDonald, M. C. (1973) A Study of *Pasteurella haemolytica* isolated from feedlot cattle. M.S. Thesis, University of California, Davis.

Melliere, A. L. and W. P. Waitt (1971) Evaluation of weight gain and feed efficiency promoting efficacy of tylosin and tylosin-sulfamethazine in swine during the years 1959-1970. Feedstuffs 43(35):23.

Paulsen, A. and M. Rahm (1979) Development of subsidiary sow-farrowing firms in Iowa. Iowa Agricultural and Home Economics Experiment Station Special Report 83. Ames, Iowa: Iowa State University.

Richmond, M. H. and K. B. Linton (1980) The use of tetracycline in the community and its possible relation to the excretion of tetracycline-resistant bacteria. Journal of Antimicrobial Chemotherapy 6:33.

Scientific Committee for Animal Nutrition (1978) Report's Final Series. Commission of the European Communities.

Smith, H. W. (1967) The effect of use of antibacterial drugs, particularly as food additives, on the emergence of drug-resistant strains of bacteria in animals. New Zealand Veterinary Journal 15(9):153.

Smith, H. W. (1977a) Antibiotic resistance in bacteria and associated problems in farm animals before and after the 1969 Swann Report. Pages 344-357, Antibiotics and Antibiosis in Agriculture with Special Reference to Synergism, edited by M. Woodbine. Boston, Mass.: Butterworths.

Smith, M. G. (1977b) Transfer of R factors from *Escherichia coli* to salmonellas in the rumen of sheep. *Journal of Medical Microbiology* 19:29.

Stemme, C., V. J. Rhodes, and G. Grimes (1978) Defining the status of large hog farms. Hog Farm Management 15(13):52.

Stemme, C., V. J. Rhodes, and G. Grimes (1979) Defining the shape of the hog industry. Hog Farm Management 16(3):44.

Stowe, C. M. (1975) Antibiotic therapy in veterinary medicine: Uses and misuses. *In* Pharmacology in the Animal Health Sector, edited by L. E. Davis and L. C. Faulkner, Fort Collins, Colorado.

Swann, M. M. et al. (1968) Report of the Joint Committee on the Use of Antibiotics in Animal Husbandry and Veterinary Medicine. London: Her Majesty's Stationery Office.

Teague, H. S. (1971) Antibiotics in swine feeds. *In* Proceedings of the American Pork Congress, March 2, 3, and 4, 1971. Des Moines, Iowa: National Pork Producers' Council.

Threlfall, E. J., G. R. Ward, and B. Stowe (1978) Epidemic spread of a Chloramphenicol-resistant strain of *Salmonella typhimurium* phage type 204, in bovine animals in Britain. Veterinary Record 130:438-444.

U.S. Bureau of the Census (1978) Census of Agriculture. Vol. II, Statistics by Subject: Livestock, Poultry, Livestock and Poultry Products, Fish. Washington, D.C.: U.S. Department of Commerce.

U.S. Department of Agriculture (1978) Economic effects of a prohibition on the use of selected animal drugs. Agr. Econ. Report No. 414. Economics, Statistics and Cooperatives Service. Washington, D.C.: U.S. Department of Agriculture.

U.S. Department of Agriculture (1979a) Cattle on Feed Reports. Economics, Statistics, and Cooperatives Service. Washington, D.C.: U.S. Department of Agriculture.

U.S. Department of Agriculture (1979b) Livestock and Meat Statistics. Economic Research Service. Washington, D.C.: U.S. Department of Agriculture.

U.S. Department of Health, Education, and Welfare/Food and Drug Administration (1972) The Use of Antibiotics in Animal Feeds. FDA Task Force Report, Bureau of Veterinary Medicine. Rockville, Md.: Food and Drug Administration.

U.S. Department of Health, Education, and Welfare/Food and Drug Administration (1978) Draft environmental impact statement: Subtherapeutic agents in animal feeds. Washington, D.C.: Food and Drug Administration, Bureau of Veterinary Medicine.

Van Arsdall, R. N. (1978) Structural characteristics of the U.S. hog production industry. Agr. Econ. Report No. 415, Economics, Statistics, and Cooperatives Service. Washington, D.C.: U.S. Department of Agriculture.

Warner, R. G. (1972) Antibiotics in veal calf and dairy replacement calf nutrition and disease control. Presentation before the FDA Task Force, Denver, Colorado, September 16-17, 1970.

Woods, W. (1970) Antibiotics in beef cattle nutrition disease control. Presentation before the FDA Task Force, Denver, Colorado, September 16-17, 1970.

Zimmerman, D. R. (1968) Antimicrobial feed additives for swine. A paper presented at the Annual Meeting of the Iowa Pork Producers, Des Moines, Iowa.